Series editor's foreword

This fourth volume in the series is concerned with the historical construction of feminity. And in both its emphasis – nineteenth-century Anglo–American pseudo-scientific and medical theories on women's health and exercise – and the detailed evidence it presents, it adds a new dimension to International Studies in the History of Sport and indeed, to Women's Studies.

Sara Delamont and Lorna Duffin, Patricia Branca, Joan Burstyn and Carol Dyhouse, among others, have written illuminatingly of the carefully prescribed image of middle-class womanhood in the nineteenth century, and the equally careful process of socialisation into femininity that accompanied it. They have all failed, however, to give due attention to exercise in the lives of women as a source of both conformity and nonconformity and they have failed to give sufficient recognition to the fact that issues of health and exercise, as Vertinsky argues, are 'central to women's emancipation'.

Other writers, including Sheila Fletcher, Martha Verbrugge and, more recently, Kathleen McCrone, for their part, have drawn our attention to the institutional function of exercise in nineteenth-century middle-class women's lives, initially as a means of restriction and subsequently, as a means of liberation as exercise slowly shifted from an improper to a proper sphere of female involvement.

Patricia Vertinsky, in this complementary study, concentrates on the nature and influence of ideologies of femininity. She raises once again, but by means of new and provocative material, the issue of exercise as a form of social control. She also reveals the lengthy, difficult and bitter struggle required to refute dominant medical theories on women and exercise and to obtain for women opportunities to define what they themselves considered appropriate and beneficial forms of recreational and competitive exercise in the pursuit of personal health and fulfilment.

Exercise, as Vertinsky makes clear, is a symbol of the broader matters of social construction, constraint and confrontation as well as an effective means of demonstrating the fallibility of 'experts' and their sometimes pompous and foolish conservatism. Finally and most appropriately in the context of the aims of this series, exercise is shown by Vertinsky to be a significant cultural phenomenon. Its consideration in this volume throws a sharply focused and bright beam of light over the wider society – its fashions, prejudices and power-structure.

J. A. Mangan

Acknowledgements

Many people have provided encouragement and support for this book. The Social Sciences and Humanities Research Council of Canada has generously supported a number of aspects of this project. I have been influenced by the fine work of female historians such as Carroll Smith-Rosenberg and Elaine Showalter who have opened up new vistas of understanding about the mental and physical health, lives and thoughts of nineteenth-century women. Roberta Park's consistently thorough documentation of nineteenth-century women's sport and physical education provides a solid grounding for new analyses of women, sport and physical activity. Tony Mangan has given ongoing inspiration and support for all phases of this work and I am particularly grateful for his commitment and enthusiasm. Brian Stoddart has also given me very valuable support and editorial help. Invaluable assistance has been obtained from numerous libraries, manuscript collections and medical society archives. Those who assisted me at the British Library went far beyond the bounds of normal duty to find the books and documents I needed. Marla Tynan, Bay Gumboc and Melodie Cook have assisted ably in preparing the technical aspects of this manuscript.

I would like to thank the editors of the *Journal of Sport History*, the *International Journal of the History of Sport* and *Women and Health* for their kind permission in allowing me to reprint the following articles, in whole or in part: 'Exercise, physical capability and the eternally wounded woman in late-nineteenth-century North America', *Journal of Sport History*, vol. 14 (1), 1987; 'Of no use without health: late nineteenth-century medical prescriptions for female exercise through the life span', *Women and Health*, vol. 14 (1), 1988; 'Escape from freedom: G. Stanley Hall's totalitarian views on female health and physical education', *International Journal of the History of Sport*, vol. 5 (1), 1988; and 'Feminist Charlotte Perkins Gilman's pursuit of health and physical fitness as a strategy for emancipation', *Journal of Sport History*, vol. 16 (1), 1989.

My family, especially my daughters Liza and Tally, have cheerfully tolerated the many hours that I have stolen from them to complete this work. To borrow Carroll Smith-Rosenberg's words, when all is said, it is to and for our daughters and their generation that we write. This book, therefore, is dedicated to Liza and Tally, who already understand the most important parts of my message.

Those who hitch their fortunes to the cultural pendulum of absolute opposites never realize that they are riding the devil's tail, not the god's own chariot to the sun.

Braun Dijkstra, Idols of Perversity (1986)

Introduction

The eternally wounded woman

The power to change the basic concepts with which people understand themselves is the power to change the world in which those people live.[1]

This book is about the historical influence of late nineteenth-century medical beliefs and values on the perceived benefits of physical activity for women across their life span. The practice of medicine and the knowledge which underpins it have never been simple and logical progressions from one truth to another. Rather, scientific knowledge, medical practice and social perception have interacted to affect views concerning what kinds and amounts of physical activity, including sport and healthful exercise, might be most appropriate for girls and women at different points in their life course. The critical aspect of these views, of course, is that they encompass far more than opinions about the potential benefits or risks of calisthenics, country walks, or various types of sports and games. Medical shibboleths about female physical activity have quite naturally reflected popular beliefs about the nature of women, their biological purpose and their social role. As agents of society, male and female physicians have demonstrated, in their practices, particular cultural values and orientations, and the importance attributed to their diagnoses and prescriptions has depended upon the active participation and collusion of members of society.[2]

Not infrequently, medically defined notions of optimal female health, individual and social wellbeing have justified the practice of viewing female physiological functions as requiring prescribed and/or delimited levels of physical activity and restricted sporting opportunities. The origins of such views and the tenacity with which they have been maintained rest on long-standing, invidious ideological assumptions about the nature of women and the assumed entitlement to medical management of the female body among the medical establishment.

1

Thus, rather than viewing the historical development of women's sport and exercise as a rational, evolutionary process spurred on by the emergence of new scientific knowledge, democratic principles and notions of equity, a review of thinking is needed in the field of socio-historical analysis concerning attitudes toward the female body and attempts to regulate female physical activity. Such analyses may generate new insights into the questions of both social control and the unevenness of progress in women's real or perceived opportunities for participating freely and fully in sports and exercise of their choice.

Implicit in women's history is the need to illuminate particular female concerns and experiences with their bodies, as well as to reappraise assumptions about categories of social analysis and theories of social change. The history of women is not the history of men, and significant turning points in history have not had the same impact for one sex as for the other.[3] Historically, perceptions of the nature of women have affected the shape of categories assigned to them which, in turn, have reinforced or remoulded these perceptions. By providing a sense both of their origins and the possibility of effecting change, women's history provides an essential tool for analysing the current difficulties of women, some of which result from faulty perceptions of female physical capabilities. The long-standing perception that 'women are the weaker sex' who cannot cope with the same level of physical activity as men remains a critical focus of historical analysis, for it manifestly continues to affect women's pursuit of lifetime involvement and expertise in sport and physical activity.[4]

The tenacity of biological determinism

The question of biology, comment Boutilier and San Giovanni, has always been central to the issue of women's involvement in exercise and sporting activities.[5] Their assumed biological differences and limitations relative to men have been and still are used as rationalizations for excluding women from sport, even though very little is known about the realities of women's biology as it relates to physical activity. Despite this lack of knowledge, in practically every generation prophets of the 'biology is destiny' argument arise – determinists invoking the tradi-tional prestige of objective science to argue in support of the biological basis of differences between the sexes and what this means for female participation in physical activity. All too often their theories have been uncritically embraced as self-confirming by those who defend the status quo and welcome its legitimization. 'The voice of the natural', notes Roland Barthes, has ever been a voice for the status quo, which is quick to claim that nature has rendered woman less able than man![6]

Cross-currents between the arenas of biological and social thought have persisted throughout the present century notwithstanding the apparent objectivity and sophistication of the modern experimental sciences.[7] Sociobiology, for example, is a particularly dramatic, contemporary version of biological determinist theories of human behaviour. Its basic premise is that human behaviour and aspects of social organization have evolved, like our bodies, through adaptations based on Darwinian selection. Interpreted by David Barash, the theory explains that though biology and culture are undoubtedly inter-related, it is tempting to speculate that our biology is somehow more important, lying unnoticed within each of us but forcefully manipulating much of our behaviour. Sociobiologists believe that men and women have different strategies and behaviour for assuring the reproduction and survival of their genes. They claim that 'because men maximize their fitness differently from women, it is perfectly good biology that business and profession tastes sweeter to them, while home and child care taste sweeter to women'.[8]

This rebirth of biological determinism in the guise of the 'science' of sociobiology, well seasoned with scientific sexism, reminds us of the dangers in assigning natural causes to phenomena of social origins, of allowing science to play handmaiden to social values. Sociobiologists reinforce stereotypes of 'woman as the lesser man', passive, dependent, maternal and physically weak, that many social scientists and feminists have vigorously tried to displace. They remind us that 'as long as there are entrenched social and political distinctions between sexes, races and classes, there will be forms of science whose main function is to rationalize and legitimize these distinctions'.[9]

This is especially so in those professions which use biology to support established professional views concerning women's bodies and to justify unequal social practices between the sexes. In particular, the physical education and medical professions have conceptualized the female body within a biological framework, viewing it as a complex biological machine to be controlled by appropriate scientific regimens. Professional discourse about health and physical activity is heavily punctuated by the use of biological categories and explanations derived from 'scientific' sources. Indeed, Michel Foucault has explained, as scientific discourse about the physical capabilities and requirements of the body expands, the human body tends to be brought increasingly within the orbit of professional power.[10] Ever present is the temptation for those dealing with the complexities of the physical body and its relationship to the social order, to legitimize personal preference and professional practice on the basis of the genetic code – to seek to edit, as Gerald Leach has suggested, the master tapes of life which carry the hereditary message, despite the fact that 'no one has read more than a paragraph or two of the hereditary bible'.[11]

Medicine as an instrument of social control

Feminists have not been slow to illustrate how much of the professional discourse about female health and exercise has traditionally been contaminated by deterministic views.[12] They rightly see health and physical expression as central to women's emancipation, and view with suspicion those professionals who have had, deliberately or not, a negative impact upon women's understanding of health and physical competence. De Beauvoir's philosophical formulation of woman as 'other' is often manifested in a health context through the perception that, since the male body is the norm, the female body is, therefore, a deviation.[13] Hence the healthy, but uniquely female functions of menstruation, pregnancy, childbirth and menopause become easily viewed as diseases or potential disorders requiring treatment.[14] Physiological functions throughout a woman's life course are thus seen to require prescribed and frequently delimited levels of physical activity because of medically defined notions of 'optimal health' for individual and social wellbeing.

Competing and conflicting medical models of the 'normal' healthy female have promoted quite different viewpoints concerning responses to and the perceived effects of vigorous physical activity, especially in relation to the reproductive function. For example, many high performance female athletes do not menstruate due to low body fat and, possibly, intensive training. Coach physicians usually insist that this state is quite reversible once training ceases, claiming that their protégés have no wish to become pregnant while training. But many medical authorities view any cessation of menstruation as problematic. Indeed the study of such problems has led to the development of a distinct medical speciality – sport gynaecology. Female athletes are warned that by being super-fit they may damage their potential for motherhood. 'How many amenorrheic athletes have a reversible problem and will be able to achieve pregnancy when they decrease their level of training?, asks Baker.[15] That pregnancy is the female athlete's overriding goal is taken for granted. In assuming so, many medical experts reconstruct the century-old debate about the impact on the female physique of competing demands of academic study and menstruation, replacing concerns about higher education (over-brain-work) with those about athletic training (over-body-work).[16]

Thus the effects of the late nineteenth-century medico-scientific concerns about female development at menarche have been far-reaching. The medical debate initially reflected the overriding concern of the age with order and scarcity, and hence with balance and moderation. Accepting Newtonian principles, doctors viewed the body as a discrete energy field containing a finite amount of vital energy. Force expended in one direction would not be available for any other function. Hence the need to husband and balance this energy for the peculiar needs of women at each stage of their life cycle was a critical underlying factor in the regulation of exercise. Of all moments in the female life course, however, adolescence was seen to be the most important, the developmental stage requiring extra amounts of precious energy to assist in the establishment of menarche. Caution and moderation in physical and intellectual pursuits were medical watchwords and have remained so to a greater or lesser extent during the twentieth century. Medical studies continue to highlight the potential ill effects of rigorous exercise, intensive training and competitive sport upon female reproductive development despite the fact that studies regarding the impact of exercise on the menstrual cycle are, at best, tentative, and without adequate controls for variables now known to influence reproductive functioning.[17]

The historical context

Concerns about women's lack of control over their own bodies, and hence control over their health and opportunities for physical activity, have led feminists to consider more closely the particular circumstances surrounding women's experiences with experts of the body, to take issue with male dominance within the medical profession, and to examine the historical context in which the development and manipulation of scientific beliefs concerning women's bodies has taken place.

In particular, attention has been drawn to the large body of medical writing on every aspect of woman's reproductive system, writing which has been used in the name of health to circumscribe female behaviour and the range and scope of 'appropriate' physical activity. The medical system and medical science have occupied and continue to occupy a central place in women's experiences of themselves as women. Such ideas, held by the medical profession about the appropriate role of exercise in women's lives must be critically re-examined from several perspectives in order to understand how conventional notions of female form, function and mobility have been validated, promoted and perpetuated. We must reconsider how scientific ideas and information about the body were absorbed into popular culture – how information about female reproduction, sexuality, health and exercise was differentially distilled, transmitted and perceived, and how far this knowledge was a stimulant to action or inaction. To assist in this venture, it is helpful to study the role of medical experts and female patients (or potential patients) in a given society, their attitude towards the human body and the valuation of health and disease at a given time. 'The scientific standard of a physician alone does not make him efficient', cautioned Sigerist. 'Society has to be ready and willing to accept his advice.'[18] Since physicians treat as well as describe and explain, medical theories are socially immanent in a way that theories of biology are not. Consequently one can expect that medical theory will ultimately reflect and be reflected by the social role of the physician.[19]

Scholars are creating new methodologies and new conceptual frameworks to deal with the significant subjects of gender roles and professional knowledge in a historical context.[20] The increased integration of medical, social and women's history to explore the relationships between medical knowledge and health and gender-related issues foreshadows a more sophisticated conceptual framework to deal with the evolution of society and women's roles within it.[21] The search to determine what Carroll Smith-Rosenberg calls the 'concatenation of factors' which have 'decreed the particular gender assumptions the Western world imposed on women' leads the social historian of women's health and perceived exercise needs to the industrializing world of the nineteenth century, the rise of the bourgeois state and the development of the professions.[22] Feminist historians especially have looked at this period from a relational point of view, i.e. relating the history of women to that of men (as Engels did in *The Origin of the Family, Private Property and the State*) by seeing, in institutional and professional development, reasons for the advance of one sex and oppression of the other.[23] Research endeavours have begun to explore those formative moments in which medical professions on both sides of the Atlantic emerged as the powerful groups and reality definers of women's bodies they continue to be.[24] The structures and practices of the developing medical profession were intimately connected to models of adult socialization, of which the acquisition of sex roles is an integral part.[25]

According to Shirley Ardener, Victorian bourgeois women were from early childhood conditioned by professional medical men to express their deepest ideas in terms of the dominant group's surface ideas, transforming their own unconscious perceptions into such conscious ideas as would accord with those generated by the dominant group.[26] Women, she suggests, can be regarded as a muted group subject to a relatively great degree of oppression, but of such a nature that they may not know of, object to, or resist their oppression.[27] Put simply, women were socialized by the medical profession to see their bodies and view their natural functions in particular ways, to discern their exercise needs and the risks and benefits they might derive from physical activity through the eyes of the Victorian doctor. Women became subject to a system intended to produce compliant beings, and the methods that encouraged compliance began in childhood.[28]

Late nineteenth-century physicians were among the first of the new experts to claim a scientific foundation for their medical pronouncements upon how women should look and behave and what they were capable of doing physically. During these years, the zealous development of medicine along Darwinian scientific lines encouraged physicians to claim expertise in solving many of society's problems. 'With claims to knowledge encompassing all of human existence, they were the first to pass judgement on the social consequences of the female anatomy and to prescribe the natural life plan of women.'[29] Promised knowledge concerning the right and scientific way to live, many middle-class women responded trustingly to a medical authority they believed was based squarely upon the latest findings of biological science.

The transformation of the medical profession, the way in which medical rhetoric was informed by contemporary scientific beliefs and the tenor of the relationships between men and women in the late nineteenth and early twentieth centuries were critical components in framing the doctor–female patient relationship, as well as the scope of medical prescriptions and advice concerning women's health and exercise needs. What physicians, from their perspective as experts and rightful knowers, had to say about women, health and physical activity had an important impact upon the lives and outlook of middle-class women and provided a legacy which has had a lasting effect throughout the twentieth century.[30] In many respects, health became almost exclusively a matter of sophisticated physical and mental intervention which could be fully understood and competently practised only by objectively trained experts. With respect to almost any conceptual or theoretical concern, the idea of health and its relationship to physical activity became decisively confiscated by the doctors and the scientists.[31]

The use of medical discourse

In constructing a portrait of medically prescribed exercise for middle-class Victorian women across their life span, the selection and inter-pretation of professional discourse is important. Everything we know about the female body, says Susan Suleiman, certainly as regards the past, exists for us in some sort of discourse which is never unmediated, never free of interpretation, never innocent.[32] Furthermore, in any historical inquiry the ways in which the evidence is selected and read matter quite as much as the ways in which the theory is built. The two are necessarily interdependent.[33]

Berger and Luckman, and Holzner and Marx point out that individuals and groups within society are continuously involved in the social construction of knowledge and belief.[34] Their theories are useful in helping us to understand the development of female perceptions concerning their bodies and their capacity for physical activity. Since the knowledge and beliefs that women have today about their physical capabilities have been partly constructed in a socio-historical framework, those images of the past that have been captured in permanent form and are known to have been widely disseminated can display unique and important clues for our understanding of this phenomena. Smith has underscored how much of our knowledge of the world is mediated to us through various documents.[35] From this point of view, many documents exist from the past that can illuminate our present understanding of the complex area of perceived female physical capability. For example, documents such as medical texts, professional journals and medical advice manuals can provide powerful evidence of a group consciousness. As Mechling notes, they represent the attempts of a group of professionals to rationalize important realms of personal behaviour.[36] Berger et al. suggest that such discourses, when linked to particular institutions and institutional processes, form a systematic description of specific constellations of consciousness.[37]

Of particular utility to the study of women and physical activity are those popular medical discourses by reputed establishment physicians which had a wide transatlantic distribution in the late nineteenth and early twentieth centuries. Most of the abundant advice about physical health in England was either written by eminent medical practitioners or influenced by their beliefs, and this was also the case in the United States after the mid-century.[38] Although it is important to recognize that 'not all medical opinions on medical or social matters emanate from a shared set of professional values or a unified set of goals for professional behaviour',[39] and that it may be risky to assume medical unanimity on any subject in nineteenth-century medical literature,[40] much evidence suggests that one can usefully regard establishment physicians as speaking as one. They were not obscure or irrelevant commentators. The discourse of a recognized group of establishment male physicians had a powerful and wide-reaching effect. Their writing in professional medical journals in America and Britain was remarkably similar and very widely diffused, and a good case has been made for regarding such writings as typical of mainstream Victorian medical thought.[41]

Although for most of the nineteenth century neither the formally trained 'regular' doctors nor the 'irregular' lay practitioners held a mono-poly on scientific truth, the future clearly lay with the regulars – the establishment – who, towards the end of the century, co-operated with , or co-opted the many non-regular physicians and came to dominate the mainstream of medicine.[42] These were the physicians who attended the better medical schools, read the best medical journals, belonged to medical societies, and in general constituted the bulwark of the reputable medical profession of the late nineteenth century. They were successful, in part, because they garnered large numbers of patients in competition with other practitioners and patent medicines, and offered services which were clearly considered worth paying for by a wealthy and influential clientele. Furthermore, the power of their writings lay in the fact that they reflected rather than caused the situations in which they found themselves.[43]

Foucault has illustrated how professional writings concerning the physical body present themselves for close investigation and analysis.[44] Broadly, discourse, for him is a kind of anthropological notion of ritua-lized stories which an entire society holds in common, usually preserved in written sources. More specifically, he has underlined the importance of investigating the discursive practices of experts in what he calls those 'dubious disciplines' which have come to be called the human sciences.

He suggests that we must analyse what experts say when they are speaking as experts through written sources such as medical manuals, pedagogical treatises and case histories. Thus, it is not everyday discourse which constitutes the object of the study, but rather 'serious speech acts' which have passed some kind of institutional test; words that a particular authority (in our case the establishment physician of repute) has written concerning what, on the basis of an accepted method, is claimed as truth. The study of the particular discursive formations or networks of experts, according to Foucault, may bring us closer to an understanding of the social reality of the time and the effects of this reality upon the perceived health and exercise needs of women and children.[45]

These networks of discursive practices are clearly moulded and influenced by social institutions, as Martha Verbrugge has ably demonstrated in her study about the health of Bostonian middle-class women.[46] The way discourses about the body are used, whether related to work, exercise or sport, and the role they play in society are thus critical questions to explore when attempting to understand how social practices are linked up with the large-scale organization of power. To Foucault, discursive practices outlining agreed upon examples of how a domain of human activity should be organized show us how our culture attempts to normalize individuals through increasingly rationalized means, by turning them into meaningful subjects and docile objects.[47] Confronted by a power that is law (or a prevailing system of expertise), the subject who is 'subjected is (s)he who obeys – a legislative power on the one side and an obedient subject on the other'.[48]

Establishment medical discourse, viewed from this perspective, has served as a mode of action to exercise power over the actions of others by establishing and encouraging systems of differentiation among age groups and between genders. It has done so by shaping the types of objectives pursued by those who act upon the actions of others, such as those which would assist in maintaining privileges and profits; by elaborating the means of effecting the power relations such as medical advice and prescriptions; by promoting certain institutional forms, such as professional regulations and types of doctor-patient relationships; and by providing greater degrees of rationalization, i.e. an increasing degree of sophistication and elaborate advice and prescriptions in pursuing professional goals. Through this constructivist model of theory-choice, discourse is viewed 'not so much as a constraint on knowledge-claims but as a producer of knowledge in the same way that the primary role of paradigms in Kuhn's sense is to provide problems for the scientist to solve, not simply narrow the sphere in which it is possible to work'.[49]

Similarly, Swindells has explored how particular gendered images were constituted through professional medical discourse in the late nineteenth century, the crucial period during which were formed the gender attitudes and practices we have inherited in the twentieth century.[50] She follows Foucault's theme that dominant categories of thought and the power to enforce these ideas can be traced to the political organization of particular occupations such as medicine. The medical profession became reality definers and organizers of dominant thought, in large part through the publicized writings of those establishment physicians highlighted in this book. This discourse signified their understanding of the way things were or should be.[51] Medical knowledge, represented in their discourse, has been viewed by some social historians as a kind of ideological capital in which the commodity produced (medical prescriptions) concealed the ideology produced (medicine as medical knowledge) which concealed the capitalist relations which had produced it. There can be a danger in this. Viewed from this perspective, a study of the discourse itself could become imprisoning, encouraging the development of what have been termed 'formularistically irreproachable conceptual categories which are empty of usable content and [can] only pass muster so long as they remain confined to their own conceptual world'.[52] More useful, perhaps, as a mode of inquiry is the notion that there existed a reciprocity of interests wherein medical discourse represented medical knowledge (ideology) to a social group, and, in doing so, represented women to themselves.[53]

Like other human action, medicine was active, interpretive work through which a particular social reality was constructed – a reality constituted by diagnosed problems and prescribed treatments.[54] Medicine took on the authority to label female complaints, or to declare women potentially sick even if they did not complain.[55] The labelling of normal female functions such as menstruation and menopause as signs of illness requiring rest and medical observation did not, in itself, *make* women sick or incapable of vigorous activity. It did, however, provide a powerful rationale to persuade them from acting in any other way. Role definitions, explains Rosenberg, 'exist on a level of prescription beyond their embodiment in the individuality and behaviour of particular historical persons. They exist rather as a formally agreed upon set of characteristics understood by and acceptable to a significant portion of the population.'[56] Thus, medical representation, through its discourse, constituted women in particular ways, and it is this constitution, in relation to women and their perceived exercise needs, with which this book is largely concerned.

Women's voices

It is also perfectly clear, as numerous feminist scholars have pointed out, that we must do more than study what we understand women were told to do or persuaded to believe by medical discourse. It is true that men, especially male doctors, published more than women about the female life cycle and played a major role in shaping the social images and stereotypes of women.[57] Stereotyping has indeed had considerable impact on both the experience and treatment of social subgroups, such as women. Yet women should not be seen simply as passive creatures acted upon by others. They are active constructors of contexts and meaning which both reflect and affect the society.[58]

Evidence of women's reaction is important, and we must, therefore, listen to women's voices, to what women said about their feelings, personal and professional beliefs and experiences, and to the stories they wrote about their own physicality and their desire for or rejection of sport and exercise experiences. All women, after all, have female bodies and experience common bodily processes such as menstruation and menopause. All are affected, in one way or another by medical and scientific views of female bodily processes.[59] The social history of health and medicine, then, must also include what the women who were most critically involved thought or tried to do for themselves and others.

An emerging group of women physicians were particularly important in this regard. In some ways,

> educated women, like the Anglo-American physician Elizabeth Blackwell and her American colleague Mary Putnam Jacobi, sought to turn the findings of biological and medical science to women's account in order to counter the much popularized evolutionary sociobiological determinism of Comte and Spencer.[60]

On the other hand, however, most early women doctors accepted and promoted the very notions of Victorian delicacy and decorum which were so strongly endorsed by their male counterparts, and which contributed to keeping women enclosed in their separate sphere. Although historical comment on female physicians and their relationship to women's health, sport and exercise has tended to accept uncritically the thesis that their professional behaviour was radically different to that of their male counterparts, this does not appear to have been necessarily the case. Morantz-Sanchez has partly exposed the fallacy of this view by examining the differing paradigms and medical practices of female and male physicians in a hospital environment, but little comparative work is evident in the area of health and exercise prescriptions.[61]

Many women physicians, rather than pressing to further women's intellectual capacity and amplify the parameters of female physical capabilities, emphasized their special qualities of female nurturance and support for maternal values. Even when the debate about exclusion versus entry to the medical profession was won, women physicians still had 'many ghosts to fight, many prejudices to overcome'.[62] Entry was not synonymous with freedom of thought or practise for the path was only nominally open to women. A female medical career was, so to speak, 'in the gift of gentlemen', and was most successful when women accepted 'traditional femininities within the convoluted ritual of professional courtship'. This, concludes Swindells, led to the ready adoption by women of secondary and servicing positions within the profession, such as public health officers and school medical inspectors, as well as ensuring their conformity to the ethos of the male-dominated profession.[63] The roles granted to them within the profession put women doctors in touch with what many cared most about in medicine: female health and the scientific management of family life which, of course, included health education and exercise. Thus the history of women and medicine can help to expose the social origins and functions of medicine, and contribute to people's confidence and ability to see through the rational, scientific disguises of power. They may then be assured that women's oppression is socially, not biologically ordained and so be able to challenge the ideologies and technologies that control us today.[64]

Just as the difficulties of penetrating and joining with the medical profession shaped the attitudes and work orientation of women doctors, so did the manner of entry to the profession of literature mould women writers and their representation of femininity and womanhood.[65] Nineteenth-century medicine and literature both relied heavily upon systems of gender differentiation and were important in constructing sexual ideology and in illuminating social perceptions of 'woman as body'. Feminist writers such as Charlotte Perkins Gilman entered into the literary profession against a powerful ideology of gender restriction. In her case, her experiences in a patriarchal society and her struggles against a restrictive medical ideology both informed her socialist treatises and pervaded her works of fiction. Analyses of women writers of Victorian novels such as those elaborated in Gilbert and Gubar's *The*

Madwoman in the Attic[66] and *No Man's Land*[67] highlight important elements of nineteenth-century sexual struggles, especially women's quest for self-definition and wholeness. Swindells, too, believes that nineteenth-century fiction was peculiarly influential in the construction of gender relations and sexual ideology.[68] Prominent in the novels of nineteenth-century authors such as Jane Austen, Mary Shelley, the Brontes, George Eliot and Emily Dickinson are angelic stepdaughters, 'extremely beautiful, inanimate *objets d'art* preserved in the glass coffin of patriarchal aesthetics', struggling against a stunted and domesticated selfhood and losing their health in the process.[69]

Mid-Victorian writers of both sexes, suggest Gilbert and Gubar, dramatized a defeat of the female in any struggle to enlarge her sphere and gain greater physical independence. By the turn of the century, however, authors such as Gilman were cautiously speculating about the possibility of women's triumph. That possibility, suggest Gilbert and Gubar, 'appears to have filled men with such dread that they had to produce specially ferocious fantasies about female defeat even though women did not elaborate fantasies about their own victory with any special confidence'.[70] One can detect such ambivalence and lack of confidence in the writings of Gilman. At the same time, the extreme anti-feminist stance adopted by psychologist G. Stanley Hall in his professional studies of female development at the turn of the century illuminates the depth of anxiety felt by many professional men over what they perceived to be inexorable female advances into a territory they believed was marked 'male'. Men's fear of the potential competition of women in the workplace, and we might also suppose on the playing field, says Dijkstra, helps explain why the amount of frightened attention women received was so intense.[71] Those who did not conform to the ideal of womanhood were 'dangerous backslider[s] in humanity's quest for evolutionary transcendence'.[72] Female energy was meant for the altruism of home and posterity, not activity of mind and body and other augmentations of her individuality.[73]

Complementary studies of both medical and women's health sources are thus necessary to document women's own concerns about physical exercise and experiences with male doctors and their advice, such as that described by Charlotte Perkins Gilman in her autobiography as well as her account of her experience of Dr Weir Mitchell's rest cure in 'The Yellow Wallpaper'.[74] Smith-Rosenberg suggests that we must search history for evidence of women's reactions (to efforts to suppress their physicality) and their efforts to assert authority and use power. If one does not accept the view of women as passive victims then there is a need, she claims, 'to identify the sources of power women used to act within a world determined to limit their power, to ignore their talents, to belittle or condemn their actions'.[75] If no one questions a role and few pressures are placed on its maintenance, then there is little reason to define it carefully or write about it. Clearly many women did challenge traditional roles and behavioural prescriptions, and they did so from a number of vantage points.

Indeed, the expanding history of women's growing participation in sport in the second half of the nineteenth century is testimony to the fact that by no means all women paid close attention to medical cautions about overuse and overstrain in sport and exercise. Many women enjoyed physical pursuits, seeing in sport and exercise the possibility of freeing themselves 'from some of the more entrenched and pervasive tenets of the Victorian ideology of femininity'.[76] New sports like tennis were taken up. Girls and women were bicycling and playing team sports. There is ample documentation to illustrate the growing numbers of sporting women on both sides of the Atlantic. The intensifying debate about the 'woman question' also pointed up the challenge by women who were chafing against traditional role prescriptions, questioning the quality of their lives and viewing vigorous physical activity as liberating. Foreshadowing today's feminists, groups of women activists argued that women must take control of their own bodies, which included liberalizing customs of female exercise and expanding women's opportunities in recreation and sports.[77]

Incorporating the experiences of particular women into our social analysis means reconsidering the fundamental ordering of social relations, institutions and power arrangements.[78] Only by listening to women's voices, continues Smith-Rosenberg, can we test the accuracy of prescriptive materials against the reality of what women actually did. Such analysis permits us to view prescription as a cultural form rather than regarding it as merely a distorted window into social realities.[79] From this perspective we can begin to construct what Kelly calls a 'conceptual vision' in order to plumb the complex interaction of norms and behaviour and the ways in which both mirror the organization of society as a whole.[80]

Methodological limitations

My primary aim in analysing late nineteenth-century establishment medical reports and literary debates about women's physical attributes and social role is to explore certain dimensions of the relationship between the professional development of medicine and women's understanding of their bodies and physical capability for exercise. This aim, however, imposes certain limitations, such as the fact that the sample of women examined was drawn solely from middle- and upper-class origins. They were, after all, the main clientele of establishment doctors.

Since historians caution that there was a diversity of opinions and issues concerning nineteenth-century attitudes towards the nature and place of women, and that these controversies must be placed carefully in their social and cultural context in order to be meaningful, it is important not to speak of women as a mass.[81] The work of qualitative sociologists and anthropologists has shown how the material conditions of individuals influence their own conception of health and physical capability, while their social location, especially their class position, contributes to both how they define responsibility for health and what they conceive health to be.[82] Women, even within the same class, do not have the same experiences and are not uniformly oppressed.[83] Though 'no topic more occupied the Victorian mind than health',[84] it was the middle-class mind that reflected on the meaning of exercise for female health and it was the woman of the 'better' classes with whom the establishment doctor was largely concerned. Literature giving these women guidance about their health and exercise behaviour was more profuse and inflexible than for working-class women, although advice for the working class increased substantially in the first two decades of the twentieth century. Poor women, who in any case had little opportunity to reflect upon the relationship between vigorous activity and their health (being often physically exhausted from unremitting toil), received scant attention from the medical profession, at least as individuals. Society doctors viewed affluent women as being in special need of protection because of their delicate nature and refined life-style, and saw working women as naturally robust and less susceptible to difficulties brought on by bodily exertion. Lower-class women were believed to be physically stronger and to feel little pain in comparison to middle-class women.

Although a number of studies are restoring working-class women to history and exploring their physical activities and perceived exercise needs as a new window into social practices, the world of nineteenth- and early twentieth-century sport and exercise for predominantly non-leisured women requires a book of its own.[85] Also, recent studies of

Victorian middle-class women have demanded a more realistic look at their subjects' life-styles and have criticized their frequent portrayal as idle creatures consumed with their own invalidism and obsessed with fashion and frivolity.[86] Many historians have mistakenly concluded that the processes of industrialization eased the burden of women's work in the home, and that the assistance of servants necessarily did the same thing. Although developing industrialization served to eliminate those types of work once assigned to men and children, in almost every aspect of household work the toil of women was left either untouched or even augmented. It was a glaring example of women's very separate sphere, for even though middle-class women were constantly advised to rest by popular medical literature, they were also expected to put in a long hard day managing both house and family activities.[87] Small wonder that so many people commented on the exhaustion and ill health of women, especially American women, during the nineteenth century.[88]

One must compare image to reality, notes Branca, through a more discriminating use of the available literature, especially the fiction concerning the daily life and health of Victorian women. It is difficult, for example, to contend that the historian should begin with novels or utilize them without a great deal of supporting evidence.[89] Certainly, as Virginia Woolf realised, the Victorian novel is a complex, even confusing source of information and must be used with the utmost care and discrimination.[90]

A further important caveat to my study of women, doctors and exercise relates to location. It is my intention to consider British and American medical discussions about female exercise needs, risks and benefits as parts of a general debate on the role and physical capabilities of late nineteenth-century women.[91] Many physicians trained, practised and lectured on both continents. Early women physicians were remarkably mobile, crossing and re-crossing the Atlantic, studying and practising in Europe and North America, developing a shared professional consensus about the roles and responsibilities of female doctors.

The underlying themes of establishment medical discourse concerning women's physical capabilities were remarkably similar in America and England, and both countries nurtured the same anxieties about women and the dangers of physical overexertion. There was a steady transatlantic traffic in medical information and popular health literature during the latter decades of the nineteenth century. As American physician Walter Taylor explained, 'the most eminent physicians both here and in England have united in deploring the state of women's health'.[92]

Harvard medical man Dr Edward Clarke's pessimistic views on the physical and mental abilities of women were as widely quoted in England as were the arguments of eminent British physicians such as Drs Clouston and Maudsley in the United States. All followed Herbert Spencer's expansive interpretation of Darwinian theory. Transatlantic agreement was also evident in Dr Mary Putnam Jacobi's reply to Clarke and Dr Elizabeth Garrett Anderson's answers to Maudsley's views in England, for both were of the same mind. British doctors freely used the opinions of American doctors on the effects of higher education despite clear differences in educational organization.[93] One might consider the 'woman question,' say Helsinger *et al.*, as MacCarthur viewed the women's trade union leagues, 'that the British movement was both grandmother and granddaughter of the American'.[94] Thus, both cultures learned and re-learned from continuous sharing of the experiences of the other, and an examination of one environment naturally entails an examination of the other.[95]

Although such an Anglo-American perspective allows a comprehensive examination of views on women which were exchanged regularly across the Atlantic, it can diminish the importance of local context and specific national environments. Showalter, while commenting that fundamental ideas about femininity and sexual difference were certainly shared by both England and the United States, also demonstrates that each society established its own moral, medical and mental boundaries around female problems.[96] Jalland and Hooper have documented how more extreme views about female infirmities were expressed in American medical texts and popular literature, and how this often led to more extreme remedies.[97] Ann Douglas Wood supports this view, commenting that nineteenth-century America was, in certain senses, more Victorian than the country from which the name was derived.[98] The bicycle debate of the 1890s, for example, though similar in many respects, was more hysterical in the United States than in England, and the recurrent nineteenth-century anxieties over the poor health of American women were couched in considerably more melodramatic terms than were British female health concerns until the very end of the century.[99]

Worries about the health of British women were publicized widely, yet medical personnel and health reformers routinely acknowledged superior British thinking and practices in the domain of female health, physical education and sport.[100] In England, reported Catharine Beecher to her American readers of *Physiology and Calisthenics for Schools and Families*, 'in matters of health and hygiene almost all women are in full perfection of womanhood ....'[101] The robust health and flushing beauty of English girls 'who think nothing of a five or ten mile walk for a constitutional', was remarked upon by Mrs Duffey in 1874.[102] Henry Slocum described in 1889 how 'the physical superiority of the English women to those of most other nations is well known due to the greater amount of exercise which they take'.[103] Could this superiority, questioned Dr Weir Mitchell, be due to the fact that for some reason mental work is more exhausting in the United States than in Europe? Perhaps, he speculated, the work of the body occasioned more strain in America than in Europe, and was followed by a greater sense of fatigue.[104]

Sara Burstall, in her evaluation of physical education practices in the United States, commented in 1894 that 'we frequently heard Americans refer to the good health of English women, and to their delight in open-air games while they regretted that such did not prevail more generally in America'.[105] By the end of the century, however, even this rhetoric was changing as commentators increasingly noted that American girls and women had finally begun to learn the advantages of those outdoor games which had traditionally been part of the middle-class English girl's education.[106]

In both national arenas local and specific concerns must necessarily be neglected in a general study such as this. There is a rich store of intimate and local studies about the experiences of particular women in relation to medical knowledge and physical culture awaiting exploration. It is a much needed part of a history of women's experiences with their bodies and I have attempted to make a start with my study of Charlotte Perkins Gilman and the particular importance she placed upon health and physical culture practices as a means of emancipation.

Finally, it is important to note that I have concentrated upon those medical and pseudo-scientific ideas about female health and exercise which were so stridently directed at late nineteenth-century women throughout their daily lives, rather than focusing upon specific institutional developments. The promotion of sport, gymnastics and health education activities in women's colleges, physical education colleges and girls' secondary schools on both sides of the Atlantic, as well as the interchange of ideas, techniques and teaching personnel among these institutions has been well documented.[107] Two recent studies related to institutional development enrich our understanding of women and exercise in the late nineteenth and early twentieth centuries by focusing upon the ideas and activities of an emergent profession of female physical educators. The collection of voluminous statistics on women's health and strength at women's colleges and co-educational institutions to appease medical fears that female health would be damaged by overwork and professional training was undertaken, not only by physicians and educators, but also by a new breed of physical education specialists committed to promoting physiological knowledge, greater exercise opportunities and a distinct sporting arena for women.[108] By documenting the particular accommodations of professional female physical educators to establishment medical views concerning properly regulated physical exercise, these studies provide a useful complement to my own study of women doctors in chapters 4 and 5.

Not surprisingly, the rationale for training women physical educators followed closely that employed by women doctors. Madame Bergman-Osterberg, initiator of the training of female physical educators in England proclaimed that 'this work we women do better, as our very success in training depends upon our having felt like women, able to calculate the possibilities of our sex, knowing our weakness, and our strength'.[109] Nor, in a patriarchal society, would one expect other than that these early institutional pioneers would tend to defer to the precepts of a double conformity, redefining rather than rejecting the Victorian feminine ideal when it came to promoting exercise and sport for girls and women.[110] As professionals, notes Mrozek, these physical educators, boosters of restraint, had an emotional commitment to reasonable behaviour 'which inclined them to a regulation of women's sport in a manner and to a degree literally impossible among men's sports'. Their effort was to maintain, through an 'alliance of results' with medical authorities, that appropriate balance of rest and moderate activity that nineteenth-century physicians articulated as necessary for improving the health of women as mothers of the race.[111]

Medical men played a significant role in enhancing beliefs among late nineteenth-century middle-class women concerning the perceived risks of physical strain engendered by higher education, professional training and vigorous exercise and sport. Medical women, in struggling to gain professional recognition, often played a supporting role. 'By virtue of being professionals, they could not help but be influenced by the growing use of the medical profession as an instrument for social control', thus their attitudes toward female health and their exercise prescriptions for women were often as conservative as those of their male establishment counterparts.[112]

Although by 1900 the cult of female invalidism was being steadily challenged by feminists promoting the beneficial effects of exercise and sport, conservative male and female doctors continued to warn an increasingly nervous public that the physical activities of the 'new woman' were going too far and that women were irresponsibly using up bodily energy that was required for healthy maternity and efficient housekeeping. These criticisms were collected and repeated uncritically to a mass audience by psychologist G. Stanley Hall, 'the publication of whose monumental *Adolescence* marked a new high-water mark of anti-feminist opinion on both sides of the Atlantic'.[113] Hall confidently assisted in popularizing and intensifying ideas about the science of society which had developed from joining Comte's positivism and Spencer's notions of human progress with Darwin's theory of natural selection, and which tended to provide a technical justification for ever-increasing levels of social inequality. Stunted by evolution, no better than children, women were increasingly expected to concentrate upon conserving their energy for their reproductive responsibility. Unable to solve her own problems, said Hall, woman was unable to be her own teacher, preacher or doctor.[114]

Female physicians were well represented in the increasing anxieties over racial improvement portrayed in that strand of social Darwinism which became the Eugenics Movement. They warned girls and women against the danger of dissipating needed energy by making a fetish of exercise.[115] Dr Arabella Kenealy accused girls' schools of impoverishing girls' bodies on the playing field and rendering them deficient for making healthy babies.[116] It was explained that excessive effort demanded by sporting pursuits, especially during menstruation, exposed girls to the risk of life-long invalidism:

> No girl can risk the strain of a match game without dangers of suffering from it sooner or later, not only because of the extreme bodily effort but because of the nervous tension arising from the excitement of competition together with the emotional disturbance inevitably attending success or defeat. These observations teach us that a woman's physical wellbeing under existing social conditions, depends largely upon her willingness to acquiesce in those moderate and proper restrictions imposed by nature upon her sex.[117]

Feminists who sought publicly to demonstrate the imprisoning nature of the physical limits imposed upon middle-class women by medical demands for a conserving, maternal life-style were often themselves rendered ambivalent about the goals and means of their own mission. Sometimes they were driven insane. Jane Addams, Eleanor Marx, Olive Shreiner, Virginia Woolf and Charlotte Perkins Gilman were all examples of feminists experiencing nervous disorders due in part to role conflict. In 'The Yellow Wallpaper' Charlotte Perkins Gilman tried convincingly to portray:

> the immediate link which existed between the male creation of (and many women's compliance with) the principles of the cult of invalidism, the physician's encouragement of that cult, and the increasing incidence of madness in women. The male world's resolute refusal to recognize the creative intelligence of women was leading many to desperate attempts to break through the pointless pattern of the wallpaper of social constriction, only to find themselves enmeshed ever more tightly in its design.[118]

Charlotte Perkins Gilman's epithet of a 'militant madonna' was not uncommon for independent women of her class advocating the development of health and strength and the struggle for independence to enlarge, if not necessarily to eliminate, the separate sphere of women's private experience.[119]

In an era where survival of the fittest had become a catchword for individual striving and progress (and when, in spite of the fact that women outlived men, men were quite obviously defined as the fittest), women were to be discouraged from entering any contest which might cause the expenditure of energy that was required for reproduction and healthy mothering. The progressive functional separation of the sexes demanded that women be socialized to become ever more feminine and to place more rather than less concentration upon their naturally ordained, primitive function of reproduction. Well-regulated sport and exercise would help in this endeavour and Dudley Allen Sargent's gymnastics system offered late nineteenth-century women, especially college women, some of the most well-designed exercise available.[120] However, the pervasive notion that should a woman step beyond this formula of correct, moderate and systematic exercise she might encounter physical, mental and moral dangers became deeply embedded in the culture of female sport and exercise. Should women become too vigorous, aggressive and competitive in their sporting activities and make the fatal mistake of entering an arena marked out as inappropriate for female endeavour, sooner or later their energy would be dissipated, their health would break down and they would be out of the race. Because they were 'eternally wounded', they were doomed to compete and lose, or not to compete at all. It was not that men and women were considered to march to different drummers, it was that many believed that men and women should not even be seen in the same parade.[121] In the competition for life, assured Dr Hughes Bennett,

22

'woman is the weaker vessel and liable to be broken when too roughly handled'.[122]

In other words man, to prove his fitness, had to exercise mind and body more than woman, and woman was advised to accept prescribed limits upon her actions, including athletic limitations, as the price for having a female body. Too active a life, she was told, contributed to the degeneration of feminine functions. Competition with men in work, play or sport wore out her body and unfitted her for maternal duties. Why did no one ask, wondered the Countess of Jersey, whether it was conceivable 'that she may sometimes like the work or sport for its own sake, without any thought of competition with the other sex?'[123] Nineteenth-century conservative doctors did not ask that question because the origin of their view of the female and her perceived health and exercise needs lay not in objective science, but in their cultural heritage which had already answered such questions in the negative. 'Happily,' said Walker, in his massive study of female physiology, and despite clear evidence to the contrary, 'the athletic temperament does not occur in women.'[124]

Organization

I have divided this book into three parts, each of which focuses upon a different facet of the broad theme elaborated so far in this introduction.

Part One examines the bases for exercise prescriptions elaborated for middle-class women during the course of their lives by nineteenth-century male establishment physicians. Conditioning of females to the laws of personal energy expenditure and to docility began early and continued throughout old age. The first three chapters outline the particular categories of exercise prescriptions which were promoted through male medical discourse for girls and women at critical developmental moments in their lives. They identify the paradigm underlying medical judgements of physical capability as they related to the perceived exercise needs of women throughout their life course.

Chapter 1 focuses upon adolescence and the relationship between medical theories of menstrual disability and medical prescriptions for exercise. Women's limited physical achievements as compared to men's were increasingly ascribed to the burden placed upon them by menstruation. From the onset of menarche till the end of their 'thirty-year pilgrimage' women were advised by doctors to treat themselves as invalids once a month, curtailing both physical and mental activity. Long-standing propositions about adolescent girls' incapacity for certain sports and strenuous exercise developed in response to late nineteenth-century physicians' interpretations of biological theories about menstruation.

Chapter 2 examines medical prescriptions for exercise during women's prime reproductive years. Exercise advice to women during pregnancy and as busy mothers is discussed, and the bicycle-riding craze among active women is examined from the point of view of the medical profession. Indeed, the medical debate concerning the risks and benefits of bicycle riding and other popular sports for women encapsulates well the anxieties of professional establishment men needing to exercise control over the female reproductive process and hence preserve the health and prosperity of society on both sides of the Atlantic. Medical images of women on bicycles (and in other physical activities) provide us with a means of exploring the general interactions of medicine, personal lives and social roles and changes.[125]

Chapter 3 explores the world of ageing and old women. It examines medical prescriptions of exercise for menopausal women; women whose 'thirty-year pilgrimage' of potential childbearing was over and whose physical and intellectual, as well as social purpose tended to be dismissed as insignificant in medical texts and advice books. This was partly because many women did not live beyond their childbearing years and partly because they were perceived to be of no further use to society. For those who did live beyond the age of forty, menopause was often regarded as a catastrophic experience, 'the death of the woman in the woman', requiring particular cautionary advice regarding health and exercise.

Part Two looks at a particular group of female actors who either fought against or fostered orthodox medicine's restrictive views concerning physical activity, and who were professionally involved in the medical debate concerning perceived exercise risks and benefits for women.

Chapter 4 describes women's struggle to enter the medical profession on both sides of the Atlantic and analyses the copious arguments advanced for and against female doctors. Aspects of the medical debate designed to restrain female professional advancement, as well as the strategies women developed to overcome establishment hurdles, are important in understanding the doctor-patient relationship developed among women and the types of therapeutic advice, including exercise prescriptions, proposed by those who became regular women doctors.

Chapter 5 examines the role played by a selection of prominent pioneer female physicians in replicating or transforming the essential tenets of the male medical debate about physical activity for women. Medical culture has a powerful socialization process and it is of interest to see how far women doctors accommodated themselves to the ethos and practices of a male-dominated profession, and in what ways they strove to preserve distinctly female values in their work. To emphasize the continuity of the transatlantic debate, the discussion centres on those influential nineteenth-century female doctors who lived and worked or studied in both America and Europe and who had a particular interest in promoting female physical culture. Elizabeth Blackwell, Elizabeth Garrett Anderson and Mary Putnam Jacobi are examples of the early pioneer tradition on both sides of the Atlantic. Eliza Mosher, Lucy Hall and Clelia Duel Mosher are examples of female physicians who worked to improve the health of girls through exercise in schools and colleges, and who wrote extensively about the physical capabilities of women. Growing concern with eugenics in the early decades of the twentieth century was shrilly reflected in the rhetoric of numerous well-known women doctors interested in female health and exercise. The writings of Arabella Kenealy, Elizabeth Sloan Chesser and Angenette Parry illuminate conservative female medical beliefs about women's physical capacity for exercise during this era.

Part Three provides two radical perspectives upon the turn-of-the-century debates over women and exercise, the powerful anti-intellectual, anti-feminist rhetoric of psychologist G. Stanley Hall, 'Darwin of the mind', and the feminist intellectual challenge of writer and utopian Charlotte Perkins Gilman.

Chapter 6 reflects upon the continuing effects of the nineteenth-century medical debate over women's physical and mental capabilities as the discussion spilled into the twentieth century. The focus of inquiry is shifted from the medical profession to the developing profession of psychology and the anti-feminist part played by its early leader in supporting, indeed edifying establishment medical views in relation to women and exercise. The chapter explores the prominent, supporting role played by psychologist G. Stanley Hall at the turn of the twentieth century in anchoring and disseminating biologically deterministic views about women's physical and mental capabilities and their exercise needs. Like many of the medical specialists he admired, Hall was an influential product of his culture's limited conception of sex roles. Although the turbulent conditions of the late nineteenth and early twentieth centuries encouraged a growing number of reformers to advocate a broader and more active sphere for women, he shared and

25

helped perpetuate the deeply rooted views of the male medical establishment concerning the 'eternally wounded woman', and the kinds of exercise which would best fit a woman for her maternal duties and her appropriate role in ensuring the survival of the race. By the first decade of the twentieth century such 'anti-feminine attitudes, often accompanied by a wholesale espousal of misogyny', had become the rule rather than the exception in both Europe and North America.[126] It is particularly important to document such views for they became deeply embedded in popular sport and in the school physical and health education curriculum. By clothing mythologies in scientific garb they have demonstrated great staying power.

Chapter 7 illustrates the growing desire of the 'new woman' to control her own body and reproductive life by pursuing health and wholeness. It examines the relationship of feminism to medical doctors and the health of middle-class women through the writings and life experiences of a socialist feminist, Charlotte Perkins Gilman. Gilman was a leading turn-of-the-century feminist whose bitter experiences with the establishment neurologist S. Weir Mitchell, and whose life-long personal pursuit of physical autonomy and creative fulfilment tell us much about the history of male opposition to female emancipation and women's desire for intellectual freedom and control over their own bodies. This chapter emphasizes the significance of biography and biographical context for understanding the debate about women, doctors and exercise. Because of the personal nature of problems and ideas connected with women's autonomy and rights, the intellectual positions of individuals who wrote on the woman question cannot be understood without reference to their life experiences.[127] The biographical details of Charlotte Gilman and analyses of her feminist writings allow a clear gaze at the immense social obstacles which the intellectual woman had to overcome and the real perceptual difficulties women had to grapple with in striving for balanced health, a sound mind in a healthy body. Charlotte Gilman's notions of mind-body relationships illustrate dominant modes of thought about female health and autonomy in the late nineteenth century.

Notes

1 Will Wright, *The Social Logic of Health*, Rutgers University Press, New Jersey, 1982, p. 24.
2 One should not forget the importance of medical efforts in caring for the sick.

Medical acts, however, have significant social consequences which demand that 'we look beyond medical boundaries in order to fully understand both the sources and consequences of particular forms of medicine'. Elliot G. Mishler, 'The health-care system: social contexts and consequences', in E.G. Mishler, L. AmaraSingham, S. Hauser, R. Liem, S. Osherson and N.E. Waxler, *Social Contexts of Health, Illness and Patient Care*, Cambridge University Press, Cambridge, 1981, p. 215.

3 Joan Kelly-Gadol, 'The social relation of the sexes: Methodological implications of women's history,' *Signs: Journal of Women in Culture and Society*, I, Summer 1976, p. 812; See also, Marjorie C. Feinson, 'Where are the women in the history of aging?' *Social Science History*, IX, no. 4, Fall 1985, pp. 429–452.

4 Indeed the 'weaker sex' perception continues to affect responses to demands for equity in the provision of competitive sporting opportunities, employment practices in jobs involving physical activity and/or strength, commercial approaches to sport, fitness and recreation, media portrayal of women exercising, at sport and in play, as well as perceptions of female health and disease and evolving public, educational, medical, and health practices and policies.

5 Mary Boutilier and Lucinda SanGiovanni, 'Women and sports: Reflections on health and policy', in Ellen Lewin and Virginia Olesen, eds., *Women, Health and Healing. Toward a New Perspective*, Tavistock Publications, New York, 1985, p. 214.

6 Roland Barthes quoted in J. Sturrock, ed., *Structuralism and Since*, Oxford University Press, Oxford, 1979, p. 60.

7 Charles Webster, ed., *Biology, Medicine and Society, 1840–1940*, Cambridge University Press, Cambridge, 1981, p. 1.

8 David Barash, *The Whisperings Within*, Harper & Row, New York, 1979, p. 114; R. Dawkins, *The Selfish Gene*, Oxford University Press, New York, 1979; E. O. Wilson, *Sociobiology: The New Synthesis*, Harvard University Press, Cambridge, MA, 1975.

9 Elizabeth Fee, 'Nineteenth century craniology: The study of the female skull', *Bulletin of the History of Medicine*, LIII, 1979, p. 433; Stephen Gould, in *The Mismeasure of Man*, talks about biological determinism and its effect upon women's lives. 'Biological determinism is, in essence, a theory of limits. It takes the current status of a group as a measure of where they should and must be... [Since] we pass through this world but once, few tragedies can be more extensive than the stunting of life; few injustices deeper than the denial of an opportunity to strive or even to hope, by a limit imposed from without, but falsely identified as lying within... We inhabit a world of human differences and predilections, but the extrapolation of these facts to theories of rigid limits is ideology.' Stephen Gould, *The Mismeasure of Man*, W.W. Norton, New York, 1981, pp. 28–29.

10 Michel Foucault, *The History of Sexuality: Volume I, An Introduction*, Vintage Books, New York, 1980.

11 Gerald Leach, *The Biocrats*, Jonathan Cape, London, 1970, p. 132.

12 See, for example, R. Hubbard and M. Lowe, eds., *Genes and Gender II: Pitfalls in Research on Sex and Gender*, Gordian Press, Staten Island, NY, 1979; M.

Lowe and R. Hubbard, eds., *Woman's Nature: Rationalizations of Inequality*, Pergamon Press, New York, 1983; R. Bleier, *Science and Gender*, Pergamon Press, New York, 1984; Anne Fausto-Sterling, *Myths of Gender*, Basic Books, New York, 1985; Ruth Hubbard, Mary Sue Henifin and Barbara Fried, eds., *Biological Woman – The Convenient Myth*, Schenkman Pub. Co., Inc., Cambridge, MA, 1982; Janet Sayers, *Biological Politics. Feminist and Anti-Feminist Perspectives*, Tavistock Publications, London, 1982. 'Critics of biological determinism', note Lewontin *et al.*, 'are like members of a fire brigade, constantly being called out in the middle of the night to put out the latest conflagration, always responding to immediate emergencies, but never with the leisure to draw up plans for a truly fireproof building. Now it is IQ and race, now criminal genes, now the biological inferiority of women, now the genetic fixity of human nature. All of these deterministic fires need to be doused with the cold water of reason before the entire intellectual neighborhood is in flames.' R. C. Lewontin, Steven Rose and Leon Kamin, *Not in Our Genes: Biology, Ideology and Human Nature*, Pantheon Press, New York, 1984, p. 265.

13 Simone de Beauvoir, *The Second Sex*, Translated by H.M. Parshley, Alfred A. Knopf, New York, 1962. (original edition, 1949).

14 Jacquelyn N. Zita, 'The premenstrual syndrome: "Dis-easing" the female cycle', *Hypatia*, III, no. 1, Spring 1988, pp. 77–99.

15 Elizabeth Renwick Baker, 'Historical perspectives of research on physical activity and the menstrual cycle', in Jacqueline L. Puhl and C. Harmon Brown, eds., *The Menstrual Cycle and Physical Activity*, Human Kinetics Publ. Inc., Champaign, IL, 1984, p. 5.

16 Dr Maudsley, the eminent British psychiatrist, was among the leaders of the late nineteenth-century movement to argue that, because of biological factors, sexual equality could only be achieved at the cost of damage to women's reproductive functions. 'When nature spends in one direction,' he wrote in a widely circulated article, 'she must economize in another.' Henry Maudsley, 'Sex in mind and education', *Fortnightly Review*, XV, 1874, p. 467.

17 Linda R. Gannon, *Menstrual Disorders and Menopause: Biological, Psychological and Cultural Research*, Praegar Scientific, New York, 1985, p. 21. Exercise physiology experts currently conceptualize exercise as MVPA i.e. moderate to vigorous physical activity, defined operationally as body weight transfer, including self-propelled movement such as running, dancing, jumping and many sports, games and calisthenics. Bruce Simons-Morton, Nancy M. O'Hara, Denise Simons-Morton and Guy S. Parcel, 'Children and fitness: A public health perspective, reaction to the reactions', *Research Quarterly for Exercise and Sport*, LIX, no. 2, June 1988, pp. 177–179. See also James F. Sallis, 'A commentary on children and fitness: A public health perspective', *Research Quarterly for Exercise and Sport*, LVIII, no. 4, 1987, pp. 326–330, and Bruce G. Simons-Morton *et al.*, 'Children and fitness: A public health perspective', *Research Quarterly for Exercise and Sport*, LVIII, no. 4, 1987, pp. 295–302.

Boutilier and SanGiovanni provide useful working definitions of exercise, fitness and sport for this book. 'We conceptualize exercise as a particular form of physical activity and use this term to refer to "reasonably vigorous" or continuous physical activity.' Physical fitness is defined as the ability to engage in fairly vigorous physical activities and includes those qualities believed essential to a person's health and wellbeing. Sport refers to human activity that involves the use of relatively complex physical skills or strenuous physical exertion and is characterized by competition occurring under formal or organized conditions. Boutilier and SanGiovanni, 'Women and sports', p. 210.

18 Henry E. Sigerist, 'The history of medicine and the history of science', *Bulletin of the History of Medicine*, IV, 1936, p. 5. See also John Woodward and David Richards, eds., *Health Care and Popular Medicine in Nineteenth Century England. Essays in the Social History of Medicine*, Croom Helm, London, 1977.

19 Ignaz Semmelweiss, *The Etiology, Concept and Prophylaxis of Childbed Fever*, translated and edited by K. Codell Carter, University of Wisconsin Press, Madison, 1983 [1861].

20 See, for example, Catherine Clinton, *The Other Civil War. American Women in the Nineteenth Century*, Hill and Wang, New York, 1984, p. 225.

21 Gerald N. Grob, 'The social history of medicine and disease in America: Problems and possibilities', *Journal of Social History*, III, Spring 1972, p. 405; Martha H. Verbrugge, 'Women and medicine in nineteenth-century America,' *Signs, Journal of Women in Culture and Society*, I, no. 4, 1976, pp. 957–973.

22 Carroll Smith-Rosenberg, *Disorderly Conduct: Visions of Gender in Victorian America*, Alfred A. Knopf, New York, 1985, p. 12.

23 Friedrich Engels, *The Origin of the Family, Private Property and the State in the Light of the Researches of Lewis H. Morgan*, International Publishers, New York, 1942 ed.; see also, Ann J. Lane, 'Woman in society: A critique of Frederick Engels,' in Berenice A. Carroll, ed., *Liberating Women's History: Theoretical and Critical Essays*, University of Illinois Press, Urbana, IL, 1976, and Mari Jo Buhle, *Women and American Socialism, 1870–1920*, University of Illinois Press, Urbana, IL, 1981; Joan Kelly, *Women, History, and Theory*, University of Chicago Press, Chicago, 1986, p. 4.

24 Julia Swindells, *Victorian Writing and Working Women. The Other Side of Silence*, University of Minnesota Press, Minneapolis, 1985, p. 3. A number of historians agree that these years represented a crucial moment in American and English social history as professional fields expanded and the emergence of new careers created a dynamic professional class. See, for example, Gloria Moldow, *Women Doctors in Gilded-Age Washington*, University of Illinois Press, Urbana, IL, 1987; Robert W. Wiebe, *The Search for Order, 1877–1920*, Hill and Wang, New York, 1967; Burton J. Bledstein, *The Culture of Professionalism: The Middle Class and the Development of Higher Education in America*, W. W. Norton, New York, 1976; Among the many studies relating the emergence of the medical profession to increased control over women's bodies number Barbara Ehrenreich and Deirdre English, *For Her Own Good. 150 Years of the Experts' Advice to Women*, Anchor Books, Garden City, NY, 1979; Anita Clair Fellman and Michael Fellman, *Making Sense of Self: Medical Advice Literature in Late Nineteenth Century America*, University of Pennsylvania Press, Philadelphia, 1981; G. J. Barker-Benfield, *The Horrors of the Half-Known Life: Male Attitudes Toward Women and Sexuality in Nineteenth*

Century America, Harper and Row, New York, 1976; Ann Douglas, *The Feminization of American Culture*, Alfred A. Knopf, New York, 1977; Linda Gordon, *Woman's Body, Woman's Right: A Social History of Birth Control in America*, Grossman, New York, 1976; Sara Delamont and Lorna Duffin, eds., *The Nineteenth-Century Woman. Her Cultural and Physical World*, Croom Helm, London, 1978; John S. Haller Jr. and Robin M. Haller, *The Physician and Sexuality in Victorian America*, University of Illinois Press, Urbana, IL, 1974; Mary Hartman and Lois Banner, eds., *Clio's Consciousness Raised. New Perspectives on the History of Women*, Octagon Books, New York, 1976; Judith Walzer Leavitt and Ronald L. Numbers, eds., *Sickness and Health in America: Readings in the History of Medicine and Public Health*, University of Wisconsin Press, 1978; Martha Vicinus, ed., *Suffer and Be Still: Women in the Victorian Age*, Indiana University Press, Bloomington, IN, 1972; Deborah Gorham, *The Victorian Girl and the Feminine Ideal*, Croom Helm, London, 1982; Joan N. Burstyn, *Victorian Education and the Ideal of Womanhood*, Croom Helm, London 1980; Mabel C. Donnelly, *The American Victorian Woman. The Myth and the Reality*. Greenwood Press, Westport, CT, 1988.

25 Virginia Olesen and Elvi W. Whittaker in Julia Swindells, *Victorian Writing*, p. 19.

26 Shirley Ardener, ed., *Perceiving Women*, Malaby, London, 1975, quoted in Delamont and Duffin, eds., *The Nineteenth-Century Woman*, p. xvii.

27 Shirley Ardener, quoted in Emily Martin, *The Woman in the Body. A Cultural Analysis of Reproduction*, Beacon Press, Boston, 1987, p. 22.

28 Donnelly, *The American Victorian Woman*, p. 9.

29 Ehrenreich and English, *For Her Own Good*, p. 4.

30 During the twentieth century, the energy balance theory was transformed into Pearl's rate-of-living theory, in which the greater the rate of energy expenditure and oxygen utilization, the shorter was the life span. Selye's general adaptation hypothesis had a further negative influence on medical and public opinion regarding the effects of exercise, particularly for women as they aged. Indeed, girls and women are still cautioned by medical advisers from entering certain sporting and exercise arenas, and social attitudes toward the sportive, fitness-oriented female remain quite ambiguous. R. Pearl, *The Rate of Living*, Knopf, New York, 1928; H. Selye and P. Prioreschi, 'Stress theory of aging', in N.W. Shock, ed., *Aging, Some Social and Biological Aspects*, American Association for the Advancement of Science, Washington, D.C., 1960.

31 Wright, *Social Logic*, p. 24.

32 Susan Rubin Suleiman, ed., *The Female Body in Western Culture. Contemporary Perspectives*, Harvard University Press, Cambridge, MA, 1986, p. 2.

33 Editorial, 'History and theory', *History Workshop*, VI, Autumn 1978, pp. 1–6.

34 Peter L. Berger and Thomas Luckman, *The Social Construction of Reality. A Treatise in the Sociology of Knowledge*, Doubleday & Company, Garden City, NY, 1966; Burkart Holzner and John A. Marx, *Knowledge Application. The Knowledge System in Society*, Allyn and Bacon, Inc., Boston, 1979.

35 Dorothy Smith, 'A social construction of documentary reality', *Sociological Inquiry*, XLIV, no. 4, 1974, pp. 257–267.

36 Jay Mechling, 'Author's response to comments on 'Advice to historians on

advice to mothers', *Journal of Social History*, X, no. 1, 1976, pp. 125–128.

37 Peter L. Berger, Brigitte Berger and Hansfried Kellner, *The Homeless Mind; Modernization and Consciousness*, Random House, New York, 1973.

38 Gorham, *The Victorian Girl*, p. 65.

39 M. Jeanne Peterson, 'Dr Acton's enemy: Medicine, sex, and society in Victorian England', *Victorian Studies*, XXIX, no. 4, 1986, p. 589.

40 Regina Markell Morantz and Sue Zschoche, 'Professionalism, feminism, and gender roles: A comparative study of nineteenth-century medical therapeutics', *Journal of American History*, LXVII, no. 3, December 1980, pp. 568–588.

41 Alex Comfort, *The Anxiety Makers: Some Curious Preoccupations of the Medical Profession*, Thomas Nelson, Camden, NJ, 1967; Peter Cominos, 'Late Victorian sexual respectability and the social system', *International Review of Social History*, VIII, 1963, pp. 19–48; Gorham, *The Victorian Girl*; Peter Gay, *The Bourgeois Experience: Victoria to Freud, Vol. 1, Education of the Senses*, Oxford University Press, Oxford, 1984.

42 Mary Roth Walsh, *Doctors Wanted: No Women Need Apply. Sexual Barriers in the Medical Profession, 1835–1975*, Yale University Press, New Haven, 1977; W. G. Rothstein, *American Physicians in the Nineteenth Century. From Sects to Science*, The Johns Hopkins University Press, Baltimore, 1972.

43 Rothstein, *American Physicians in the Nineteenth Century*, p. 25.

44 Foucault, *The History of Sexuality*; see also a very recent discussion of feminism, the body and Foucault in Susan R. Bordo, 'The body and the reproduction of femininity: a feminist appropriation of Foucault', *Gender/ Body/Knowledge*, Alison M. Jaggar and Susan R. Bordo, eds., Rutgers University Press, New Brunswick, 1989, pp. 13–33.

45 Elinor Shaffer, Review of *The History of Sexuality, Vol. 1: An Introduction* by Michel Foucault. Trans. Robert Hurley, Pantheon Books, New York, 1978, *Signs, Journal of Women in Culture and Society*, V, no. 4, 1980, p. 814.

46 Martha H. Verbrugge, *Able-Bodied Womanhood: Personal Health and Social Change in Nineteenth-Century Boston*, Oxford University Press, Oxford, 1988, p. 9.

47 Hubert L. Dreyfus and Paul Rabinow, *Michel Foucault. Beyond Structuralism and Hermeneutics*, 2nd ed., University of Chicago Press, Chicago, 1983, p. xxvii.

48 Foucault, *History of Sexuality*, p. 85.

49 Linda Alcoff, 'Justifying feminist social science', *Hypatia*, II, no. 3, Fall 1987, p. 115.

50 Swindells, *Victorian Writing*, p. 23.

51 Swindells, *Victorian Writing*, p. 4.

52 Editorial, *History Workshop*, p. 3.

53 Swindells, *Victorian Writing*, p. 32.

54 Samuel Osherson and Lorna AmaraSingham, 'The machine and metaphor in medicine', in Mishler *et al.*, *Social Contexts of Health, Illness and Patient Care*, p. 163.

55 Ivan Illich, *Medical Nemesis. The Expropriation of Health*, New York, Bantam Books, 1977, pp. 36–8.

56 Charles E. Rosenberg, *No Other Gods, On Science and American Social Thought*,

Johns Hopkins University Press, Baltimore, 1976, p. 54.

57 Pat Jalland and John Hooper, eds., *Women From Birth to Death. The Female Life Cycle in Britain 1830–1914*, The Harvester Press, Brighton, Sussex, 1986, p. ix.

58 Angus Maclaren, *Reproductive Rituals*, Methuen & Co., New York, 1984.

59 Martin, *The Woman in the Body*, p. 5.

60 Susan Groag Bell and Karen M. Offen, *Women, the Family and Freedom: The Debate in Documents, Vol. 2, 1880–1950*, Stanford University Press, Stanford, 1983, p. 5.

61 Regina Markell Morantz-Sanchez, *Sympathy and Science. Women Physicians in American Medicine*, Oxford University Press, Oxford, 1985.

62 Virginia Woolf quoted in Swindells, *Victorian Writing*, p. 23.

63 Swindells, *Victorian Writing*, p. 26.

64 Verbrugge, 'Women and medicine', p. 968; see also Barbara Ehrenreich and Deirdre English, *Complaints and Disorders: The Sexual Politics of Sickness*, The Feminist Press, Old Westbury, NY, 1973, pp. 9, 89.

65 William Leach, *True Love and Perfect Union. The Feminist Reform of Sex and Society*, Basic Books Inc., New York, 1980, p. 172.

66 Sandra M. Gilbert and Susan Gubar, *The Madwoman in the Attic: The Woman Writer and the Nineteenth Century Imagination*, Yale University Press, New Haven, CT, 1979.

67 Sandra M. Gilbert and Susan Gubar, *No Man's Land. The Place of the Woman Writer in the Twentieth Century, Vol. 1, The War of the Words*, Yale University Press, New Haven, CT, 1988.

68 Swindells, *Victorian Writing*, p. 117.

69 Mary Jacobus, 'Book review of "The Madwoman in the Attic" ', *Signs, Journal of Women in Culture and Society*, VI, no. 3, Spring 1981, pp. 518–523.

70 Gilbert and Gubar, *No Man's Land*, p. 4.

71 Bram Dijkstra, *Idols of Perversity. Fantasies of Feminine Evil in Fin-de-Siecle Culture*, Oxford University Press, Oxford, 1986, p. 215.

72 Dijkstra, *Idols*, p. 216.

73 G. Stanley Hall, *Adolescence, Its Psychology and its Relation to Physiology, Anthropology, Sociology, Sex, Crime, Religion and Education*, Vol. 2, D. Appleton & Co., New York, 1904, p. 588.

74 Charlotte Perkins Gilman, *The Living of Charlotte Perkins Gilman. An Autobiography*, D. Appleton and Co., New York, 1935; Charlotte Perkins Stetson, 'The yellow wallpaper', *New England Magazine*, V, May 1892, pp. 647–659.

75 Smith-Rosenberg, *Disorderly Conduct*, p. 17.

76 Kathleen E. McCrone, *Sport and the Physical Emancipation of English Women 1870–1914*, Routledge, London, 1988, p. 2.

77 Verbrugge, *Able-Bodied Womanhood*, p. 123.

78 Smith-Rosenberg, *Disorderly Conduct*, p. 19.

79 Smith-Rosenberg, *Disorderly Conduct*, p. 29.

80 Kelly, *Women, History and Theory*, p. xx.

81 Elizabeth K. Helsinger, Robin Lauterbach Sheets and William Veeder, *The Woman Question. Defining Voices, 1837–1883*, Vol I., Garland Publishing Inc., New York, 1983, p. xii.

82 Lewin and Olesen, *Women, Health and Healing*, p. 7.

83 Ehrenreich and English, *Complaints and Disorders*, p. 11.

84 Bruce Haley, *The Healthy Body and Victorian Culture*, Harvard University Press, Cambridge, MA, 1978, p. 3.

85 An excellent contribution has been made by Kathy Piess in *Cheap Amusements. Working Women and Leisure in Turn-of-the-Century New York*, especially her study of dance madness among young and single working women. In the commercial dance halls of New York, she explains, spieling and tough dancing allowed young women to use their bodies to express sexual desire and individual pleasure in movement that would have been unacceptable in any other arena. Kathy Piess, *Cheap Amusements: Working Women and Leisure in Turn-of-the-Century New York*, Temple University Press, Philadelphia, 1986, p. 102.

86 See, for example, Patricia Branca, 'Image and reality: The myth of the idle Victorian woman', in Hartman and Banner, eds., *Clio's Consciousness*, pp. 179–191; It would be quite wrong, says Stage, to imply that all middle-class women were idle and pampered toys. Sarah Stage, *Female Complaints. Lydia Pinkham and the Business of Women's Medicine*, W. W. Norton & Company, New York, 1979, p. 66.

87 Ruth Schwartz Cowan, *More Work for Mother*, Basic Books Inc., New York, 1983, p. 64; To manage a household, says Filene, was, for many, an exhausting job that dragged from early morning to bedtime. Peter J. Filene, *Him/Her/Self: Sex Roles in Modern America*, 2nd ed., The Johns Hopkins University Press, Baltimore, 1986, p. 8.

88 See for example, Dio Lewis, Elizabeth Cady Stanton, James Read Chadwick, 'The health of American women', *North American Review*, CXXXV, no. 313, December 1882, pp. 503–524; Nor did the presence of domestic servants necessarily allow the 'comfortably situated housewife' to be a lady of leisure, for servants were becoming increasingly scarce as the century wore on. Filene, *Him/Her/Self*, p. 66.

89 Branca, 'Image and reality', p. 182.

90 Virginia Woolf quoted in Patricia Otto Klaus, 'Women in the mirror: Using novels to study Victorian women', in Barbara Kanner, ed., *The Women of England from Anglo-Saxon Times to the Present*, Archon Books, Hamden, CT, 1979, p. 296.

91 Helsinger, Sheets and Veeder, *Defining Voices*, Vol I., p. xiii.

92 Walter C. Taylor, M.D., *A Physician's Counsels to Woman in Health and Disease*, W. J. Holland, Springfield, 1872, in the author's preface.

93 Joan N. Burstyn, 'Education and sex: The medical case against higher education for women in England 1870–1900', in *Proceedings of the American Philosophical Society*, CXVII, no. 2, April 1973, p. 82.

94 Elizabeth K. Helsinger, Robin L. Sheets and William Veeder, *The Woman Question. Social Issues 1837–1883*, Vol II, Garland Publishing, Inc., New York, 1983, p. xiii.

95 Park supports the view that middle-class Victorian concepts of women, their perceived physical abilities as well as their opportunities for sport and exercise were remarkably similar on both sides of the Atlantic. Such similarities were reinforced, she explains, by a shared language, common popular literature (though more often of British origin) conveying scientific, medical and educational ideas about the body and physical culture, and continued

contact between the two countries. Roberta J. Park, 'Sport, gender and society in a transatlantic Victorian perspective', in J. A. Mangan and Roberta J. Park, eds., *From 'Fair Sex' to Feminism. Sport and the Socialization of Women in the Industrial and Post-industrial Eras,* Cass Publications, London, 1987, pp. 58, 62.

96 Elaine Showalter, *The Female Malady. Women, Madness and English Culture, 1830–1980,* Penguin Books, New York, 1985, p. 6.

97 Jalland and Hooper, *Women from Birth,* p. 7; See also Showalter, *The Female Malady.*

98 Ann Douglas Wood, ' "The fashionable diseases": Women's complaints and their treatment in nineteenth-century America', in Hartman and Banner, eds., *Clio's Consciousness,* p. 3.

99 Cynthia Epstein, *Woman's Place,* University of California Press, Berkeley, 1971, p. 41; American women everywhere were afflicted with weakness and disease, wrote Abba Gould Woolson in *Women in American Society* in 1873. Girls and women who formerly indulged in out-door sports and jollity had abandoned them, shunning air and sunlight. Abba Gould Woolson, *Women in American Society,* New York, 1873, pp. 203, 208.

100 Mrs. E. Lynn Linton, for example, roundly condemned the increasing lack of vigour of English women in *The Girl of the Period, and Other Social Essays,* Vol I, Richard Bentley & Son, London, 1883.

101 Catharine E. Beecher, *Physiology and Calisthenics for Schools and Families,* Harper and Bros., New York, 1856, p. 11.

102 Eliza Brisbee Duffey, *No Sex in Education, or an Equal Chance for Both Boys and Girls,* J. M. Stoddart, Philadelphia, 1874, p. 31.

103 Henry W. Slocum, Jr., 'Lawn tennis as a game for women', *Outing,* XIV, April–September 1889, p. 289.

104 S. Weir Mitchell, *Wear and Tear, or Hints for the Overworked,* J.B. Lippincott, Philadelphia, 1871, pp. 58, 61; In Mary Beedy's comparison of girls and women in England and America, she pointed out the thin, unhealthy-looking physique and nervous sensibility of Americans compared to the English who were the finest physical race in the world. The superiority of British women was due to the great national importance placed upon health and the family, the athletic habits of the people and the large amount of out-of-door exercise. Mary E. Beedy, 'Girls and women in England and America', in Anna C. Brackett, ed., *The Education of American Girls Considered in a Series of Essays,* G. P. Putnam's Sons, New York, 1874, pp. 213–214.

105 Sara A. Burstall, *The Education of Girls in the United States,* Macmillan & Co., New York, 1894.

106 Sophia Foster Richardson, 'Tendencies in athletics for women in colleges and universities', *Popular Science Monthly,* L, February 1897, pp. 517–526.

107 Verbrugge, *Able-Bodied Womanhood;* Kathleen E. McCrone, 'The "lady blue": Sport at the Oxbridge women's colleges from their foundation to 1914', *British Journal of Sports History,* III, no. 2, September 1986, pp. 191–215; Sheila Fletcher, *Women First. The Female Tradition in English Physical Education, 1880–1980,* The Athlone Press, London, 1984; Paul Atkinson, 'The feminist physique: Physical education and the medicalization of women's education', Mangan and Park, eds., *Fair Sex,* pp. 38–57; Jennifer Hargreaves,

'Playing like gentlemen while behaving like ladies: Contradictory features of the formative years of women's sport', *British Journal of Sports History*, II, no. 1, May 1985, pp. 40–52.

Paul Atkinson, for example, has described how in both nineteenth-century Britain and America the provision of academically sound education for young ladies became inextricably involved with issues of health, fitness and forms of physical activity, in part to accommodate medical shibboleths for the protection and conservation of female energy for reproduction. Paul Atkinson, 'Strong minds and weak bodies: Sports, gymnastics and the medicalization of women's education', *British Journal of Sports History*, II, no. 1, May 1985, p. 63.

Health and physical activities at Cheltenham Ladies, Rodean, and the North London Collegiate were paralleled in the United States at women's colleges such as Vassar, Wellesley and Smith, and several studies have documented the ways in which these and many other ladies' colleges in the United States came to view health and fitness through sport and exercise as paramount objectives. Thomas Woody's *History of Women's Education in the United States* and Dorothy Ainsworth's *History of Physical Education in Colleges for Women* are two of the classics in this regard, detailing the close attention given to hygiene, physiology, gymnastics and outdoor games at educational institutions for middle class girls and women. Thomas Woody, *A History of Women's Education in the United States*, Vol. II, Octagon Books, New York, 1974; Dorothy Ainsworth, *History of Physical Education in Colleges for Women*, A. S. Barnes & Company Inc., New York, 1930.

In her excellent study of the Oxbridge women's colleges, Kathleen McCrone has shown how games and exercise at Girton, Newnham, Lady Margaret Hall and Somerville College came to be viewed as appropriate mechanisms to support the potentially physically debilitating pursuit of higher learning. Estimating the significance of these exercise and sporting opportunities to college women of the time, McCrone notes that attending a woman's college in the late 1800s 'brought a plethora of unique new experiences and the opportunity to think, achieve and take genuine exercise; and to some at least it brought an awareness of the potential and reality of mental and physical power'. On the other hand, she reminds us that collegiate sports were the experience of very few and that the female collegian was compelled to accept numerous limitations on the playing field and in other physical endeavours invoked largely as a result of medical views concerning female physical weakness and appropriate ladylike behaviour. Kathleen E. McCrone, 'The "lady blue" ', p. 209.

108 Sheila Fletcher and Martha Verbrugge have made insightful analyses of the attributes and accomplishments of these pioneer physical educators in England and Boston respectively. Fletcher, *Women First*; Verbrugge, *Able-Bodied Womanhood*.

109 Madame Bergman-Osterberg, 'Physical training as a profession', *Women's International Congress*, 1899, p. V.

110 Fletcher, *Women First*, p. 2.

111 Donald J. Mrozek, *Sport and American Mentality, 1880–1910*, University of Tennessee Press, Knoxville, TN, 1983, p. 153.

The eternally wounded woman

112 Morantz-Sanchez, *Sympathy and Science*, p. 209.
113 Paul Atkinson, 'Fitness, feminism and schooling', Delamont and Duffin, eds., *Nineteenth-Century Woman*, p. 124.
114 Hall, *Adolescence* II, p. 634; see also, Janice Law Trecker, 'Sex, science and education', *American Quarterly*, XXVI, 1974, pp. 352–366.
115 Dr. Jane Walker quoted in Sara Burstall, *English High Schools for Girls. Their Aims, Organization and Management*, Longmans, London, 1911, p. 99.
116 Arabella Kenealy, 'Woman as an athlete', *The Living Age*, III, May 1899, pp. 363–70.
117 Caroline Wormeley Latimer, M.D., *Girl and Woman. A Book for Mothers and Daughters*, D. Appleton & Co., New York, 1910, pp. xiii–xiv.
118 Dijkstra, *Idols of Perversity*, p. 36.
119 Mary A. Hill, *Charlotte Perkins Gilman. The Making of A Radical Feminist, 1860–1896*, Temple University Press, Philadelphia, 1980.
120 Dudley Allen Sargent, 'The physical development of women', *Scribner's Magazine*, V, February 1889, pp. 172–185.
121 M. Mackie, 'Gender relations', R. Hagedorn, ed., *Sociology*, 3rd ed., Holt, Rinehart and Winston, Toronto, 1986, p. 100.
122 A. Hughes Bennett, M.D., 'Hygiene in the higher education of women', *Popular Science Monthly*, XVI, February 1880, p. 529.
123 Countess of Jersey, 'Ourselves and our foremothers', *Nineteenth Century*, XXVII no. 15, January 1890, pp. 56–57.
124 Alexander Walker, *Beauty in Woman, Analysed and Classified*, Simpkin, Marshall & Co., London, 1892, p. 199.
125 Verbrugge, 'Women and medicine', p. 965.
126 Dijkstra, *Idols of Perversity*, p. 389.
127 Bell and Offen, *Women, The Family and Freedom*, p. 7.

Part One

Male medical discourse: women and exercise across the life span

1

Menstrual disability and female physical capability

As a body who practise among women, we have constituted ourselves, as it were the guardians of their interests, and – in many cases – the custodians of their honour. We are, in fact, the stronger and they the weaker. They are obliged to believe all that we tell them and we, therefore, may be said to have them at our mercy. . .[1]

During the late nineteenth century arguments about women's limited physical and mental capacity and the centrality of the reproductive process for understanding women's bodies increasingly defined medical views of women's health and the productive boundaries of their lives. Ostensibly basing their views upon new scientific evidence influential medical practitioners, many of whom were men, utilized pseudo-scientific theories about the effects of the reproductive life cycle upon women's physical capabilities in order to rationalize the life choices of middle-class women and define limits for their activities.

Although women were held to be victims of their entire reproductive experience, the onset of menstruation and its recurring cycle were believed to be the cause of particular handicap. Women's limited physical achievements as compared to men's were increasingly ascribed to the burden placed upon them by their reproductive apparatus, especially menstruation. The onset of menses was considered an illness to be weathered only with particular care. For the next thirty years of life's pilgrimage, women were advised to treat themselves as invalids once a month, curtailing both physical and mental activity during the 'catamenial week' lest they succumb to accidents, disease and loss of fertility.

The widespread notion that women were chronically weak and had only finite mental and physical energy because of menstruation had a strong effect upon the medical profession's and consequently the public's attitude towards female exercise and sport. Victorian doctors readily imputed invalidism to menstruating women who were simply displaying normal symptoms and regarded the male body as the norm and the female as a deviation.[2] Furthermore, these attitudes have persisted throughout the twentieth century despite accumulating scientific and medical evidence that menstruation need not affect physical performance.

In a recent summary of the scientific literature related to exercise and menstruation, Wells notes that misinformation and traditional views concerning the menstrual function are major blocks to the active participation of girls and women in competitive sports. Until quite recently, for example, the International Olympic Committee believed that sports training and competition were detrimental to proper reproductive functioning in women and used these beliefs to exclude female participation in certain sports.[3] Female athletes and feminists have had to work hard even to begin dispelling such myths.[4]

It is important, then, to explore how long-standing propositions about adolescent girls' capacity for sport and strenuous exercise developed in response to late nineteenth-century physicians' interpretations of biological theories about menstruation. In issuing popular medical advice to middle class girls and women in the last three decades of the nineteenth century, establishment physicians on both sides of the Atlantic promoted a theory of menstrual disability that deepened the stereotyping of women as both the weaker and a periodically weakened sex. In their professional and popular writings and in their medical practice, these physicians disseminated their beliefs about the menstrual function and offered their notions of the therapies and life-style behaviours required to help women cope with the 'illness' of menstruation with its baneful and limiting effects upon female physical capabilities.

Looked upon as an 'eternal wound', an illness and as a shortcoming, menstruation came to be seen as a process requiring certain kinds of moderate physical activity, suitable open air exercises and sports appropriate for physical renewal. Perceived as a pathological condition, however, it provided cause for exclusion of women from vigorous and competitive sports and from any physical exertion which the medical experts considered overtaxing. Thus, although requirements for certain exercises were among the most frequent prescriptions for combatting the recurring drain of menstruation, constraints were increasingly imposed upon the extent and nature of female participation in exercise and sporting activities. Medical advice concerning exercise and physical activity reflected and perpetuated understandings about woman's abiding sense of physical weakness and the unchangeable nature of her physical inferiority.

Increasingly, medico-biological arguments concerning menstruation were generalized to buttress the dominance of establishment physicians as arbiters of female physical behaviour, legitimizing doctor's claims that women required constant medical guardianship. Doctors judged who was physically fit and who was not, with these judgements carrying implications of being fit or unfit for particular tasks, physical activities and certain types of sports.

A study of how medical reasoning about the menstrual function developed to define and delimit the parameters of female physical activity is instructive in helping understand the shaping of popular scientific thought by a dominant group of physicians operating within the technical and ideological framework of their era. For many perceived disorders, the labelling of disease or disability, the delimiting of disease characteristics and the choices made among possible therapies depend heavily upon social and professional convention (and/or convenience). Furthermore, 'there are complex ambiguities in the application of medical models and practices to chronic disorders and especially to normal processes'.[5] In attempting to root views of womenkind in biology, late nineteenth-century regular medical practitioners became human engineers by conditioning middle-class females to view their normal menstrual function as pathological, thus distorting female perceptions of their own vigour and physical abilities.

Theories of menstruation: myth, magic and science

The widespread notion that women were rendered physically disabled due to the recurring fact of menstruation was not a creation of the nineteenth century because it had deep roots in magical, religious and medical mythologies. Menstrual taboos are among the most inviolate in many societies. Indeed, few taboos 'evoke as forceful and as universal a response as those surrounding menstruation'.[6]

The cyclical character of menstruation has generated long-standing beliefs. Primitive society connected the rhythm of menstruation with the cycles of the moon, the seasons and the rhythm of tides. Many ancient legends relate the cyclic occurrence of the moon to the recurring menses. Fluhman, in his treatise on menstrual disorders, noted the persistence of the saying in ancient treatises, 'luna vetus vetulas, juvenes nova luna repurgat' (The old moon repurifies old women, the new moon (repurifies) young women).[7] Aristotle considered the moon to be female since 'the menstrual flux and the waning of the moon both take place towards the end of the month, and after the wane and the discharge, both become whole again'.[8] Centuries later, one of King George II's physicians explained that 'the ancients observed, and everyone knows, how great a share the moon has in forwarding those evacuations of the weaker sex. . . . In countries nearest the equator where we have proved lunar action to be strongest, these monthly secretions are in much greater quantity than in those near the poles where the force is weakest.'[9] In the nineteenth century Darwin perpetuated the imagined link between menstruation and the moon, suggesting that the connection was directly formed at a very remote period of zoological evolution and that the periodicity then impressed upon the organism had survived until the present day.[10]

Many traditional beliefs reflected a fear of the powers of menstrual blood whereby the menstruating woman, albeit weakened, was also seen as a contaminating agent.[11] Thus many taboos developed around female contact with food and people, especially men. Sometimes seen as a healing agent, menstrual blood was more often believed to have destructive powers. Contact with it, said Pliny the Roman, 'turns new wine sour – hives of bees die – to taste it drives dogs mad and infects their bite with an incurable poison'.[12] Many primitive societies excluded menstruating females from public life, especially from food gathering and preparation so that they would not contaminate members of the tribe.

Taboos also extended to intercourse during menstruation. In the Judeo-Christian scriptures, the rule was underscored in Leviticus: 'And if a woman have issue, and her issue in her flesh be blood, she shall be put apart seven days: and whoever toucheth her shall be unclean until the even.'[13] Christianity clung to the Old Testament belief in the imperfect nature of woman which in turn was believed to be, in part, a consequence of the menstrual flow.[14]

Thomas Aquinas described woman as 'defective and misbegotten', a result of a defect in the active power of the male seed or some external influence such as a moist south wind.[15] To early monks, woman was impure as a result of the pollution of menstruation and was forbidden to take communion in the early Christian churches. Orthodox Jews insisted upon Niddah, a minimum of twelve days' separation of wife and husband during and after the menses with strict prohibitions about food handling and intimate practices.[16]

Suggestions that menstruating women contaminated things they came in contact with increased in currency during the nineteenth century. John Elliotson wrote in 1840 that menstruating women must be regarded as unclean, for they could not cure meat at such a time.[17] Thirty-eight years later the *British Medical Journal* published extensive correspondence concerning whether or not a menstruating woman could contaminate the food she touched. One contributor extended the argument to oppose medical education for women. 'If such bad results accrue from a woman curing dead meat whilst she is menstruating, what would result, under similar conditions, from her attempt to cure living flesh in her midwifery or surgical practice?'[18]

Two general propositions dominated medical thought about menstruation. On the one hand, the condition was seen as a regular release of accumulated excess blood and body impurities – a form of purification. The second proposition related to the reproductive process. During pregnancy the accumulated blood was believed to be a nutritive source for the foetus, this being the female contribution to reproduction. Aristotle had observed that menstruation was the outward sign of female inferiority, a result of the passive part played by women in reproduction. The active male was believed capable of generating heat to transform matter into semen. The colder female could not transform matter, hence had to discharge the residue of useless nourishment from her blood vessels each month unless she was pregnant.[19] Hippocrates and Pliny shared the belief which persisted for centuries. Pliny wrote that 'women who do not menstruate are incapable of bearing children because it is of this substance that the infant is formed. The seed of the male, acting as a sort of leaven, causes it to unite and assume a form, and in due time it acquires life and assumes a bodily shape.'[20]

Other theorists agreed with the unique need of women to periodically shed extra blood, though for different reasons. In the second century A.D., Galen believed that menstruation consisted of fluids accumulated from leading an idle life, which were thus regularly evacuated for the body's relief.[21] Soranus felt that both men and women generated surplus matter; women eliminated it as menses, men through athletics.[22] Smellie, in 1766, concurred that 'the catamenia is no more than a periodic discharge of that superfluous blood which is collected through the month'.[23]

Medical theorists later focused upon the mode of evacuation. Avicenna, an eleventh-century Arab physician, suggested that menstrual blood was eliminated through the womb because that organ had been the last formed and was therefore the weakest.[24] His idea was further developed in the seventeenth century by Regnier de Graaf who likened the escape of blood from the weakened uterus to fermented wine or beer seeping out of a defective barrel.[25]

The demonstration of the Graafian follicle by Dr Graaf and others was predicated upon the notion that ovulation occurred at the time of conception. Subsequently a number of physicians began to suspect that ovulation may be a spontaneous process and that menstruation was intimately connected with the ovarian function. In 1793 Dr John Beale Davidge, a prominent Maryland surgeon, wrote a dissertation arguing that the menstrual flow was a uterine secretion under control of the ovaries. In 1812, John Power of London further enunciated the relationship between menstruation and specific ovarian changes, and studies of the ovulation process appeared increasingly in the first half of the nineteenth century.[26]

By 1865, Pfluger was arguing that the development of the Graafian follicle produced an irritation of the ovarian nerve leading to a reflex stimulation which resulted in simultaneous ovulation and menstruation.[27] Pfluger's theory that nervous stimulation triggered menstruation was widely accepted by American physicians in the last three decades of the nineteenth century despite several studies which suggested that such a view might be mistaken.[28] Graaf's theory of ferment, or 'vehement effervescence', laid the basis for the Stephenson wave theory expounded in 1882. Stephenson, a physician, understood menstruation to be related to cyclical waves of vital energy, shown in the body temperature, daily urine and pulse rate. In his view menstruation coincided with average body temperature changes and sought the weakest exit (the womb) when excessive nutritive material and vital energy were not required for reproduction.[29] Stephenson's theory also explained vicarious menstruation, for he believed that if there was an obstruction anywhere in the body the resulting wave would be thrown to the weakest part of the system. G. Stanley Hall later used Stephenson's theory to explain why every trouble in a woman demanded special attention to the pelvis.[30]

Stephenson based his wave principle on the experimental findings of Mary Putnam Jacobi and John Goodman . . . a Louisville physician, which were essentially a reformulation of Galen's plethoric theory.[31] Goodman claimed that menstruation was presided over by a law of monthly periodicity, a menstrual wave which affected the entire female and rendered her periodically unstable and liable to serious derangement.

Mary Putnam Jacobi explained that women experienced a rhythmic wave of nutrition, such nutritive material being expelled in menstruation when not used for reproduction. This caused a perturbation of the female system periodically and could, she admitted, lead to hysteria.[32] Though she criticized those who considered menstruation to be a morbid circumstance, she reported evidence which suggested that women might be unfit because of menstruation to bear the physical fatigue and mental anxieties of such activities as obstetrical practice.[33] Dr King went further than Goodman to claim that menstruation was abnormal and must logically be an interference with nature.[34] Dr King maintained that menstruation must be unnatural since although conception occurred at that time, the intercourse necessary to cause conception might cause gonorrhea in the male. Dr Gardner, author of *Conjugal Sins*, warned that menstrual blood was corrupt and virulent, threatening an unwitting penis with 'disease, excoriations and blenorrhagias'.[35] John Cowan predicted that the foetus might be damaged should intercourse take place at menstruation. 'Do not, I pray you, . . . do this unclean thing. . . while a new body is being developed.'[36] King's cure for the menstrual disease was to repress it altogether through continual pregnancies, since in her primitive state woman was constantly conceiving and menstruation was therefore rare.

The timing of ovulation was a matter of guesswork. Thomas Addis Emmet, surgeon-in-chief to the Woman's Hospital of the State of New York, wrote that 'impregnation frequently takes place in early married life just before the menstrual flow, or even while it exists'. However, he explained that the chances of impregnation lessened rapidly after the first year of marriage 'since we are likely to have disease of the body and ovarian irritation established in the course of time, as nature's protest at the childless condition of the married female'.[37]

Such views cemented the picture of the female as somehow 'driven by the tidal currents of her cyclical reproductive system, a cycle. . . reinforced each month by her recurrent menstrual flow'.[38] Each month, for a woman's thirty-year pilgrimage, menstruation presented itself as a trauma – a morbid and unnatural activity, a disease requiring specific therapies.[39] It was a circumstance over which a woman had little control yet which shaped her personality and physical ability to respond to life's demands. As Dr Van de Warker explained, women's limited physical achievements as compared with men's stemmed from the menstrual cycle which rendered her 'periodically susceptible to accidents and hysteria'.[40] Menstruation, some physicians warned, could drive a woman temporarily insane.[41]

Not until 1896 was the reflex nerve irritation theory refuted by Westphalen who described the cyclical changes in the uterine lining and the continual process of building up and breaking down of that lining. Important discoveries about the endocrine function in menstrual physiology came only after 1900 when the cycle of changes in the endometrium and the role of ovarian hormones in triggering the cycle became more clearly understood.[42]

Explaining menstrual disability

No woman ever passed through life without being ill. She suffers from 'the custom of women' or she does not. In either case, she is normally or abnormally ill. Thus, every woman is, according to temperament and other circumstances, always more or less an invalid. Therefore, no woman can pursue uninterrupted physical or mental labour. Nature disables the whole sex, single as well as married, from competing on equal terms with men. . .[43]

Though clearly hampered by a lack of knowledge about the precise functioning of the menstrual system, late nineteenth-century male physicians developed a remarkably elaborate set of explanations and accompanying prescriptions to offset what they insisted were the deleterious effects of recurring menstruation. Dr Edward Clarke considered neglect of the periodical function to be the principal source of disease among women, its repression or over-production to be equally fatal to health.[44] Michelet, whose writings on women had a huge readership in both England and America,[45] referred to the menstrual function as 'the cause of the whole drama'.[46] Hayes called it 'an internal wound, the real cause of all this tragedy'.[47]

Underlying the perceived need to regulate girls' and women's behaviour during menstruation was an overriding concern with order and with scarcity. The anxieties of physicians (and other health advisers) produced calls for obedience to the laws of nature lest loss of control, disorder and disease follow. Perceived as a discrete energy field, the body was believed to contain a specific amount of vital energy. If excess energy was used in one direction, less would be available for another. Energy had to be husbanded for the needs of mind and body. Furthermore, one's quota of energy for the life span had to be spent carefully. Since what was spent in one period was bound to be missed in another, energy had to be apportioned carefully. Overuse could well be billed to future generations who would pay for it from their own limited supply. This belief in a limited energy pool was a kind of 'mercantilism of self' for, 'in the great economy of nature, force answers to force and everything must be paid'.[48] 'Nature,' warned Herbert Spencer, 'is a strict accountant . . . and if you demand of her in one direction more than she is prepared to lay out, she balances the account by making a deduction elsewhere.'[49]

Herbert Spencer's writings were enormously influential in popularizing the supposed physical disabilities of women. Spencer was perhaps the supreme ideologue of the Victorian period, his prolific work reflecting the dominant middle-class ideas and values.[50] In North America his main forum was the *Popular Science Monthly*, a serious and widely read journal initially founded as a forum for his ideas.[51] In his numerous books and articles Spencer delineated the relationship of women to both evolutionary theory and the social and physical energy scheme. His argument went as follows. Men have always been physically stronger than women. Though primitive women nearly approached the physical status of civilized men, evolution freed women from the necessity of hard physical work. In the process they lost their physical strength, for the Lamarckian mechanism decrees that disease develops when organs are not used.[52] Though males and females both need physical strength for growth and development, girls develop more rapidly than boys and use up their available strength quota faster.[53] Thus not only do they start with less strength and lose it more quickly, women are subsequently 'taxed' with the special energy demand necessitated by menstruation and reproduction. This is a biological and social tax, because women are obliged to pay the price for the preservation of society. Such a 'reproductive sacrifice' limits individual development but is necessary in preserving the fitness of the race.

Spencer therefore established the central argument against female emancipation by elucidating the conflict between self-development and reproduction. To social theorists of his ilk, self-development for females had to be formulated as self-sacrifice, since women were required to spend their cache of physical and mental energy at the motherhood bank. There simply was not enough vital force left over from the demands of reproduction for women to develop their intellects.[54]

Boys and men, too, were warned about excessive or imbalanced use of physical and mental activity. In their case intellectual activity was not considered a drain upon physical energy. What could debilitate was excessive sexual vigour and the deliberate loss of sperm, which led to mental disability and disease.[55] Parsons has argued that late nineteenth-century physicians also considered males to be victims of their reproductive systems, equating at times the prostate with the uterus.[56] Certainly the loss of seminal fluid was considered as detrimental to body and brain as the loss of blood.[57] Also certain energetic exercises were thought to be provocative of masturbation and hence loss of vital fluid; 'those in which the whole weight of the body [is] sustained by the hands' would be better excluded from the gymnasium, said Dr Howe in 1883.[58] However, males could use force of will to prevent loss of fluids, while females could not. A life-style of self-denial could turn away weakness and disease from the male, whereas women's blood loss was spontaneous, ungovernable and required for the sake of the race.

The constant and increasing emphasis upon the need for race betterment at this time focused the physician's spotlight upon the menstrual disability theory. A woman who consumed her vital force in brain work depleted her energy stock required by the reproductive system, especially during menstruation or pregnancy. Male physicians saw no possible competition between the pursuit of culture and the demands of nature. Women could not do two things well at the same time. 'We would rather err on the safe side and keep the mental part of the human machine back a little, while we would encourage bulk, and fat and bone and muscular strength. . . This applies to the female sex. . . more than to the male [since] women's chief work [is] to the future of the world.'[59]

Since a woman's chief function was motherhood, the laws of nature demanded that not only should a bountiful energy supply be reserved for reproductive demands, but that more energy still should be earmarked to compensate for the monthly menstrual drain. As Dr A. Hughes Bennett explained, even under the best of circumstances the frequently recurring menstrual processes rendered a woman 'specially liable to derangements of her general health . . . under adverse conditions she is almost certain to fall a victim'.[60] Dr Taylor concurred in *A Physician's Counsels to Women in Health and Disease*.

> We cannot too emphatically urge the importance of regarding these monthly returns as periods of ill health, as days when the ordinary occupations are to be suspended or modified . . . . Every woman should look upon herself as an invalid once a month since the monthly flow exaggerates any existing affection of the womb and readily rekindles the expiring flames of disease.[61]

Notions of menstrual disability became widespread in Europe and North America. Dr Tilt was an eminent and widely read authority in

England. 'For thirty years,' he wrote in the *Lancet*, woman is 'thrown into a state of haemorrhagic and other orgasm every month.'[62] At such time, explained a supporting authority, they are 'unfit for any great mental or physical labour. . ..They suffer under a languor and depression which disqualify them from thought or action.'[63] Michelet, in *L'Amour*, explained that for fifteen or twenty days out of twenty-eight the woman was 'not only an invalid, but a wounded one. It was woman's plight to ceaselessly suffer love's eternal wound.'[64] From Germany Dr Runge insisted that 'since a woman needs protection during menstruation all demands on her strength must be remitted. Every month for several days she is enfeebled, if not downright ill.'[65] In 1904 G. Stanley Hall summed up many of these medical arguments in his monumental treatise, *Adolescence*. At this time, he said, 'girls and women can do less work with mind and body [and] make less accurate and energetic movements'.[66]

Although women had to expect to be disabled by menstruation for thirty of their best years, the onset of menarche was believed to be particularly taxing physically because the entire developing female organism was thrown into turmoil. Adolescence was the period of maximum growth when all energies were to be conserved. Puberty for boys marked the onset of strength and enhanced vigour; for girls it marked the onset of prolonged and periodic weaknesses of womanhood. The years between ten and fourteen are full of import to a girl, wrote William Potter, for 'during them she lays the foundation for future weal or woe'.[67] George Austin warned girls that when menstruation appeared special dangers awaited, all of them due to sexual functions.[68] J.H. Kellogg wrote repeatedly that the first occurrence of menstruation was critical for a female, each subsequent recurrence rendering her more 'susceptible to morbid influences and liable to serious derangements'.[69] When the first flow appeared, absolute mental and physical rest was advised. Nineteenth-century physicians recalled Hippocrates' analysis that 'nubile virgins, particularly about the menstrual periods, are affected with paroxysms, apoplexies'.[70] Many were sure that the onset of menarche made a girl ripe for disease and so special precautions were necessary.

Adolescence: life-style prescriptions for coping with menstrual disability

Adolescence is the most important period of a woman's life, the period during which the foundations of future health are laid.[71]

The protection of pubertal girls from excessive mental and physical activity at menarche became a campaign among the proponents of menstrual disability. Girls of the better classes, said Thomas Emmet in a widely quoted medical textbook, should spend the year before and two years after puberty at rest. 'Each menstrual period should be passed in the recumbent position until her system becomes accustomed to the new order of life.'[72]

John Thorburn feared 'disproportion between development of muscle and of nerve in women'. Agreeing with Emmet, he insisted that girls should do little steady work for the three years surrounding puberty. Furthermore, they should 'plan to lie fallow' about a quarter of the time. 'Girls,' he continued, 'should develop the dignity and efficiency of going slow.'[73] The best medical specialists, concluded G. Stanley Hall, agreed that a girl should be 'turned out to grass' and be withdrawn from other activities to 'let nature do its beautiful work of inflorescence'. 'Periodicity, perhaps the deepest law of the cosmos, celebrates its highest triumphs in woman's life.' Once regular menstruation was established, he added, 'the paradise of stated rest should be revisited in the monthly sabbath'. Idleness should be cultivated and woman, realizing that ' "to be" is greater than "to do" should step reverendly aside from her daily routine and let Lord Nature work'.[74]

Hall's volumes on *Adolescence* confirmed medical concerns about appropriate life-style behaviour for girls and young women. In various public arenas he declared that every girl should be educated not to become self-supporting but 'primarily to become a wife and mother'.[75] Education for adolescent girls should consist of courses in 'heroalogy' – the teaching of the noble lesson of service to the people wherein women, as bearers of the race, would be the conduit through which 'mansoul' would some day become 'supermansoul'.[76] Since efficient reproduction was the raison d'etre of woman's existence, the explanation and prescription of appropriate adolescent female activities were considered crucial. Hall used the fact that American girls had their first menses, on average, at fourteen years of age (rather than at fifteen and a half as in Europe) to support medical claims that American girls were too precocious. This precocity he blamed upon 'mentality and nerve stimulation' resulting especially from inappropriate female education.[77] He thus buttressed the popular medical feeling that 'there are, in the physiological life of women, disqualifications for continuous labor of the mind'.[78]

The precise physiological disqualifications of young women were elaborated most clearly by Dr Edward Clarke in 1873. His treatise on *Sex and Education* (which ran through seventeen editions in thirteen years) mounted a major attack upon the educational and professional aspirations of late nineteenth-century middle-class women, and his chief weapon was the theory of menstrual disability. 'Let the fact be accepted,' he declared, 'that there is nothing to be ashamed of in a woman's organization, and let her whole education and life be guided by the divine requirements of her system.' A professor of medicine at Harvard, Clarke was convinced that girls between twelve and twenty should concentrate solely upon developing their reproductive systems. Energy expended upon mental activity (i.e. female education) could only deplete the energy required for full physical development. Mental activity during the catamenial week destroyed feminine capabilities and might well interfere with ovulation and arrest reproductive development. Studying forced the brain to use the blood and energy needed to get the menstrual process functioning efficiently. Indeed, Clarke warned, if a girl 'puts as much force into her brain education as a boy, . . . the special apparatus will suffer'.[79] Dr William Goodell, Professor of Clinical and Didactic Gynecology at the University of Pennsylvania, embellished the arguments of Clarke in 1882, deploring the pale and sickly women of the time and complaining that:

> too much brain-work and too little body-work is the crying evil in this land. The fact is that our girls are over-educated. . .Energy is withdrawn from the trophic and reproductive centres, and physical development is arrested. Precocious cleverness is attainable only at the cost of physical and sexual development.[80]

Dr Clouston went further, attributing stunted growth, nervousness, headaches, hysteria and insanity to overstimulation of the female brain.[81] Potter protested that 'nerve-tire' would result from overwork, leading to a disastrous reaction upon the pelvic organs of the young girl. Brain cramming, he said, could turn 'a ruddy robust healthy girl of fourteen into a hysterical, moody invalid in less than two years'.[82] Maudsley drew upon Clarke's portraits of the ill effects of education upon young women to describe the girl who:

> enters upon the hard work of school or college at the age of fifteen or thereabouts, when the function of her sex has perhaps been fairly established; ambitious to stand high in class she . . . [allows] herself no days of relaxation or rest . . . paying no attention to the periodical tides of her organization, unheeding a drain that would make the stroke oar of the University crew falter . . . In the long run nature asserts its powers. . . [She] leaves college a good

scholar but a delicate and ailing woman, whose future is one of more or less suffering.[83]

Dr Kellogg agreed. 'There is no doubt,' he said, 'that many young women have permanently injured their constitutions while at school by excessive mental taxation during the catamenial period.'[84]

Although there were a number of immediate objections to its implications, the menstrual disability theory of Clarke and his physician contemporaries in Europe and North America became widely accepted. Julia Ward Howe, a leading critic of Dr Clarke's thesis, provided other explanations for the potentially debilitating effects of menstruation. 'Despite Dr Clarke's prominent position in this community,' she wrote in a collection of essays by leading public figures, 'we do not feel compelled to regard him as the supreme authority on the subjects of which he treats.' In seeking to disprove his thesis that you cannot feed a woman's brain without starving her body, she pointed instead to the powerful influence of climate upon the health of American women, as well as to the young female's need for special guardianship. 'Many young women,' she insisted,

> are periodically kept from all violent exercise and fatigue so far as the vigilance of elders can accomplish this . . . [but] . . . a single ride on horseback, a single wetting of the feet . . . may entail lifelong misery . . . I have known of repeated instances of incurable disease and even of death arising from rides on horseback taken at the critical period.[85]

While exonerating educators from shouldering all the blame for exacerbating female weakness, she and other critics of Clarke did not challenge the notion that the periodic function was a potentially debilitating condition requiring specific life-style precautions and prescriptions.

Instead, given the number of studies pointing out the excellent health of many college women, they attributed menstrual disability problems more to a school or household regimen which provided insufficient rest and careful exercise during menstruation than to the actual physical drain of studying.[86] W. LeC. Stevens collected data from the Presidents of Cornell, Michigan and Wesleyan that suggested that education need not endanger the health of women students if proper care was taken.[87] The resident physician from Vassar, for example, claimed that all possible precautions were taken not to overtax Vassar girls during the critical period. All students

> are carefully instructed regarding precautions which are periodically necessary for them . . . . They are positively forbidden to take gymnastics at all

during the first two days of their period . . . They are also forbidden to ride on horseback then; and . . . strongly advised not to dance, nor run up and down stairs, nor do anything else that gives sudden and successive . . . shocks to the trunk. They are encouraged to go out of doors for quiet walks or drives, or boating and to do whatever they can to steady the nervous irritation.[88]

Indeed, the evils of going up and down flights of stairs were mentioned frequently by medical men as reason to keep girls away from schools with buildings more than two storeys high.

Arguments about the ramifications of the menstrual disability theory upon adolescent education took a similar tack in England. Although rebuking Henry Maudsley for his exaggerated conclusion that women could not compete with men since 'for one quarter of each month during the best years of life [they were] . . . more or less sick and unfit for hard work', Dr Elizabeth Garrett Anderson encouraged teachers to protect adolescent girls from mental fatigue and violent physical activities such as long walks, riding, dancing, or lifting heavy weights. Instead, she advocated gymnastics, active games, daily baths and other hygienic reforms for female students in order that their physical condition might be improved.[89]

The onset of menarche thus confronted the adolescent girl and her guardians with the need to concentrate upon the regulation of her menses and the honing of her reproductive capacity. The family doctor was expected to take a major role in assisting the adolescent. Indeed, said Dr Wilson in 1885, 'such is the tendency of most American girls . . . towards functional disorders, that to inaugurate a proper hygiene that should lead to healthy and vigorous womanhood in most cases needs nothing less than medical supervision'.[90] While vigorous activity was frowned upon and periods of rest strongly encouraged, regulated healthy exercise was definitely indicated. Caution was the watchword, however, since muscular exercise was assumed to expend energy required for developing complete womanhood. Restricted activity was much less necessary for a pubescent boy than for his adolescent sister because 'greater and more costly constructions are afoot in her case than her brother's'.[91] Physicians, then, elaborated for young women a detailed regimen which blended rest and restorative exercise.

Exercise for young girls and adolescents

Clearly, the argument for appropriate physical activity had to be care-fully construed. On the one hand, definitions of femininity and the menstrual disability theory implied a lack of physical vigour and robustness, and a recurring energy drain which prevented participation in education and hard labour. On the other hand, the development of physical strength and health was a necessary attribute of a robust, productive mother.[92] There was a difficulty, then, says Smith-Rosenberg, of providing the appropriate regimen to smooth the path taken by the dependent, fragile girl en route to the demanding responsibilities of motherhood.[93]

Some experts, such as Dr Kellogg, advocated a more active childhood, including outdoor play and exercise for young prepubertal girls. He advised mothers to treat their daughters like sons and encourage both in outdoor play and vigorous exercise.[94] An active tomboy would surely develop, through boyish sports, the physical health for future motherhood, he reasoned.[95] Dr Weir Mitchell agreed that, 'to run, to climb, to swim, to ride, to play violent games, ought to be as natural to the girl as to the boy'.[96] 'Girls should be encouraged to take much active exercise. . . It is as good for little girls to run and jump, to ramble in the woods, to go boating, to ride and drive, to play and have fun generally as for little boys.'[97] Thus, childhood tomboyism would assist the young girl in developing the health and strength needed for motherhood as well as provide fresh air and exercise to build resistance to the dangerous childhood diseases. Dr Rice underscored the physiological merits of these elements in helping prevent disease, and explained how good health was contingent upon the normal functional activity of all organs (since functional derangements and their consequences constituted a large percentage of all diseases). By developing the organs during childhood with the powerful assistance of muscular exercise, he continued, good health would be secured. And in order that muscular exercise would result in good physical development, it had to be carried out systematically throughout childhood. Play, gymnastics and calisthenics were to be supplemented by outdoor games. As long as physical exercise was neglected, concluded Dr Rice, disease would continue in abundance.[98] Indeed, for children, games were to be considered more beneficial than drill and calisthenics.[99]

The Lamarckian notion that physical traits acquired at an early age would be transmitted to future generations further supported the promotion of vigorous childhood activity for young girls. Exercise habits, organized and internalized, would become long-term instruments for social improvement.[100] Letting girls join their brothers in their athletic sports would, said Dr Oswald, allow the regenerative tendency of nature to assert itself.[101] Healthy outdoor games and activities, commented Dr Anderson, would ensure more durable good health for feeble schoolgirls.[102] The most important advantage of all to be derived from fresh air and frolic in girlhood was the storing of energy 'for the future, for woman's work of the future, for motherhood, for the race of the future. . . '.[103]

Although childhood was regarded as the time to rear little girls with a view to storing up enough vital energy for perfect physical development, at the first sign of menarche the carefree romping and vigorous activity had to cease. Appropriate activity could then be obtained in the kitchen, the washroom, and the garden – 'nature's gymnasia for adolescent girls'.[104] Rest and carefully regulated exercise were to be the norm in the abrupt transition from activity to relative passivity. The sportive competitiveness which could be encouraged in childhood was to give way to selfless femininity. Indeed, after puberty, women were never to compete, for that would challenge the notion of complementary spheres of influence and competence. Competition should be deplored in girls, said Saleeby, since they were liable to overstrain and apt to take trifles to heart.[105] Nor were girls to be encouraged to achieve mastery in such masculine areas as physical skill, strength and courage.[106] 'Certain games, like football and boxing, girls cannot play', said Hall.[107] Rather, girls were to understand that from puberty on all bodily strength should be dedicated to the ceaseless routine of maternity and caring for others, most notably, husband and children. Indeed, every time menstruation occurred, rest of mind and body was to be sought.[108]

Menarche, then, abruptly ushered girls toward their predetermined vocation and they 'were exempted from the necessity of engaging in violent exercises'.[109] Bodily changes associated with menarche also dictated an alteration in exercise prescription. At puberty, said Dr Roberts, the 'pelvis alters its shape. . . and the effect . . . is to bring the knees closer together, and to produce a weak-kneed condition and awkward running gait peculiar to women. Much walking or standing should be avoided and short but vigorous gymnastic exercises substituted, and when possible the recumbent position assumed.'[110] Drs Allen and McGrigor explained that during the monthly periods:

> violent exercise is injurious; iced drinks and acid beverages are improper; and bathing in the sea, and bathing in cold water, and cold baths, are dangerous; indeed, at such times as these, no risks should be run. . . The monthly periods are times not to be trifled with, or woe betide the unfortunate trifler.[111]

Dr Clouston summed up the general attitudes of the establishment medical profession toward physical education for adolescent girls. The right kind, he explained, is 'that which hardens the muscles, adds to the fat, softens the skin, enriches the blood, promotes but does not over-stimulate the bodily functions'.[112] To exercise the muscles, romping and play, especially out of doors, were the perfect answer.[113] Gymnastic exercises, if well selected and proportioned, would promote muscular development, grace and vigour, but were easily carried to extremes where they could break down the constitution.[114] Excessive muscular development was unfavourable to maternity since it increased the difficulties of giving birth. Most suitable, then, were calisthenics or other movements with light elastic apparatus, said Anderson, which promoted grace and symmetry. If an hour each day were set apart for developing the physique at this critical stage of life, a hardier race of mothers would develop.[115]

Dr Madison Taylor proposed that the 'enfeeblement, so common among pubescent girls should be combated by romping, ball, beanbags, battledore, hoops, running, golf, tennis, bicycling, self-bathing in cold water and deep breathing exercises once or twice a day, rather than by systematic physical culture'.[116] Especially appropriate, reminded Alice Tweedy, were 'homely gymnastics', or in other words, housework.[117] Nellie Whitaker suggested that housework might be profitably taught by mothers under the name of physical culture.[118] Dr Howard from Baltimore had much to say about the importance of medically directed physical exercise for girls and young women:

> Woman is physiologically other than man and no proper education can change her, but false education can pervert her, and misdirected physical exercise can injure her beyond recovery. The man who best realizes this is the physician (for) the scientific medical man deeply realizes that woman has characteristic differences from man in every organ and tissue.[119]

Girls, he noted, should do no physical work except walking and swimming for the first year after puberty. 'Walking is normal, body developing exercise and should be done regularly, in the country if possible and with hill climbing to open the cells of the lungs.' Fencing, he continued, 'is excellent for the fully developed woman but inadvisable for the girl'. Furthermore, 'any form of exercise that causes undue psychic excitement such as personal contests or basketball games is too great a strain for the nervous system especially for the nerve-tensioned American girl'. The result of such excitement could be 'a riotous rebellion in some part of the girl's physiological functions'. It may be delayed until later life, he said, but it will come, 'for Nature never forgives robbery or insult'.[120] The normal woman, he concluded, 'was not intended by nature to be a high jumper or a performer on the trapeze, but to be a wife and mother, and with such a glorious future she should be so educated that her physical condition is always a pleasure to herself and a blessing to her husband'.[121]

In relation to exercise, physicians also worried about the female adolescent's diet. To develop fat, 'that most essential concomitant of female adolescence', the blood needed enrichment by good nutrition. 'Fat is to the body what fun is to the mind', explained Clouston. It is 'an indication of spare power for future use'.[122] Though physicians did not understand the exact relationship between the onset of menarche and a critical level of body fat, they did worry about anorexia scolastica, a debilitating thinness and weakness that they believed to result from too much mental stimulus, especially during menstruation.[123] They were also acutely aware of the linkage between the body changes of puberty and chlorosis, a common form of anaemia named for the greenish tinge that often marked the skin of young women.[124] Chlorosis was linked variously to poor diet, lack of exercise, lack of fresh air, impoverished blood and mental effort.[125] The menstrual function was almost always implicated. Its derangement resulted in anaemic and chlorotic girls, some of whom manifested amenorrhea, while others showed increased blood volume which was interpreted as a promise of fecundity.[126] Loss of strength and appetite were the most frequently reported symptoms of the condition and medical guides noted that common characteristics of chlorotic girls included menstrual problems, a distaste for meat and low tolerance for physical activity.[127] Physicians prescribed a combination of rest, moderate exercise in the fresh air, blood and nerve remedies, iron pills and the eating of red meat to combat what they perceived as the crisis evoked by the establishment of periodicity.[128]

Life-style prescriptions for the adolescent girl thus became a set of signposts erected to assist her passage from girlhood to womanhood. 'Puberty for a girl,' concluded Hall, 'is like floating down a broadening river into an open sea. . . (where) . . . the currents are more complex and the phenomena of tides make new conditions and new dangers.'[129] In a similar vein, Dr Tilt warned that:

> Instead of flowing on in smooth tranquillity from the cradle to the grave, the stream of life is marked by rapids which have been called critical, metamorphic or developmental epochs. . . The object of each successive critical readjustment of our frame is to ensure the greatest possible amount of health

for each subsequent period of life.[130]

The metaphorical use of tides and currents in relation to the periodic crises of menstruation indicated the generalized fear of late nineteenth-century authorities that social order and well-being were being threatened by waves of uncontrollable elements – among them, demands by the 'new woman' to break out of the separate sphere defined for her. Establishment physicians saw themselves as stemming the tide of female demands for higher education, entrance to the professions, new bodily freedoms such as birth control and competitive sporting activities. The doctors did so by invoking scientific authority to assert broader control over women's bodies. We must not 'abet women as a sex in rebelling against maternity, or in quarrelling with the constitution of the solar system'.[131] 'We must protect them from being dashed to pieces on the rock of childbirth, ground on the ever-recurring shallows of menstruation.'[132] We must warn them of 'the effeminacy of wealth, the new woman movement and foeticide'.[133] We must not countenance these women who 'strive to theoretically ignore and practically escape the monthly function'.[134]

Establishment medical opinion confirmed that women's periods must be more respected, and reiterated the role that physicians must assume as medical guardians, almost moral directors of the intimate, personal behaviour of females. The same mechanistic, closed model of a finite store of nervous energy served equally to account for incidences of fragility and disorderliness in social and moral affairs.[135] To many late nineteenth-century male doctors increasingly anxious about the tensions of urban industrial life, moderation was the key to the desired equilibrium. Excess was morally and physiologically foolhardy. Energy-discharging activities must always be compensated for by energy-conserving ones. Activity must be countered with rest and relaxation, indoor work balanced by activity in the open air, and so on. 'With a peculiar appropriateness,' says Rosenberg, 'science provided a vocabulary and a sense of imagery to express and support these beliefs, and from among them, physicians selected those scientific plausibilities which fitted most conveniently into their professional paradigm.'[136]

Those who supported most staunchly the menstrual disability theory were the most uneasy about the dangers of feminine excess and lack of balance whether it be in study, professional work or sports and exercise. Not necessarily considering themselves conservative in their attitudes toward women, they nevertheless were convinced that medical evidence demonstrated the physiological undesirability of strenuous and prolonged exertion in mental and physical activities. 'When we thus look the matter honestly in the face,' said Maudsley:

> it would seem plain that women are marked out by Nature for very different offices in life from those of men, and that the healthy performance of her ... special functions renders it improbable she will succeed, and unwise for her to persevere, in running over the same course at the same pace with him. For such a race she is certainly weighted unfairly ... Women cannot rebel successfully against the tyranny of their organization. This is not the expression of prejudice nor of false statement, it is the plain statement of a physiological fact.[137]

Sporting activities as well as educational pursuits had to be compatible with female physiology and to be focused upon health and balance rather than the irresponsibility of inactivity or the recklessness of unregulated competition. The demands of periodicity were monthly reminders that nineteenth-century women could not and should not play the game like men.[138] The burgeoning demands of the 'new woman' at the end of the century, however, suggested that, in athletics as well as in other endeavours of the male sphere, women were not unanimously committed to the notion that they were eternally wounded.[139]

Notes

1 'The Obstetrical Society meeting to consider the proposition of the council for the removal of Mr. I.B. Brown', *British Medical Journal* (i), 1867, p. 396.
2 Brian Harrison, *Separate Spheres. The Opposition to Women's Suffrage in Britain*, Croom Helm, London, 1978, p. 61; McCrone, *Sport and the Physical Emanicipation of English Women*, p. 193.
3 Christine L. Wells, *Women, Sport and Performance: A Physiological Perspective*, Human Kinetics Pubs., Champaign, IL, 1985.
4 See, for example, M. Ann Hall and Dorothy A. Richardson, *Fair Ball: Towards Sex Equality in Canadian Sport*, The Canadian Advisory Council on the Status of Women, Ottawa 1982; Carole A. Oglesby, ed., *Women and Sport, From Myth to Reality*, Lea and Febiger, Philadelphia, 1978. Mary C. Boutilier and Lucinda San Giovanni, *The Sporting Woman*, Human Kinetics Pub., Champaign, IL, 1983. G. Pfister has described how, in Germany, female doctors and athletes have had to battle against prejudice and discrimination generated by the scientific assertions of male physicians that the female body was naturally inferior. 'The influence of women doctors on the origins of women's sports in Germany', *Medicine and Sport*, XIV, 1981, pp. 58–65.
5 Eric Holtzman, 'Science, philosophy and society', *International Journal of Health Services*, XI, no. 1, 1981, p. 125.

6 Menstrual taboos are discussed by Elaine and English Showalter in 'Victorian women and menstruation', *Victorian Studies*, XIV, no. 1, 1970, pp. 83–89; Vern Bullough and Martha Voght, 'Women, menstruation, and nineteenth-century medicine', *Bulletin of the History of Medicine*, XLVII, no.1, January–February 1973, pp. 66–82; Janice Delaney, Mary Jane Lupton and Emily Toth, *The Curse: A Cultural History of Menstruation*, E.P. Dutton, New York, 1976; E. Novak, The superstition and folklore of menstruation', *Johns Hopkins Hospital Bulletin*, XXVII, 1916.
A major national study on menstruation, *The Tampax Report*, published in 1981 notes that menstruation still remains a taboo subject for most Americans. Of the 1,034 men and women interviewed by a Research Consortium, the majority thought that menstruation affected women physically and emotionally, and one third believed that women should restrict their physical activities. *The Tampax Report*, Tambrands, Inc., New York, 1981.

7 C. Frederic Fluhman, *Menstrual Disorders, Pathology, Diagnosis and Treatment*, W.B. Saunders, Philadelphia, 1939, p. 18.

8 Aristotle, quoted in R. Crawford, Editorial, *The Lancet*, II, 1915, p. 1331.

9 Richard Mead, *The Medical Works*, Edinburgh, 1765 quoted in Fluhman, *Menstrual Disorders*, p. 18; Some nineteenth century physicians remained convinced that climate affected menstruation, especially the age of menarche. According to the research of Dr. Pye Henry Chavasse, girls in warm climates menstruated at 10 or 11 but those in Russia might wait till they were 20 to 30 years old, and even then only menstruate a few times a year. Pye Henry Chavasse, *Woman as a Wife and Mother*, Philadelphia, 1871, pp. 90–91.

10 Quoted in Havelock Ellis, *Man and Woman*, London, 1894, p. 282.

11 See Freud, for example, who saw in man's fear of blood an ambivalence toward women as both sacred and cursed, both pure and unclean. Sigmund Freud, *Civilization and its Discontents*, W.W. Norton, New York, 1962 (first pub. 1930). Devereux discusses examples of the central theme of the psychoanalytic approach to menstruation which is the menstruating woman as 'witch' possessing special dangers and powers. He concludes that taboos on menstruation reflect women's real power as propogators of men. G. Devereux, 'The psychology of feminine genital bleeding', *The International Journal of Psycho-Analysis*, XXXI, 1950, pp. 252–253. Bruno Bettleheim, in *Symbolic Wounds*, The Free Press, Glencoe, IL, 1954, discusses psychoanalytic interpretations of male envy and fear of female menstruation and the taboos and ceremonies which developed around these beliefs. Psychoanalysts have contributed to notions that menstruation is a monthly neurosis fraught with numerous psychic fears. According to Karen Horney, man devalues woman's functions in order to keep her out of his domain, creating an ideology that will keep him powerful and her inferior. By viewing the menarche and menstruation as problematic, the male can see the female as biologically incapable of assuming positions of power. Karen Horney, 'The problems of feminine masochism', *Feminine Psychology*, Norton, NY., 1967.

12 Cajus Plinius Secundus, *Natural History*, Book 7, trans. H. Rackham. Harvard University Press, Cambridge, MA, 1961, p. 549.

13 Leviticus 15:19, New Revised Standard Translation.
14 Mary Douglas explains that much of Leviticus is taken up with outlining the physical perfection and completeness required in being holy and, therefore, blessed. The idea of holiness was given an external, physical expression in the wholeness of the body, seen as a perfect container. Natural functions producing bodily waste, especially menstruation, degraded this notion of completeness and rendered women somehow less able to conform to the holiness essential for gaining God's blessing. Thus, a polluting person was always seen as marginal, and a source of weakness to the social unit. *Purity and Danger: An Analysis of the Concepts of Pollution and Taboo*, Routledge and Kegan Paul, Boston, 1966.
15 Anton C. Pegis, ed., *Basic Writings of St. Thomas Aquinas*, Random House, New York, 1948, p. 880.
16 Though Orthodox Jews believe these laws to have originated from the time of Adam and Eve, when Eve was punished by God with menstruation and pain in labour for bringing mortality to Adam, Genesis Rabbah 17:13, and to be underscored in the writings of Leviticus, a book, *Baraita de Niddah*, published by a heretical Jewish sect in 1890, reinforced a number of traditional taboos concerning menstruation. See Cora Goldberg Marks, 'In purity and love. An introduction to the Jewish attitudes towards marriage', *Lifestyles*, XIII, 1986, pp. 98–106; see also, Nancy Datan, 'Corpses, lepers and menstruating women: Tradition, transition and the sociology of knowledge', *Sex Roles*, XIV, 1986, pp. 693–703.
17 John Elliotson, *Human Physiology*, 5th ed. London, 1840, pp. 770–771.
18 W. Storey, *British Medical Journal*, 1878, p. 324. The correspondence columns of the *British Medical Journal* debating menstruation and contamination are discussed in detail in Ronald Pearson, *The Worm in the Bud. The World of Victorian Sexuality*, Penguin Books, London, 1969 .
19 Aristotle, *On the Generation of Animals*, trans. A.L. Peck, Heinemann, London, 1943, pp. 2, 4, 185. See also, Elizabeth Gasking, *Investigations into Generation. 1651–1828*, Johns Hopkins University Press, Baltimore, 1967; Nancy Tuana, 'The weaker seed. The sexist bias of reproductive theory', *Hypatia*, Vol. III, no. 1, Spring 1988, pp. 35–59.
20 Cajus Plinius Secundus, *Natural History*, pp. 7, 13.
21 Fluhman, *Menstrual disorders*, p. 19; Galen, quoted by John Freind, *Emmenologia*. trans. Thomas Dale, London, 1729 , pp. 19, 67.
22 Soranus, *Gynecology*, trans. Oswei Temkin, Johns Hopkins University Press, Baltimore, 1956 , p. 23.
23 W. Smellie, *A Treatise on the Theory and Practice of Midwifery*, 5th ed. London, 1766, p. 14.
24 Fritz Vosselmann, *La Menstruation, Legendes, Coutumes, et Superstitions*, Lyon, 1935, pp. 16–17.
25 Regnier de Graaf, *Histoire Anatomique des Parties Genitales de L'homme et de La Femme*, Paris, 1699 .
26 John Power, *Essays on the Female Economy*, Burgess] Hill, London, 1831 C. Negrier, *Recherches sur les Ovaries*, Paris, 1840 .
27 E.P.F. Pflüger, *Uber die Bedeutung und Ursache der Menstruation*, Berlin, 1865, cited in Fluhman, *Menstrual Disorders*, p. 24.

28 J. Williams, *Obstetrical Journal of Britain and Ireland*, III, 1875–76, p. 496.

29 W. Stephenson, *American Journal of Obstetrics*, XV, 1882, pp. 287–294; also in an 1879 article in *The Lancet*, Dr Aldridge George similarly argued that the excess of blood shed during puberty was used during pregnancy to build the foetus. 'When conception has taken place,' he wrote, 'there is an outlet for the surplus nutritive income over expenditure in the growth of the foetus and uterus, and a similar outlet also exists during lactation, so the occurrence of menses during lactation is a comparatively rare event.' Both are quoted by Fraser Harrison, *The Dark Angel. Aspects of Victorian Sexuality*, Sheldon Press, London, 1977, p. 56.

30 Hall, *Adolescence*, 1, 487.

31 J. Goodman, 'The cyclical theory of menstruation', *American Journal of Obstetrics*, XI, no. 67, 1878 , pp. 3–44; Mary Putnam Jacobi, *The Question of Rest for Women During Menstruation*, Boylston Prize Essay of Harvard University for 1876, G.P. Putnam's Sons, New York, 1877 .

32 Mary Putnamn Jacobi, 'Hysterical fever', *Journal of Nervous and Mental Disease*, XV, 1890 , pp. 373–388.

33 Quoted by Mary Putnam Jacobi from an address to the Obstetrical Society of London in 1874, reported in the *British Medical Journal*, (ii), January 1875. See Showalter and Showalter, 1970, p.85.

34 A.F.A. King, 'A new basis for uterine pathology', *American Journal of Obstetrics*, VIII, 1875, p. 237.

35 Augustus Kinsley Gardner, *Conjugal Sins: Against the Laws of Life and Health and Their Effects Upon the Father, Mother and Child*, J.S. Redfield, New York, 1870, pp. 17, 145–146.

36 John Cowan, *The Science of a New Life*, Cowan and Co., New York, 1871, p. 29.

37 Thomas Addis Emmet, 'Transactions of the American Gynecological Society, first annual meeting', quoted in Harold Speert, *Obstetrics and Gynecology in America: A History*, Waverly Press, Inc., Baltimore, 1980, p. 41.

38 Smith-Rosenberg, 'Puberty to menopause: The cycle of femininity in nineteenth-century America', *Disorderly Conduct*, p. 183.

39 W.W. Bliss, *Woman and Her Thirty Year Pilgrimage*, William M. Littell, New York, 1869.

40 Ely Van De Warker, 'The genesis of women', *Popular Science Monthly*, V, June 1874, p. 276.

41 Edward Tilt, *The Change of Life in Health and Disease*, 4th ed. Bermingham and Co., New York, 1882, pp. 16, 39, 94–95; and, *On the Preservation of the Health of Women at the Critical Periods of Life*, London, 1851; P.J. Moebius, *Uber den Physiologischen Schwachsinn des Weibes*, Berlin, 1908; P.S. Icard, in *La Femme Pendant la Période Menstruelle*, Paris, 1890 , was widely quoted as stating, 'The menstrual function may … induce sympathethically a mental state varying from a slight psychosis to absolute irresponsibility.'

42 R. Leonardo, *History of Gynecology* Froben, New York, 1944; see also, E. Novak, *Menstruation and Its Disorders*, D. Appleton & Co., New York, 1921. New theories did not mean, however, that medical opinions were quick to cast off traditional ideas. *New York Times*, on 28 March, 1912 commented, 'No doctor can ever lose sight of the fact that the mind of a woman is always

threatened with danger from the reverberations of her physiological emergencies.' See also Speert, *Obstetrics and Gynecology in America: A History*, Ch. 4.

43 J.M. Allan, 'On the real differences in the minds of men and women', *Transactions of the Anthropological Society of London*, VII, 1869, p. cxcix.

44 Edward H. Clarke, *Sex in Education; or A Fair Chance for Girls*, James R. Osgood and Co., Boston, 1873, pp 37–38.

45 Dijkstra, *Idols of Perversity*, p. 26.

46 Jules Michelet, *L'Amour*, Paris, 1859. He stated, 'Woman is forever suffering from cicatrisation of an interior wound which is the cause of the whole drama', p. 48.

47 Albert Hayes, *Physiology of Women*, Peabody Medical Institute, Boston, 1869, pp. 84–85.

48 J.S. Jewell, 'Influence of our present civilization in the production of nervous and mental energy', *Journal of Nervous and Mental Disease*, I, January, 1874, quoted by Fellman and Fellman, *Making Sense of Self*, pp 70–71.

49 Herbert Spencer, *Education: Intellectual, Moral and Physical*, Williams and Norgate, London, 1861, p. 179.

50 For a discussion of Spencer's views on women and biological determinism, see Louise Michele Newman ed., *Men's Ideas/Women's Realities; Popular Science, 1870–1915*, Pergamon Press, New York, 1985, pp. 1–11; Delamont and Duffin, *The Nineteenth Century Woman*; Haller and Haller, *The Physician and Sexuality*.

51 E.L. Youmans started *Popular Science Monthly* in part to bring Spencer's ideas to America. See Robert C. Banister, *Social Darwinism: Science and Myth in Anglo-American Thought*, Philadelphia, 1979; and Susan Sleeth Mosedale, 'Science corrupted: Victorian biologists consider the woman question', *Journal of the History of Biology*, XI, no.1 Spring 1978, pp. 9.

52 The Lamarckian mechanism explained that the use of an organ resulted in its development, and disuse resulted in its degeneration over time. Due to prolonged disuse, women lacked a number of abilities that men had developed, especially abstract thought and reason. Female brains were thus marred by disuse and Darwin considered 'catch up' to be impossible for the female since the male was advancing so rapidly. Woman, in short, was less completely evolved than the male, and was likely to remain so for male traits were strengthened by use somewhat differently than were those of the female. Charles Darwin, *The Descent of Man and Selection in Relation to Sex*, 2nd ed., Werner, Akron, 1874, pp. 576–577. This kind of reasoning, David Ritchie noted in 1890, was tantamount to shutting up a bird in a narrow cage and then pointing out that it was incapable of flying. David Ritchie, *Darwinism and Politics*, 2nd ed., Mosedale, London, 1890; reprinted, Charles Scribner's and Sons, New York, 1909, pp. 68–69.

53 A note in *Popular Science Monthly*, XVII, July 1880, p. 431, suggested that Delaunay had advanced the opinion that precocity was a sign of biological inferiority and that in all domestic animals the female was formed before the male. Furthermore, the precocity of organs and organisms was in an inverse ratio to the extent of their evolution. See, also, G. Delaunay, 'Equality and inequality in sex', *Popular Science Monthly*, XX, December 1881.

54 Susan Sleeth Mosedale, in 'Science corrupted', analyses Spencer's and other's arguments about the mental and physical capacities of women.

55 Ben Barker-Benfield, 'The spermatic economy: A nineteenth century view of sexuality', *Feminist Studies*, I, no. I, Summer 1972, pp. 45–74.

56 Robert Ultzman, *The Neuroses of the Genito-Urinary System in the Male, with Sterility and Impotence*, Philadelphia, 1890, p. 11. See Gail Pat Parsons, 'Equal treatment for all: American medical remedies for male sexual problems, 1850–1900', *Journal of the History of Medicine*, XXXII, January 1977, pp. 55–71.

57 G.B.H. Swayze, 'Spermatorrhea', *Medical Surgery Report*, XXXIII, Philadelphia, 1875, p. 61.

58 Joseph W. Howe, M.D., *Excessive Venery, Masturbation and Continence*, New York, 1883 , pp. 63–66.

59 T.S. Clouston, 'Female education from a medical point of view', *Popular Science Monthly*, XXIV, January 1884b, p. 325.

60 Hughes Bennett, 'Hygiene in the higher education of women', p. 521.

61 Taylor, *A Physician's Counsels to Woman*, quoted in Barbara Ehrenreich and Deirdre English, *Complaints and Disorders: The Sexual Politics of Sickness*, The Feminist Press, New York, 1973 , p. 21.

62 Dr Tilt, *The Lancet*, XI, 1862, p. 480, quoted by Lorna Duffin, 'The conspicious consumptive: Woman as an invalid', Delamont and Duffin, *The Nineteenth Century Woman*, p. 32.

63 Allan, 'On the real differences', p. cxcviii.

64 Michelet, *L'Amour*, p. 48.

65 Max Runge, *Das Weib in Seiner Geschlechtliche Eigenart*, Berlin, 1900 , p. 3.

66 Hall, *Adolescence*, I, p. 472.

67 William Warren Potter, M.D., 'How should girls be educated?', *The New York Medical Journal*, LIII, 21 March 1891, p. 321.

68 George L. Austin, *Perils of American Womanhood, or a Doctor's Talk with Maiden, Wife and Mother*, Lee & Shepard, Boston, 1883 , p. 150.

69 J.H. Kellogg, *Plain Facts for Old and Young*, I.F. Segner, Burlington, Iowa, 1889 , p. 183.

70 Robert Barnes, 'Lumleian lectures: The convulsive diseases of women', *The Lancet*, I, 1873, p. 514.

71 George Engelmann, 'The American girl of to-day: The influence of modern education on functional development', President's Address, *American Gynecological Society*, XXV, 1901, pp. 8–45.

72 Thomas E. Addis Emmet, M.D., *The Principles and Practice of Gynecology*, Philadelphia, 1879, p. 21.

73 John Thorburn, M.D., *Female Education from a Medical Point of View*, Manchester, 1884 .

74 Hall, *Adolescence*, I, pp. 618, 639.

75 G. Stanley Hall, 'The ideal school as based on child study', *The Forum*, XXXII, September, 1901 , p. 35.

76 Clarence J. Karier, 'G. Stanley Hall: A priestly prophet of a new dispensation', *Journal of Libertarian Studies*, Spring 1983, p. 54.

77 Hall, *Adolescence*, I, p. 478.

78 Silas Weir Mitchell, *Lectures on Diseases of the Nervous System Especially in Women*, Lea Bros. and Co., Philadelphia, 1885 , p. 15. Dr Mitchell was

famous for his rest cures for women who had become, he claimed, nervous and hysterical due to improper lifestyles. For an excellent analysis, see Ellen L. Bassuk, ' The rest cure: Repetition or resolution of Victorian women's conflicts?' *Poetics Today*, VI, no. 1, 1985, pp. 245–257.

79 Clarke, *Sex in Education*; pp. 40–42.

80 William Goodell, M.D., *The Dangers and the Duty of the Hour*, S.M. Miller, Medical Publishers, Philadelphia, 1882, pp. 18, 8.

81 T.S. Clouston, M.D., 'Female Education from a Medical Point of View', *Popular Science Monthly*, XXIV, December 1883, pp. 214–228.

82 Potter, 'How should girls be educated?', p. 323.

83 Maudsley, 'Sex in mind', p. 475.

84 Kellogg, *Plain Facts*, p. 83.

85 Julia Ward Howe, ed., *Sex and Education: A Reply to Dr. Clarke's Sex in Education*, Roberts Brothers, Boston, 1874, Reprinted Arno Press, New York, 1972, pp. 8, 15, 18–19.

86 The Association of Collegiate Alumnae, Health Statistics of Women College Graduates, 1885. See also Leta Stetter Hollingworth, *Functional Periodicity: An Experimental Study of the Mental and Motor Abilities of Women During Menstruation*, Columbia University, New York, 1914, and John Dewey, 'Health and sex in higher education', *Popular Science Monthly*, XXIX, March 1886, pp. 606–615.

87 W. LeC. Stevens, *The Admission of Women to Universities*, Boston, 1883.

88 Alida C. Avery, Testimony from Colleges, Vassar, 1873, in Julia Ward Howe, *Sex and Education*, rpt. ed., 1972 [1874], p. 193.

89 Elizabeth Garrett Anderson, 'Sex in mind and education. A reply', *Fortnightly Review*, XV, 1874, p. 503. She and other female physicians such as Mary Jacobi did attempt to counter the belief that rest was necessary or even desirable for women who menstruated normally. Jacobi, *The Question of Rest*; Clelia Mosher also pointed out that the tradition that women must be incapacitated at periods tended to increase the idea that efficiency was impaired. Clelia Mosher, 'Normal menstruation and some of the factors modifying it', *Johns Hopkins Hospital Bulletin*, April–May, June 1901, p. 178.

90 J.T. Wilson, M.D., 'Menstrual disorder in school girls', *The Texas Sanitarium*, June 1885, p. 19.

91 C.W. Saleeby, *Woman and Womanhood*, Mitchell Kennerley, New York, 1911, p. 102.

92 The female role in reproduction, note Ehrenreich and English, required stamina and if you counted in the activities of child raising and running a household, it required full-blown energetic health. *For Her Own Good*, p. 134. Such stamina appeared to many physicians in the latter part of the nine-teenth century to be palpably lacking among white, Anglo-Saxon, middle-class American women. They pointed to an alarming drop in the birth rate among the 'native stock' and challenged women to do their duty and improve their health or accept a 'new rape of the Sabines' to save the race. See, for example, Hall, *Adolescence*, II, pp. 561–647.

93 Smith-Rosenberg, 'The hysterical woman', *Disorderly Conduct*, p. 658.

94 J.H. Kellogg, *Ladies' Guide in Health and Disease, Girlhood, Maidenhood, Wifehood, Motherhood*, Des Moines, IA, 1883, p. 118.

95 Kellogg, *Ladies' Guide*, p. 188. For a discussion concerning the integration of tomboyism with a traditional view of women's domestic role, see Sharon O'Brien, 'Tomboyism and adolescent conflict: Three nineteenth-century case studies', Mary Kelley, ed., *Woman's Being, Woman's Place: Female Identity and Vocation in American History*, G.K. Hall & Co., Boston, 1979, pp. 351–372.

96 S. Weir Mitchell, M.D., *Doctor and Patient*, Mitchell Kennerly, Philadelphia, 1888, p. 141.

97 M. L. Holbrook, *Parturition Without Pain: A Code of Directions for Escaping From the Primal Curse*, Wood & Holbrook, New York, 1875, p. 22.

98 J. M. Rice, M.D., 'Physiology and the prevention of disease', *Popular Science Monthly*, XLI, 1892, pp. 309–313.

99 J.W. Wainwright, M.D., 'Exercise', *Medical Record*, 5 May 1906, p. 707.

100 George W. Stocking, Jr., 'Lamarckianism in American social science: 1890–1915', *Journal of the History of Ideas*, XXIII, 1962, pp. 239–259.

101 Felix Oswald, M.D., 'Physical education', *Popular Science Monthly*, XIX, May 1881, p. 24.

102 W.E. Anderson, M.D., *The Physical Side of Education*, Wisconsin State Board of Health Report, 1887. Quoted in 'Out-door play for school-girls', *Popular Science Monthly*, XXXII, April 1888, p. 856.

103 Clouston, 'Female education', 1884b, p. 324.

104 Kellogg, *Ladies' Guide*, p. 188.

105 Saleeby, *Woman*, p. 109.

106 Smith-Rosenberg, 'The Hysterical Woman', p. 212.

107 Hall, *Adolescence*, I, p. 615.

108 Thorburn, *Female education*, 1884.

109 Oswald, 'Physical education', p. 23.

110 C. Roberts, M.D., 'Bodily deformities in girlhood', *Popular Science Monthly*, XXII, January 1883, p. 324.

111 M.B. Allen and A.C. McGrigor, M.D., *The Glory of Woman*, Elliott Publishing Co., Philadelphia, 1896, p. 87. It should be noted that one of the authors of *The Glory of Woman* was a female doctor.

112 Clouston, 'Female education', 1883, p. 227. Clouston echoed Clarke that physical education for girls was to be stressed only as it connected with the duties of maternity.

113 Clouston, 'Female education', 1884b, p. 320.

114 Henry Ling Taylor, M.D., 'Exercise as a remedy', *Popular Science Monthly*, XVIII, March 1896, p. 630.

115 William G. Anderson, M.D., *Anderson's Physical Education*, A.D. Dana, New York, 1897.

116 J. Madison Taylor, M.D. 'Puberty in girls and certain of its disturbances', *Pediatrics*, 15 July 1896.

117 Alice B. Tweedy, 'Homely gymnastics', *Popular Science Monthly*, XL, February 1892.

118 N.C. Whitaker, 'The health of American girls', *Popular Science Monthly*, LXXI, September 1907, p. 243; Carol Dyhouse, 'Good wives and little mothers: Social anxieties and the schoolgirl's curriculum, 1890–1920', *Oxford Review of Education*, III, no. 1, 1977, pp. 21–35.

119 William Lee Howard, M.D., 'Athletics for young women', *New York Medical

Journal, LXXXIII, 3 February 1906, p. 239.

120 Howard, 'Athletics', p. 239.

121 Howard, 'Athletics', pp. 239–240.

122 Clouston, 'Female education', 1884b, p. 323.

123 M.G. Van Rensselaer, M.D., 'The waste of woman's intellectual force', *Forum*, 1892, p. 616; Although S. Weir Mitchell admitted he did not understand the relationship between fat and health, gaining weight, he felt, improved the blood and made the skin ruddy, which was a certain sign of physical health. Mitchell, *Wear and Tear*.

124 R.P. Hudson, 'The biography of disease: Lessons from chlorosis', *Bulletin of the History of Medicine*, LI, 1977, pp. 440–463; A.C. Siddall, 'Chlorosis: Etiology reconsidered', *Bulletin of the History of Medicine*, LVI, 1982, pp. 254–260; T. Clifford Allbutt, 'Chlorosis', *A System of Medicine*, T.C. Allbutt, ed., Macmillan, New York, 1905 ; R.L. Tait, *Disorders of Women*, Lea, Philadelphia, 1889 .

125 Joan Jacobs Brumberg, 'Chlorotic girls 1870–1920: A historical perspective on female adolescence', Judith Walzer Leavitt, ed., *Women and Health in America*, The University of Wisconsin Press, Madison, 1984, p. 188.

126 L. Warner, *A Treatise on the Functions and Diseases of Women*, Manhattan, New York, 1875; Taylor, 'Puberty in girls'.

127 E.L. Jones, *Chlorosis: The Special Anemia of Young Women*, Balliere and Tindall, London, 1897; Allbutt, 'Chlorosis'. See also Dr. Matthews Duncan quoted by William Withers Moore, President, British Medical Association, *The Lancet*, II, 1886, p. 315.

128 As many commentators on nineteenth century nutritional practices have noted, it was not surprising that Victorian adolescents eschewed or were not offered red meat, for the link between animal flesh and rampant sexuality had been well established by numerous physicians and health reformers. See, for example, Haller and Haller, *The Physician and Sexuality*; James C. Whorton, *Crusaders for Fitness: The History of American Health Reformers*, Princeton University Press, New Jersey, 1982 ; Bullough and Voght, 'Women, menstruation and nineteenth century medicine'.

129 Hall, *Adolescence*, 1, pp. 507–508.

130 Tilt, *The Change of Life*, 4th ed., 1882, p. 10.

131 Grant Allen, 'Plain words on the woman question', *Popular Science Monthly*, XXXVI, December 1889, p. 181.

132 Engelman, 'The American girl of today', p. 9.

133 Havelock Ellis, M.D., *Determinants of Puritan Stock and Its Causes*, New York, 1894.

134 Hall, *Adolescence*, 1, p. 609.

135 In their analysis of the medical advice literature of the late nineteenth century, the Fellmans note that 'a general sense that the world outside is coming undone is frequently related to the haunting fear that the body and the mind are fragile structures. The imperiled body is both metaphor and ideological focus.' Fellmans, *Making Sense of Self*, p. 138.

136 Charles E. Rosenberg, 'Science and American social thought', David D. Van Tassel and Michael G. Hall, eds., *Science and Society in the United States*, The Dorsey Press, Illinois, 1966, p. 139.

137 Maudsley, 'Sex in mind', p. 468.
138 James Whorton has described the debate about the medical consequences of athletics for men and the effect it had upon the formation of public attitudes toward strenuous exertion and competitiveness in sport. Those physicians fearful about the squandering of bodily reserve power by young men in their battle for victory pointed to cardiac hypertrophy, emphysema, kidney damage and insanity. James C. Whorton, 'Athlete's heart: The medical debate over athleticism, 1870–1920', *Journal of Sport History*, IX, no. 1, Spring 1982, pp. 30–52; The debate over athlete's heart, was well over by the time of World War I. The debates about the medical implications of female sport, however, especially during menstruation, have been more enduring.
139 See, for example, Carroll Smith-Rosenberg, 'The new woman as androgyne: Social disorder and gender crisis, 1870–1936', *Disorderly Conduct*, pp. 245–296; and Mrozek, *Sport and American Mentality*.

2

The thirty-year pilgrimage: exercise in the prime of life

> The hygiene and the rules suitable for a man do not apply in the case of a woman. She has duties thrown on her in life and special capacities to do them entirely different from man . . . Her periods of periodic illness necessarily handicap her in many ways. . . . Her peculiar duties of childbearing and nursing are attended, at least in civilized life, by dangers and risks of exhaustion and disease.[1]

The periodic draining of a woman's energy which began at menarche and continued through multiple pregnancies was regarded by many physicians as a 'thirty-year pilgrimage' which disqualified women from all but the main task of maternity. The earliest years of this pilgrimage were admittedly of critical importance. Dr Napheys contended that 'the two years which change the girl to the woman often seal forever the happiness or the hopeless misery of her whole life. They decide whether she is to become a healthy, hopeful, cheerful wife and mother, or a languid, complaining invalid to whom marriage is a curse, children an affliction and life itself a burden.'[2] Only when a girl had been safely guided through the breakers of puberty was there good reason to hope for on-going health, and this had to be carefully husbanded by the physician.[3]

Menarche was only the beginning of a journey, doctors realized, and the conditions surrounding women's continuing reproductive functioning became an ongoing focus of medical concern. The perceived need for women to rest while menstruating did not cease once menstruation had become established. Because of the energy drain from menstruation and maternity, a woman was often considered to be a natural invalid for most of her adult life, lacking the strength for sustained physical or mental effort. In 1895, August Strindberg saw this pilgrimage as necessarily debilitating. 'A human body cannot develop in a normal fashion if it is deprived in this way of such a significant quantity of nutritive fluid. . . These periodical bleedings are in part to blame for the arrest in growth and development of women . . . indeed, this anaemia of necessity serves to atrophy the brain.' He considered it appropriate, therefore, to designate the normal physical and mental condition of the grown woman as that of a 'sick child'.[4]

The notion that the brain was permanently deprived of blood lost through years of menstruation was also posited by Romanes in 'Mental differences between men and women'.[5] Not only was the grey matter of the female brain shallower than that of the male in the first place, it was further reduced by menstruation. Woman was, therefore, deemed to be perpetually and increasingly brain-drained as she matured.

'Whether they come to be mothers or not,' said Henry Maudsley in 1874, 'they cannot dispense with those physiological functions of their nature that have reference to that aim, however much they might wish it, and they cannot disregard them in the labour of life without injury to their health.'[6] Thus, even if a woman was celibate, the labour of potential procreation still occupied a quarter of the time of her life between her twelfth or fourteenth year to somewhere around her forty-fifth.[7]

Just as precautionary exercise was extolled by physicians as an important mechanism at menarche to balance the weakness meted out by the 'monthly sickness', a woman learned that she should continue to comply with a medical regimen throughout her productive childbearing years. During her thirty or more fertile years, she was told, the constant threat of disease and nervous disorder must be held at bay by exercising those life-style habits which would best ensure the smooth functioning of her reproductive organs and the careful expenditure of scarce energy.[8] Engrossing literary pursuits, no less than anxiety, care or an overtaxed physical system were all to be avoided since they interfered with procreation. The successful rearing of noble boys and girls was seen to be the greatest work of all.[9] Thus, from adolescence until she was forty years old, at least 20 per cent of a woman's energy had to be diverted for the maintenance of maternity and its attendant functions.[10] This estimate was based upon the supposition that, in addition to the monthly menstrual drain of energy, at each birth a portion of a woman's vital energy was transformed and imparted to the newborn child. As each child was born, the mother experienced a physical loss to her already over-drained body. As a prominent physiologist explained, 'in mankind, as in other animals, to procreate is in effect to die to oneself and to leave one's life to posterity'.[11]

Those convinced by Galton's theories agreed that women should be persuaded to become mothers of at least four children in order to preserve the race (since fifty per cent of those born would not be expected to attain maturity).[12] Some encouraged more births, believing that the quality of children improved, within reason, by practice, thus allowing nature a chance to do her best. Add to the energy expenditure of at least four births the recurring monthly drain of menstruation, running a household, rearing children and ministering to a husband, then it was clear that little energy could be available for any but the main function, and that life-style habits must be concentrated upon supporting the special and debilitating burden of motherhood. 'With women it is very much the same as fruit trees', commented Dr Currier. A period of bearing had to be succeeded by a period of rest. If the boughs were heavily laden with fruit year after year, the vitality of the tree would soon be exhausted.[13] Indeed, complained a female physician, the drain of maternity was such that relatively few women who entered the marriage state blooming and vigorous remained that way.[14]

Since childbearing and childrearing consumed most of a married woman's adult life, there was little time available for exercise during these years.[15] As Dr Bennett admitted:

> many years of the most vigorous and active period of a woman's life are spent in germinating and suckling her offspring, during which time she is physically capable of little else. . . The whole sexual system of woman has a profound influence on her physical nature . . . Indeed her natural muscular feebleness and delicacy of constitution render violent exercise . . . distasteful to her.[16]

At the same time, married women were frequently warned not to neglect the healthful exercise needed to maintain their vitality. It was suggested that middle-class women obtained neither enough fresh air nor sufficient exercise and that many of them habitually neglected exercise and generated large amounts of reserve materials 'in the shape of fat which became burdensome by its bulk'.[17] Endurance exercises and those designed to assist the respiratory system were considered to be the most suitable for burning up this surplus and improving health.[18] Unlike adolescence, doctors felt that when a woman was mature she could partly compensate for overtaxing the mental function by resting, although she needed to maintain her muscular strength with a certain amount of modest exercise. 'After a good muscular system has been developed in childhood and youth,' said Dr Richards, 'a comparatively small amount of time judiciously devoted to exercise will keep a person in healthy working order till near the age of forty.'[19] Edwin Checkley, in his *Natural Method of Physical Training*, agreed that sufficient health and strength could generally be obtained 'in the ordinary activities of life, if these activities, however meagre, are carried on in obedience to right laws'.[20]

Elisabeth Scovil, in her *Preparation for Motherhood Manual*, echoed the cautionary advice of the establishment physicians. Although fresh air was absolutely essential for health, she commented:

> most women get sufficient exercise in moving about their households, and a long walk does not bring sufficient compensation for the fatigue it causes. Sitting on the piazza, or lying in the hammock, in summer, will often be more beneficial than keeping on one's feet to walk. In winter, wrapping up warmly and moving slowly about a room with the window open answers the purpose of a constitutional, and is not nearly as tiring.[21]

Pregnancy was regarded as needing special exercises, close medical advice and supervision. The expectant woman had to conserve her resources. She was living for two and the child's future depended on the mother's conduct during pregnancy. In *Parturition Without Pain*, Dr Holbrook explained that exercise was central to the medical supervision of pregnancy. 'From the beginning of pregnancy, even more care than usual should be taken to use regular, abundant and healthful (n.b. not excessive nor violent) exercise.' The forenoon is the best part of the day for exercise, said Dr. Holbrook, 'the afternoon the second best only; the evening the worst; and early going to bed highly expedient'. Exercise in the morning, he explained further, would secure two advantages. First, 'the use of the best physical strength, thus avoiding the additional risks from exertion when the body is . . . fatigued with the results of the day's occupation; and second, the use of the best of the sunshine and air'.[22] 'Every woman with child . . . should take moderate exercise', said Dr Pierce in his medical advice book,[23] and Dr Napheys recommended very moderate exercise in the open air during the entire pregnancy but never so active or prolonged as to induce fatigue.[24]

Walking in the open air was consistently promoted as the most suitable activity for pregnant women, though never to be taken to extremes. Walking could be replaced by driving in the latter weeks as movement became difficult. It is sometimes difficult, noted Dr Green, to induce women to take sufficient open-air exercise, but there is no question that most women benefit from such exercise and have easier labour in consequence. 'Women should be willing to train themselves in some

degree for their labour, as an athlete would train himself for a race.'
'Fortunately,' he said, demonstrating the ideological underpinnings of
many doctors' arguments, 'most women are engaged in house-keeping
duties, and except for the want of open air, housework is probably the
healthiest occupation a woman can have.'[25] For the most part,
household tasks were considered quite appropriate for pregnant
women though some doctors did warn against fatiguing housework
such as a heavy washing, sweeping or going up and down stairs.[26] Dr
Galabin also recommended a 'reasonable amount of exercise in the open
air during pregnancy as well as the avoidance of excessive fatigue,
strains and the lifting of heavy weights'.[27] Dr Thomas Bull, an English
obstetrician, cautioned against all agitating exercise such as 'riding in a
carriage with rapidity on uneven roads, dancing much and frequently,
. . ..; in short, all masculine and fatiguing employments whatever'.[28]
'Do not run; do not jump, do not drive unsafe horses, give up dancing
and riding, do not plunge into cold water', said another.[29] Moderate,
gentle, daily exercise was thus to be the rule, in the open air if possible,
but always including a share of housework.

Certainly, it was agreed that it was important for the expectant
mother that every muscle be in good working order in able to perform its
proper work. Judicious exercise would do this.[30] Thus, during
pregnancy, those accustomed to regular physical exercise might
continue it while those unaccustomed to it should commence.[31] One
precaution, however, was critical. No violent exercise, or indeed any
bodily exercise was to be taken at the time that would have been the
menstrual period under ordinary conditions. This rule had to be
implicitly observed, since its neglect could cause the loss of the child's
life and serious injury to the mother.[32] Indiscreet exertion at this time,
cautioned Dr Green in the *Boston Medical and Surgical Journal*, 'can cause
miscarriage and other unfortunate results, thus in these days, exercise
should be restricted'.[33] Just as the monthly period was considered to
exacerbate the tendency towards convulsive fits and 'kindle the flames
of disease',[34] so during pregnancy the body and mind remained at risk
every month at that point in the cycle where the woman would have
menstruated.[35]

During and after childbirth itself orthodox doctors were generally
committed to forbidding exercise for some time, preferring to keep
women horizontal for at least three or four days. Resting time was
longer for delicate women, to guard against ligament strain and
prolapse of the womb.[36]

The consensus among establishment physicians concerning appropriate moderate exercise for women of childbearing age was apparent in 'A Symposium of eminent doctors on how to be healthy at all ages', published in *Strand Magazine* in the early years of the twentieth century.[37] Several English establishment doctors, mostly from London, were asked about the best means of conserving the constitution of women and about their recommendations for general exercise in all weathers and all seasons of the year. Their replies were unanimous:

Dr Robert Bell of Surrey, author of *Woman in Health and Sickness*:

> What is required for preserving the health and beauty of women are, first, a strict observance of hygienic laws, especially . . . plenty of open-air exercise and gymnastics to a moderate extent. Any amusement that necessitates a good amount of walking in the open air . . . is a good general exercise. In a word, walking is the best all-round exercise we can take.

Dr Joseph Kidd of London, author of *The Laws of Therapeutics* and physician to Lord Beaconsfield:

> Daily open-air exercise is among the best preservatives of the health and beauty of women. The best exercise for all weathers and all seasons of the year is regular steady walking in the open air

Dr F. Needham of London, author of *Brain Exhaustion*:

> I know of no exercise which is universally applicable and suited to all seasons of the year, so good as walking.

Dr J. Milson Rhodes of Manchester:

> Exercise is like food, it should be mixed, and I do not mind what the form takes so long as there is plenty of fresh air with it.

Dr C.W. Saleeby of London, author of *The Cycle of Life*:

> As regards exercise, the main consideration is that it be such exercise as can and must be taken in pure air. The only exercise worth a straw is that which takes one into the open air.

Dr W.K. Sibley of London:

> Women's health and beauty are largely preserved by leading a natural and not artificial life. Women were intended by nature to be mothers of families and to devote their time and attention to their children and homes. Regular habits, simple but properly-cooked food, early hours, sleeping with open windows these are the best preservatives of comeliness. . . .. Laziness in all classes is the malady of the age. For exercise for the young ... the hygienic advantages of the old fashioned skipping rope have never been superseded even by the recent physical culture exercises 'made in Germany'.

Dr Andrew Wilson, popular medical writer on health subjects:

> Certainly there are special conditions to be reckoned with in the case of girls, but I regard the greater attention paid today to women's exercise and calisthenics, as an admirable aid to their better physical development. . . . I feel convinced a good walk, with part of it uphill, is as excellent a form of exercise as anybody can take. It encourages deep breathing, braces the muscles, tones up the heart, and promotes the action of the skin, all excellent results of natural exercise.

Dr Yorke-Davies of Harley Street, author of *Health and Condition in the Active and Sedentary*:

> Outdoor exercise is undoubtedly essential to robust health and in all cases, when taken regularly and with discretion, tends to increase strength and improve condition.

Summarizing the doctors' discussions, the symposium compiler noted unkindly that 'their views in regard to women's health are well worth considering in spite of the fact that we may be sure they will not be followed except perhaps by one here and there'.[38]

Many establishment physicians clearly regarded some exercise for women as essential for preserving health and preventing disease, particularly outdoor walking and other 'natural' forms of exercise, and felt that mature women needed to be assisted by their doctors in monitoring the required balance of rest and exercise for a life dedicated to healthy reproduction. Dr Ling Taylor explained the challenge for physicians to be not merely the prescription of exercise, 'but rather such proportioning and contrasting of the muscular activity to periods of rest that the total result shall be beneficial'.[39] J. William White MD claimed that 'exercise was the most important therapeutic and hygienic agency at the command of the physician'.[40]

Since physicians agreed that the amount of exercise required was to be determined by the needs of the female body at each stage of reproductive development, and that doctors were well placed to advise women on all facets of exercise, they felt compelled to comment on a new exercise craze which emerged in the 1890s with imagined risks and benefits to female health – bicycle riding.[41] That 'no woman should ride a bicycle without first consulting her medical man' became a popular phrase in establishment medical journals, which increasingly portrayed the pros and cons of bicycle riding upon female health in that decade.[42] It stands to reason, noted the *British Medical Journal* in a ten-part series concerning bicycling and health in 1896, that:

the introduction of a new and fascinating form of exercise, and one which has likely been in many cases adopted by those who have not been accustomed to physical exertion from their youth upwards, must have a marked effect on the health of those who indulge in it, and it therefore behooves the guardians of the public health to study its effects . . . [and] to regulate its use . . .[43]

The medical debate over female exercise and the bicycle

Exercise is conducive to health when intelligently employed; otherwise, it is injurious and sinful.[44]

No study of nineteenth-century women and exercise can ignore the 1890s and the role of the bicycle in expanding women's views concerning their potential for physical mobility or in promoting a stream of cautionary and often contradictory advice from establishment physicians. The establishment medical debate concerning the health risks and benefits of bicycling for women encapsulated the anxieties held by a prestigious group of professional men concerning the need to control the female reproductive process and to guard the health and prosperity of society on both sides of the Atlantic. 'As prosaic and trivial as it may first appear,' says Whorton, 'the 1890s debate over the bicycle offers an informative capsule view of the pressure imposed by cultural preoccupation on medical deliberation.'[45]

Initially the improved safety bicycle with pneumatic tyres appeared to offer a reasonable solution to the sedentary life of middle-class women criticized so frequently by physicians. The emergence of a safe, light and comfortable machine overcame earlier suspicion of the wheel, and the bicycle was soon touted as a revolutionary social force.[46] Although all social levels were touched by the emergent bicycle boom, it was in many respects a middle-class enthusiasm 'fuelled largely by visions of improved health'.[47] Feminists and physicians alike argued over the bicycle's potential for improving the physique and health of middle-class women. In England, where the craze followed that in France and the United States, the Countess of Malmesbury called the sport 'one of the greatest blessings given to modern women'[48] and championed, with Viscountess Harberton, the rationalization of dress necessary for unencumbered riding and physical mobility.[49] 'Physically rather weaker than men we undoubtedly are,' said Viscountess Harberton,

but why exaggerate this weakness by literally so tying ourselves up in clothing that the muscles in some parts of the body dwindle till they become useless? We should realize the harm we are doing ourselves and the race by habitually lowering our powers of life and energy in such a manner.[50]

Elizabeth Cady Stanton championed a similar cause in the United States.[51] It was the means, she said, by which health would be restored to an ever increasing number of nervous, overwrought women.[52] Rational dress was popularized in America by numerous female reformers who complained that long skirts, heavy materials and corsets not only endangered women's health but 'recklessly cursed the unborn'. Bloomers, knickerbockers and other bicycling costumes were promoted by female riders and became enormously popular before eventually being discarded in favour of shorter, lighter skirts.[53] Frances Willard, for example, developed a cycling costume with a skirt three inches off the ground, claiming that no one with common sense could take exception to such a modest suit.[54]

At its peak of popularity in the late 1890s, cycling promised liberal-minded middle-class women, the emergent 'new women', the potential benefits of healthy, active recreation as well as a new sense of liberty from restrictive dress and chaperonage. Louise Jeye extolled:

> There is a new dawn, a dawn of emancipation, and it is brought about by the cycle. Free to wheel, free to spin out into the glorious country, unhampered by chaperon or even more dispiriting male admirer, the young girl of today can feel the real independence of herself, and while she is building up her better constitution, she is developing her better mind.[55]

The initial consensus among establishment physicians was that bicycling could be more useful in strengthening and exercising female bodies, young and old, than most other sports or recreations. 'Bicycling per se,' said Dr Hatch in 1897, 'appears void of offence.'[56]

When Dr Prendergast suggested that 'it is almost universally conceded that any form of exercise that will bring women and girls into the open air must be of great value', he was alluding particularly to tricycling and bicycling.[57] After two years of intensive study, he said, he had decided that bicycle riding for women of all ages would be 'productive, of great value to the present generation, while in the next its benefits will be seen in the form of better health, finer physical development and more stable nervous systems'. Thus 'we have in the bicycle an agent which will accomplish an enormous amount of good for women'.[58]

Dr Fenton claimed in the *Nineteenth Century* that thousands of women qualifying for general invalidism had been rescued by cycling.[59] A marked decline in female deaths from consumption in Massachusetts over five years was attributed to the invigorating exercise of bicycling.[60]

As a therapeutic agent, bicycling was extolled for encouraging exercise of the large muscle masses, invigorating the respiratory system, improving digestion, purifying the blood as well as generally refreshing mind and body.[61] Cycling might encourage women to discard their damaging corsets, said a number of doctors, allowing them to strengthen their abdominal muscles through exercise. Used by women with direction and sense, doctors claimed, cycling produced more stable nerves, easier labours and healthy children.[62] More specifically, some believed that bicycling would strengthen the muscle bundles of the uterus so that childbirth might be made easier (this in contrast to horseback riding which Dr Garrigues believed was apt to produce a funnel-shaped pelvis posing difficulties for childbirth).[63] It was further argued that strengthened leg muscles would stimulate pelvic tone, strengthening the pelvis and restoring reproductive normalcy.[64]

Cycling, it appeared, had come along just in time to rehabilitate British and American women.[65] Not only would it fortify women during their childbearing years, it could also bring much needed benefits to those middle-aged spinsters 'passing through a period of mental fermentation and physical irritability of varying degree'. Nervous disorders set up by the irritability engendered by a dissatisfied life could be eased, it was suggested, by the exhilaration brought on by riding on a bicycle in the open air, providing a much needed mental and nerve tonic.[66]

The very popularity of bicycling, however, soon alarmed many doctors. Excessive activity was said to be the problem as too many women abandoned the law of moderation. The wheel, warned Dr Love, 'is like alcohol, good in some cases if used very temperately, but the trouble is that the temptation is great to use both to excess'.[67] The bicycle, it seemed, could be 'a double-edged instrument which might cut through debility caused by slothfulness and poor living habits' only to produce a new debility from overexertion.[68] Having initially advocated certain kinds of games and exercise to counteract the increasing sedentariness of an industrialized society, once athletics and games became popular and vigorously competitive the doctors worried that moderation was being overthrown. Many doctors became staunch foes of the very athletic trends initiated and encouraged with considerable eagerness by the medical profession itself.[69] They worried about the effects of overstrain upon the heart, spinal deformities from unbalanced exercise, sore joints and strained body parts. Some claimed that the vast majority of women were unable to carry weight on their wrists or develop the ability to sustain their weight on the pedals. Avid female bicycle riders were said to develop 'bicycle-face', which included wild staring eyes, a strained expression, a projecting jaw and a 'general focusing of all the features toward the centre, a sort of physiognomic implosion'.[70]

The most vigorous medical debates, of course, concerned the supposed damage caused to female reproductive health by bicycle riding. British and American doctors heeded warnings by French colleagues at the Medical Academy in Paris: no one should become a habitual cyclist without medical authorization, and all cyclists should be content with a moderate pace and distance.[71] There are times, said Dr Stables, when no girl should cycle much. 'If, instead of enjoying the scenery and the fresh air, you only try how far and how fast you can go, ten to one the run will do you little good and may do incalculable harm.'[72]

Furthermore, many physicians began enumerating the diseases caused by cycling and debating the acute and chronic conditions diagnosed among those female patients who had overstepped moderation. Dr Prendergast worried that a number of his women patients had become prostrated by unduly strenuous long bicycle rides. Damage appeared to be occurring in precisely those areas which had earlier promised the most benefits. Jarring and jolting were said to cause uterine displacement and spinal shock. The pelvic organs and overstrain and hardening of the abdominal muscles were especially targeted for the problems they might cause in labour.[73]

Dr Longaker identified faulty saddles as a particular problem. They were too hard, too long and too narrow and consequently injured the perineum and vulva.[74] Bicycle manufacturers worked to develop broader and softer saddles for women's bicycles, and the invention of a soft 'Komphy' pad worn under the skirt was said to help.[75] Alarmists were worried more by the potential for masturbation caused by friction from the bicycle saddle, though many establishment doctors admitted this to be an exaggerated concern.[76] Dr Turner, writing in the *British Medical Journal*, agreed with a French physician in claiming to treat this subject, that the woman, not the bicycle was at fault in this instance. Masturbation was a most unlikely consequence of bicycle riding and healthy open-air exercise could be trusted to minimize such excessive behaviour. For Turner excessive speed and competition were the real dangers 'the physiological crimes' posed by cycling, as was riding during the menstrual period, while pregnant or for three months after confinement. Moreover, whenever any 'pelvic mischief' was apparent, riding was contra-indicated. Old people too were warned to avoid the strain of bicycle riding upon their brittle vessels and degenerate muscles, as well as the almost certain danger of falls.[77]

These attempts to involve the bicycle in the aetiology of female disease illustrated the continued uneasiness felt by male physicians about the effects of physical exertion on women's health and strength. It is difficult, also, to avoid the conjecture that many physicians were nervous not only about the effects of physical exertion on women's health and strength but also about the freedom, physical liberty and new female ambitions that bicycling appeared to represent. 'Speaking of women and the bicycle,' said Dr Love misogynously, 'I sometimes think when I see a bifurcated bloomer on the wheel, that the fool-killer neglects his business.'[78] Other doctors claimed that women were behaving mannishly and avoiding their responsibilities to home and family.[79] Yet in his major report on bicycling and health, Dr Turner emphasized the establishment position that, with care, mothers of many children could ride daily and be rewarded with renewed and increasing health. After all, he continued, one cannot dismiss the exhilaration of the balanced wheel and 'the gift of improved nerve tone which experience shows a course of judiciously regulated bicycle riding confers on the weaker sex'.[80]

Although the bicycle did more, perhaps, than any other activity to form new conceptions of what it was possible for females to do and be and to engage women in health-related exercise, other sports too were increasingly accepted by establishment physicians as a means of using carefully managed activity to strengthen women for childbirth and as a tonic to revive their enthusiasm for their housewifely duties. The type of outdoor girl popularized in newspapers and magazines at the turn of the century 'supported the views of conservatives who reasoned that their daughters should cultivate an excellent physique as insurance for a stable society founded on sound motherhood'.[81] Sportsman Edwyn Sandys drew up medically acceptable guidelines for those sports that improved women's childbearing abilities and counselled against those which jeopardized reproductive health. Riding, hunting, tennis, rowing and golf were all on the former list. Rowing was thought to be good for the health, provided it was moderate and non-competitive. It hardened the muscles, strengthened the back and increased the breathing power of the lungs. Canoeing also was seen to be an appropriate female activity since:

> the lightness of the sport puts it easily into woman's kingdom. All the movements are to round the body out and forward, and to expand the lungs at every stroke . . . The training is rhythmical and natural, asking less of a

woman than the insistent golf ball.[82]

Swimming and golf were health-engendering if not performed to excess.[83] (In the case of golf, this sometimes meant leaving driving to the men while women confined themselves to putting.)[84] When women did drive, they were advised to drive with a half or threequarter swing.[85] John S. White explained that tennis was a safe activity for women because the strain was so short in the effort to reach and return the ball that internal damage was unlikely.[86] Even versatile sportswomen advised women tennis players to serve underhand and to play mixed doubles rather than the more fatiguing singles. Tennis as played by a woman, said Maud Marshall, was a very different thing from the man's game and she counselled against the use of 'forward or volleying tactics.'[87] In *Outing*, the late nineteenth-century journal which often discussed the sporting activities of well-to-do women, Henry Slocum Jr extolled tennis as 'the one athletic game which a woman may enjoy'. 'It must be conceded,' he continued, 'that lawn tennis is a game wonderfully well fitted to be a medium of exercise for women,' though 'it is a game which, when too violently played, becomes as severe a strain upon the muscles and produces as serious an effect upon the action of the heart and lungs as any of the more exhausting athletic sports.'[88] Women were often perceived to be in danger of overtaxing themselves at tennis, becoming overheated, straining weak muscles, or developing big knotty biceps on one arm and a broadened palm.

Similarly horse-riding for women was both extolled and cautioned against. 'If indulged in with moderation, there isn't a finer exercise in the world for women, nor one that affords more pleasure', said a commentator in *Outing*.[89] Charles Clay, while complaining that the leisured classes 'are not in as healthy physical condition to sustain the burdens of maternity and its consequent strain upon the system as they ought to be', believed that there was not an exercise so thoroughly enjoyable and useful as the practice of fencing. 'It ought really,' he said, 'be an indispensable necessity of a young lady's complete physical education,' particularly 'since the sport does not abnormally develop one set of muscles to the detriment of others, as in the case of lawn tennis'.[90] In fencing, claimed Margaret Bisland, there were 'what a physician would call strictly physical advantages to be gained such as no other exercise offers'. Good posture, strong muscles and finer contours were all advantages to be gained, as well as release from nervous irritability, while physical exhaustion was never brought on. 'Nervous prostration . . . may be vanquished at the blade's point . . . Nothing violent to further deplete the jaded system, but enough muscular exertion to stimulate and interest.'[91]

The medical profession thus endorsed the participation of leisured women in numerous recreational sports which offered the promise of increased health and reduced mental strain. Although few women could actually swim, swimming came to be extolled as an excellent sport, always provided that the exercise was not too violent and the bathing costume was modest. From the health and character points of view, cold bathing was regarded as a particularly good tonic for the circulation. Sea bathing came to be medically recommended to women with menstruation pains and as a means of increasing fertility.[92] With its educative effects of cultivating the willpower, its predicted possibilities of increasing fertility, the opportunity for developing muscular strength and endurance, and the added bonus of cleanliness, recreational swimming epitomized medically appropriate sportive exercise for the modern woman.

Yet the depth and breadth of medical anxiety, and pessimism and fears about the implications of women's increasing physical mobility and independence continued to be demonstrated in establishment medical discourse. With the advent of the automobile at the turn of the century, the bicycle lost its popularity, and a number of women cyclists became motor enthusiasts. Sure enough, before long, doctors began to worry about the 'quite formidable array of troubles, nervous and otherwise, which have been charged against motoring, and which point to the fact that the sport at best is a somewhat strenuous one for women'.[93] In addition to auto-eye, conjunctival inflammation, auto-leg, abortion inducement and pulmonary diseases, young women who motored extensively were thought to be in danger of a 'sequelae of nerve strain and exhaustion, such as hysteria and neurasthenia'.[94]

Although car manufacturers were learning to build cars designed to suit feminine abilities and limitations, noted the *Journal of the American Medical Association*, women were not seen to be as fit as men to meet the exigencies of motoring. Hence for women the 'exercise of motoring' was to be kept within reasonable limits, speeding eschewed and motoring confined to 'areas outside the crowded portion of the larger cities'. The latter point was advisable since 'women are in general more excitable and of less steady judgement than men, shortcomings which may prove disastrous in emergencies'.[95] Properly used, then, the car was seen as a valuable therapeutic agent.[96] Doctors, however, stood ready to define for women the appropriate limits of the activity:

> . . . All women absorbed in motoring should from time to time consult their physicians.[97]

Notes

1 T. S. Clouston, *The Hygiene of the Mind*, Methuen & Co., London, 1906, p. 208.
2 George Henry Napheys, M.D., *The Physical Life of Women; Advice to the Maiden, Wife and Mother*, G. Maclean, Philadelphia, 1870, p. 24.
3 Whitaker, 'The health of American girls', p. 241.
4 W.W. Bliss coined the term 'thirty-year pilgrimage,' in *Woman and Her Thirty-Year Pilgrimage*, William M. Littell, New York, 1869; It was further explicated in August Strindberg, 'De l'inferiorite de la femme', *La Revue Blanche*, January 1895, pp. 13–14.
5 George John Romanes, 'Mental differences between men and women', *The Nineteenth Century*, XXI, no. 123, May 1887, p. 657.
6 Henry Maudsley, 'Sex in mind', p. 466.
7 Strindberg, 'De l'infériorité de la femme'.
8 James Read Chadwick calculated in 1882 that the duration of fertility for English women was 31.35 years, and for Americans, 31.85 years. James Read Chadwick, 'The health of American women', *North American Review*, CCCXIII, December 1882, pp. 505–524.
9 Holbrook, *Parturition Without Pain*, p. 8.
10 M. A. Hardaker, 'Science and the woman question', *Popular Science Monthly*, XX, March 1882, p. 521.
11 Walker, *Beauty in Women*, p. 51.
12 Grant Allen, 'Plain words on the woman question', p. 170.
13 Andrew F. Currier, *The Menopause*, D. Appleton and Company, New York, 1897, p. 144.
14 Eliza M. Mosher, 'The health of American women', in Benjamin Austin, ed., *Woman: Her Character, Culture and Calling*, Book and Bible House, Brantford, 1898, pp. 235–345.
15 See, for example, Mary Jo Bain, *Here to Stay: American Families in the Twentieth Century*, Basic Books, New York, 1976, pp. 24–27; Robert V. Wells, 'Women's lives transformed: Demographic and family patterns in America, 1600–1970', Carol Ruth Berkin and Mary B. Norton, eds., *Women of America. A History*, Houghton Mifflin Co., Boston, 1979.
16 Bennett, 'Hygiene in the higher education of women', p. 520.
17 Wainwright, 'Exercise', p. 707.
18 Henry Ling Taylor, 'Exercise as a remedy', *Popular Science Monthly*, XLVIII, 1896, p. 635.
19 Eugene Richards, 'The influence of exercise upon health', *Popular Science Monthly*, XXIX, July 1886, p. 333.
20 Edwin Checkley, *A Natural Method of Physical Training: A Practical Description of the Checkley System of Physioculture*, W. C. Bryant, Brooklyn, NY, 1890, p. 36.
21 Elisabeth Robinson Scovil, *Preparation for Motherhood Manual*, Henry Altemus,

Philadelphia, 1889, p. 39.
22 Holbrook, *Parturition Without Pain*, pp. 29 and 32.
23 R. V. Pierce, *The People's Common Sense Medical Advisor*, new edition, World's Dispensary Medical Association, Buffalo, New York, 1908, p. 201.
24 Napheys, *The Physical Life of Women*, p. 168.
25 Charles M. Green, 'The care of women in pregnancy', *Boston Medical and Surgical Journal*, CXXVI, no. 8, February 25, 1892, p. 188.
26 Pierce, *Common Sense*, p. 200.
27 A. L. Galabin, M.D., *A Manual of Midwifery*, London, 1900, p. 138.
28 Dr Thomas Bull, English obstetrician, quoted in Holbrook, *Parturition without Pain*, p. 30.
29 Dr Verdi, *Maternity* quoted in Holbrook, *ibid*, p. 31.
30 Scovil, *Preparation for Motherhood*, p. 114.
31 Scovil, *Preparation for Motherhood*, p. 116; See also Pierce, *Common Sense*, p. 201.
32 Scovil, *Preparation for Motherhood*, p. 117.
33 Green, 'Women in pregnancy', pp. 188,8.
34 Taylor, *A Physician's Counsels to Women*, p. 29; Barnes, 'Lumleian lectures', p. 622.
35 George Engelmann, M.D., 'The American Girl of Today', *American Journal of Obstetrics* XLII, no. 8, December 1900, p. 769.
36 S. Pancoast, M.D., *Ladies Medical Guide to Mothers and Daughters of the United States of America*. Discussed in *The Lancet*, 2 November 1872. Originally published by Keystone Publishing Co., Philadelphia, 1859, p. 416. This argument, that vigorous exercise might strain ligaments of the uterus, has been invoked many times to restrain women in sport. Too many labours was probably the reason for the frequent prolapse of the womb in nineteenth-century women. F.B. Smith, *The People's Health, 1830–1910*, Croom Helm, London, 1979, pp. 26–27.
37 'A symposium of eminent doctors on how to be healthy at all ages', *Strand Magazine*, XXXI, February 1906, pp. 297–308.
38 'A symposium', p. 308.
39 Taylor, 'Exercise as a remedy', p. 626.
40 J. William White, 'A physician's view of exercise and athletics', *Lippincott's Magazine*, XXXIX, 1887, p. 1008.
41 Wendy Mitchinson, 'Causes of disease in women. The case of late 19th century English Canada', Charles G. Roland, ed., *Health, Disease and Medicine*, Hannah Institute for the History of Medicine, Toronto, 1984, pp. 381–395. See also Charles K. Mills, 'The treatment of nervous and mental disease by systematized active exercises', *The New York Medical Journal*, XLVII, 1888, pp. 129–137; Alexander Skene, *Medical Gynecology*, D. Appleton & Company, New York, 1895; Henry Garrigues, *A Textbook of the Diseases of Women*, W. B. Saunders, Philadelphia, 1894; Paul Munde, *A Practical Treatise on the Diseases of Women*, Philadelphia, 1891.
42 *Dominion Medical Monthly and Ontario Medical Journal*, VII, 1896, pp. 504 and 11; 1898; pp. 28 and 30. See Mitchinson, 'Causes of disease', p. 389.
43 E.B. Turner, 'A report on cycling in health and disease', *British Medical Journal*, (i) May 9, 1896, p. 1158.

44 William C. Hatch, 'Women and the bicycle', *Massachusetts Medical Journal*, XVII, 1897, p. 10.
45 James C. Whorton, 'The hygiene of the wheel: An episode in Victorian sanitary science', *Bulletin of the History of Medicine*, LII, no. 1, Spring 1978, p. 62.
46 *New York Times*, June 21, 1896, p. 4; Richard Harmond, 'Progress and flight: An interpretation of the American cycle craze of the 1890's', *Journal of Social History*, V, no. 2, 1971–72, pp. 235–257; *Scientific American*, LXXIV, January–June 1896, pp. 2, 4 and 185.
47 Whorton, 'Hygiene of the wheel', p. 307. The working-class desire to cycle was inevitably inhibited by cost, long working hours, lack of paid holidays and the disinclination for physical exertion of those who had laboured all day. See David Rubinstein, 'Cycling in the 1890's', *Victorian Studies*, XXI, no. 1, Autumn 1977, pp. 47–71.
48 H. Graves, G. L. Hillier and Susan, Countess of Malmesbury, *Cycling*, Lawrence and Bullen, London, 1898, p. 96.
49 The Rational Dress League was founded in 1898 to encourage dress reform for bicycling and promoted its view through the *Rational Dress Gazette*.
50 Florence Pomeroy, Viscountess Harberton, 'Rational dress for women', *Macmillan's Magazine*, 1882, quoted in Janet H. Murray, *Strong-Minded Women*, Pantheon Books, New York, 1982, p. 70.
51 Elizabeth Cady Stanton, *Minneapolis Tribune*, August 10, 1895; See also Robert A. Smith, *A Social History of the Bicycle*, American Heritage Press, New York, Chapter 5, 1972.
52 Elizabeth Cady Stanton quoted in Susan, Countess of Malmesbury, 'Bicycling for women', H. Peek and F. G. Aflulo, eds., *The Encyclopedia of Sport*, The Standard Edition A–EEL, Lawrence and Bullen Ltd., London, 1900, p. 290.
53 Robert A. Smith, *A Social History of the Bicycle. Its Early Life and Times in America*, American Heritage Press, New York, 1972, Ch. 5.
54 Frances Willard, *A Wheel Within a Wheel*, Boston, 1895, p. 11.
55 Louise Jeye, *Lady Cyclist*, August 1895, p. 224.
56 Hatch, 'Women and the bicycle', p. 10.
57 J. F. Prendergast, 'The bicycle for women', *American Journal of Obstetrics*, XXXIV, no. 2, August 1896, p. 245.
58 Prendergast, 'The bicycle for women', pp. 245, 252.
59 W. H. Fenton, 'A medical view of cycling for ladies', *Nineteenth Century*, XXXIX, 1896, p. 797.
60 Whorton, 'Hygiene of the wheel', p. 308; Editorial, 'The bicycle and phthisis', *Medical News*, LXXI, 1897, p. 535.
61 Luther Halsey Gulick, 'The bicycle as a therapeutic agent', *Boston Medical and Surgical Journal*, CL, no. 2, January 14, 1904, pp. 40–43; Henry J. Garrigues, 'Women and the bicycle', *The Forum*, XX, 1896; J. James, 'The beneficial effects of cycling as an orthopaedic agent', *British Medical Journal*, (ii), 1896, p. 947; See also Pierce, *Common Sense*, p. 275.
62 Prendergast, 'The bicycle for women', p. 253.
63 Garrigues, 'Women and the bicycle', p. 579.
64 Robert L. Dickinson, 'Bicycling for women from the standpoint of the gynecologist', *American Journal of Obstetrics*, 1895, p. 25.

65 *New York Herald*, June 27, 1897; 'The sanitary aspect of cycling for ladies', *British Medical Journal*, (i), 1896, p. 681.

66 A. L. Benedict, 'Dangers and benefits of the bicycle', *Century Magazine*, July 1897, pp. 471–473.

67 I.N. Love, M.D., 'From a doctor's sentimental standpoint', *Journal of the American Medical Association*, 1899, p. 1026.

68 Whorton, 'Hygiene of the wheel', p. 69.

69 Whorton, 'Athlete's heart', p. 30.

70 *Minneapolis Tribune*, July 20, 1895.

71 'Precepts for cyclists', *The Lancet*, October 5, 1895, pp. 857–858.

72 Gordon Stables, M.D., 'Health', *Girls Own Paper*, August 1901, p. 4.

73 Fenton, 'Medical view', p. 799; Thomas R. Evans, 'Harmful effects of the bicycle upon the girls' pelvis', *American Journal of Obstetrics*, XXXIII, 1896, p. 554.

74 Dr Longaker quoted in Prendergast, 'The bicycle for women', p. 263; James Chadwick, 'Bicycle saddles for women', *Boston Medical and Surgical Journal*, CXXXII, 1895, pp. 595–596.

75 Harvey Green Smith, *Fit For America: Health, Fitness, Sport and American Society*, Pantheon Books, New York, 1986, p. 232.

76 Dickinson, 'Bicycling for women', pp. 33–34; Prendergast, 'The bicycle for women', p. 250; Bernard Talmey, M.D., *Woman*, Stanley Press, New York, 1906, p. 158; See discussion in Haller and Haller, *The Physician and Sexuality*, pp. 175–187; Graeme M. Hammond, 'The influence of the bicycle in health and disease', *Medical Record*, 1895, pp. 131–132.

77 E. B. Turner, MD, 'A report on cycling in health and disease', *British Medical Journal* (i), May 9, 1896, p. 1399; Turner, 'Report on cycling', *British Medical Journal* (iii), June 27, 1896, p. 1564.

78 Love, 'From a doctor's sentimental standpoint', 1899, pp. 1026–1027.

79 Francis Smith Nash, M.D., 'A plea for the new woman and the bicycle', *American Journal of Obstetrics*, XXXIII, 1896a, pp. 556–560.

80 Turner, 'Report on cycling', May 30, 1896, p. 1337.

81 Martha Banta, *Imaging American Women: Ideas and Ideals in Cultural History*, Columbia University Press, New York, 1987, p. 88.

82 L.G. Peabody, 'The canoe and the woman ', *Outing*, XXXVIII, April–Sept. 1901, p. 534.

83 Edwyn Sandys, 'The place that woman occupies in sport', *The Illustrated Sporting News* II, 21 November 1903, p. 11.

84 'Golf', *Girls' Own Paper*, June 1890.

85 Louie Mackern and M. Boys (ed), *Our Lady of the Green*, Lawrence and Bullen, London, 1899, p. 68.

86 John S. White, 'The New Athletics', Proceedings of the American Association for the Advancement of Physical Education, III, 1889, pp. 46–52.

87 Maud Marshall, 'Lawn Tennis', in Frances E. Slaughter, (ed.), *The Sportswoman's Library*, II, Archibald Constable, London, 1898, pp. 315–317.

88 Henry Slocum Jr., 'Lawn tennis as a game for women', *Outing*, XIV, April–Sept. 1889, p. 289.

89 Lizzie A. Tompkins, 'Habit and saddle for ladies', *Outing*, XIV, April–Sept. 1889, p. 104.

90 Charles E. Clay, 'Mask and foil for ladies', *Outing*, XIII, Oct. 1888, p. 313.
91 Margaret Bisland, 'Fencing for women', *Outing*, XV, Oct. 1889–March 1890, p. 346.
92 'Effects of Seabathing', *The Practitioner*, VIII, December 1895, p. 205; 'Hints on swimming for women', *Outing*, XII, April–Sept. 1888, pp. 431–2.
93 'Women motorists', *Public Health Journal*, IV, Toronto, April 1913, p. 248. (reprinted from the *Journal of the American Medical Association*).
94 'Women motorists', p. 249; J.C. Edgar, 'The influence of the automobile on obstetric and gynecologic conditions', *American Journal of Obstetrics*, June 1911, p. 1084.
95 'Women motorists', p. 248.
96 G.B. Delavan, 'The influence of the use of the automobile on the upper air passages, *Medical Record*, Aug. 20, 1910, quoted in 'Women Motorists', p. 249.
97 'Women motorists', p. 249.

3

Menopause, old age and exercise

Menopause is a period forming an isthmus between growth and decay, a lull between flowing and ebbing tides, a milestone to mark the end of a definite period of existence.[1]

The importance placed by Victorian doctors upon honing the female reproductive process and preserving the health and strength of women for maternity was bound to affect their attitude towards menopause and old age. Conceptions of the ageing female body in the latter part of the nineteenth century were profoundly influenced by the machine paradigm and the idea that an old and less efficient apparatus was of little use to society.[2] 'A time comes at length,' explained Dr Humphry 'when, in the course of the descending developmental process, the several components of the machine slowly, and much, though equally weakened, fail to answer one another's call.'[3]

It followed that representations of the menopause often equated that period of transition from fertility to infertility as the passage to becoming an 'unperson'. Since menopause marked the end of fertility, attitudes towards it reflected the social status of women, and the value attached to their reproductive capacity.[4] For a woman, the physical stigma of ageing were often seen not only as the harbinger of infertility but also the end of social usefulness. Partly because of such attitudes, notes Stearns, female old age still remains as unheeded in historical literature as it may be in life.[5] Furthermore, it is ironic, says Posner, that ageing women who have been most oppressed can find the least support in the burgeoning feminist social sciences. Until very recently, although many social historians have focused upon the experiences of ageing white men, ageing women have been neglected by establishment scholars and feminists alike. Roebuck, for example, claims that 'the invisible woman in history has been the little old lady'.[6]

Studies examining the role of medical theory and practice in shaping and limiting the options and roles available to late nineteenth-century women, have tended to focus upon popular medical advice designed to improve the functional childbearing and childrearing capacities of young women and mothers. Much less is known about those women 'beyond reach of sexual storms',[7] women whose thirty-year pilgrimage of potential childbearing was over and whose physical and intellectual, as well as social purpose tended to be dismissed as insignificant by medical texts and advice books. A major reason for this was probably that many women did not live to an old age, or indeed much beyond their childbearing years. For those who did, however, medical advice about appropriate physical behaviour, including exercise, embodied fixed ideas about the ageing body and its decreasing physical usefulness to society as women grew older. Indeed, if the primary meaning of a woman's life was achieved through maternity, then once her childbearing capacity was lost a woman's world was characterized by a loss of meaning. Menopause meant an end to womanhood, an end to productive life and to a primary sexual identity that was inextricably linked with motherhood. In many ways culture rather than biology was the decisive influence on the Victorian view of the menopause, and on the ways in which women adjusted to both the change of life and to medical views of appropriate behaviour for ageing women.[8] Men were perceived to be old when they could no longer perform their work (and the age at which men were thought to make their major contributions to society fell towards the end of the nineteenth century). Women were regarded as old when their work of childbearing and rearing was done.[9]

In the late nineteenth century only about 15 per cent of women lived beyond their fertile years. Many physicians claimed that after forty years of age the prime of life declined rapidly into old age.[10] Although the evidence is inexact, life expectancy for middle-class white American women at the end of the nineteenth century has been calculated at 51·08 years. (Men could expect to live for 48·23 years). Only four of every 100 Americans reached sixty-five.[11] In England female life expectancy was similar although the class distribution of longevity is difficult to estimate.[12] Data on expectation of life at birth for women in England between 1839 and 1900, for example, show a gain of six years to 47·77 years.[13] Shorter explains that despite a slight female advantage in life expectancy, girls between five and twenty had a significantly higher mortality rate than boys (often due to tuberculosis) and married women in their thirties stood perhaps a twenty-five per cent greater risk of dying than their husbands (probably as a result of childbirth-related difficulties).[14] Death from puerperal fever after childbirth increased steadily in the latter part of the nineteenth century, accounting for half the total maternal mortality. The general morbidity/mortality patterns, therefore, illustrate higher mortality rates for women at younger ages, though female survivors have a slightly longer life-span than men.[15] Although female longevity data shows that since at least the middle of the nineteenth century, women were doing better than men in many aspects of being old, the belief persisted that women aged and became useless sooner than men.[16] Declines in fertility as well as mortality rates during the nineteenth century meant that maternal retirement began to occur at an earlier age. The impact of this event was deepened by its tendency to coincide with the physiological changes of menopause.

Women who survived beyond forty often believed that 'menopause marked the beginning of a period of depression, of heightened disease incidence and of early death'.[17] For many late nineteenth-century women the onset of menopause between forty and forty-five years of age was the gateway to old age and, in all probability an event which took place shortly before death.[18] Dr R.V. Pierce agreed that in temperate climates menses generally ceased at the forty-fifth year.[19] In line with the belief that disorders of the reproductive system were the source of almost every female disease, physical and mental, some establishment physicians blamed most diseases associated with ageing upon the menopause. Physical decline, bodily and mental disorders and diminished functions were often emphasized as the general characteristics of menopausal development. There were few expectations for women whose vitality was viewed as having already largely ebbed away through repeated menses, pregnancies and childbirths.[20] Referring to the manifestations of the shock from losing menstruation, a leading gynecologist explained that the system was so thoroughly accustomed to this drain that once it stopped, especially if suddenly, 'we would naturally suppose "that event" to be followed by untoward consequences. This we find in reality to be the case.'[21]

Above all, then, the arrival of menopause was equated with crisis and loss, even though medical authorities could not help but observe that women often lived through it, lived longer than men and generally survived in better health than their elderly male counterparts. Especially in the female sex, noted Dr Clouston, better health can be enjoyed at this nondescript period of life.[22] 'After the change has been completed we generally find her system improved. . . She becomes more capable of rendering herself useful . . . [and] . . . passes on to old age better than men.'[23] The superiority of female longevity was well known, explained Dr Humphry obliquely, 'as a result of the smaller machinery of her frame'.[24] He was referring to a dubious hypothesis of Dr Walker that the shorter stature of women meant a smaller demand upon the vital system, even after giving birth several times.[25]

Menopause itself was often referred to as a catastrophic experience in medical discourse on both sides of the Atlantic. The eminent British authority Dr Tilt viewed menopause, like menstruation, as a potentially pathological condition through which a woman passed at peril of her life and from which emanated the threat of numerous diseases such as severe depression, hysteria, melancholy, dyspepsia, diarrhoea, vaginitis, prolapsed uterus, rheumatic pains, paralysis, apoplexy, uterine haemorrhaging, tumours, breast and uterine cancer, tuberculosis, scrofula and diabetes. Listing 120 infirmities subdivided into seven distinct modes of suffering related to the menopause, he went on to claim that the management of these menopausal problems taxed the ingenuity of the medical confidant. 'If he be not prepared to be at once a divine, a moralist, and a philosopher, without ceasing to be a physician, his medicines will, in some cases, be of little use.'[26] To his nineteenth-century pioneering studies were added those of Barnes, who noted that:

> the climacteric perturbation is often even more severe and more marked than what is observed at any previous period of life. . . . It is a stage of transition and of trial for all. . . . Many women may have passed through the trials of puberty and of child bearing without serious nervous disorder and will break down at menopause.[27]

In 1893 Dr Galabin attributed the nervous disorders accompanying menopause to the outward expenditure of energy, haemorrhaging and hot flashes being two frequent examples. The result was hysteria, headaches, irritability or depression, pelvic disorder, indigestion and sometimes a resort to alcohol. The tendency to corpulence and fat deposits, he believed, led to a neglect of outdoor exercise and an exacerbation of digestive disturbances.[28] Other physicians blamed menopausal disorders for driving women to violence or suicidal tendencies, drugs and strong drink, or perhaps an increased sexual intensity.[29] At the change, remarked Tilt, an unhinged nervous system could cause ladies to desert husband and children, or even to have their children removed for fear of murdering them.[30]

All intelligent physicians, claimed Dr Napheys, knew that the change of life was particularly dangerous to women. 'There is in very many cases a most unpleasant train of symptoms which characterize this epoch in the physical life of woman. They are alarming, painful, often entailing sad consequences. . .' One must remember, he continued, that every month for some thirty years of her life the woman of forty-five has been moderately bled, and for that reason 'we need not wonder that suddenly to break off this long habit would bring about plethora, which would in turn be the source of manifold inconveniences to the whole system'.[31] Dr Pierce believed that once the flow of blood was diverted from the uterus, it could be directed to the head and cause 'morbid tendencies'.[32] The death of the reproductive faculty, wrote one physician, 'is accompanied by struggles which implicate every organ and every function of the body'.[33]

The widely read Dr Currier was not quite so pessimistic. Overviewing the relevant nineteenth-century literature in his own widely disseminated treatise, *The Menopause*, he was less inclined than Dr Tilt to accept unconditionally the view of menopause as a dangerous and critical time. Less than 1 per cent of menopausal women who died in the United States between 1870 and 1880, he noted, had died from cancer of the genital organs, so the menopause was hardly to be feared on that account. Physicians may have been unduly influenced, he speculated, by unscientific, ancient observations about the serious consequences of menopause. Hippocrates, for example, had recorded that

> exculcerations, violent and even scirrhous tumours of the uterus are sometimes produced by cessation of the menses. Neither do the external parts of the body escape the fatal consequences of such suppression, since . . . they are frequently affected with the itch, the elephantiasis, boils, erysipelatous disorders.[34]

On the other hand, Currier noted, menopause excited most attention and disturbance among highly bred, tenderly raised women of civilized life and it was not infrequently associated with a more general breaking up of the vital forces of the individual.[35] Not surprisingly, menopausal disorders were believed more serious among women who had violated physiological laws and adopted unfeminine activities in their earlier years. If women had not taken care of themselves during their youth, they would pay the price in their menopausal years.[36] As Tilt put it, 'if the seeds of destruction have been slumbering for years within her, the change of life will give them increased activity'.[37] Indiscretions in earlier life, some doctors noted, included efforts at birth control, abortion, too much education or a heightened sexuality.[38] Currier considered that 'irregular and unwomanly occupations' and excessive sexual activity could cause early menopause. Excessive indulgence was followed sometimes by disastrous results.[39] The woman who transgressed nature's laws, said Kellogg, would find menopause 'a veritable Pandora's box of ills and may well look forward to it with apprehension and foreboding'. Furthermore, 'it is the nervous and hysterical woman who has a hard time at menopause (or at any rate she thinks she has) and this is often due to faulty education, to want of restriction during childhood and young womanhood'.[40] Many doctors assumed that once a woman reached menopause her sexual drive and physical attractiveness would cease. Indeed, some warned that menopausal sexuality should be regarded as a sure indicator of disease.[41] Marriage at this time was certainly to be avoided, said Dr Tilt. 'It is most imprudent for women to marry at this epoch without having obtained the sanction of a medical man.'[42]

With the climacteric, said the doctors, came defeminization, a loss of womanly function and declining feminine grace. Post-menopausal women were seen as both increasingly masculinized (drooping breasts, sunken bones, fleshy skin, facial hair) and regressing to childish ways. Dr Hicks called it the beginning of a neutral man-woman state.[43] Dr Skene thought that after menopause there was an apparent female mental tendency to become more like the male.[44] The anatomical differences of male and female, wrote Delauney in the *Popular Science Monthly*,

> bring on intellectual and moral differences that explain why, in higher societies, the two sexes, after sharing each other's sports in infancy, become separated during the age of maturity, and become again more alike in old age. Skeletons are feminine till men differentiate at puberty, [but] . . . at about forty-five years the distinctions begin to attenuate, and the sexes end by resembling each other in advanced age, when the characteristics are rather masculine.[45]

Ideas about older women being either childish or masculine underscored late nineteenth-century notions that the centrality of female reproductive capability was almost overwhelming, and that it was based (as has been mentioned earlier) upon far more than simple biological theory.[46] Once the female lost her capacity to reproduce she was perceived to be at the mercy of the pathological nature of menopause. Her body had run its course and begun its final decline.[47] When a woman's usefulness was seen to be ended, she was described as 'less of the woman she was than a man is a man at the same time of life'.[48] Sometimes described in the medical literature as a terminal illness, menopause became viewed as the 'death of the woman in the woman'.[49]

Toward senescence

The climacteric marked the division between maturity and senescence, and demanded that the female slowly adjust to her new stage of life and manner of living. Medical literature sometimes gave the impression that the years after menopause could be seen as a deathwatch made endurable by solace in religion, routine and attention to the soul: 'old women merely existed, their long senescence a tragedy redeemed only by quiet and undemanding piety'.[50] Even household duties were considered of diminishing importance as an old woman's physical degeneration led to diminishing competence.

> The body itself does not long delay entering into decrepitude, and soon we see the woman once so favoured by nature when she was charged with the duty of reproducing the species degraded to the level of a being who has no further duty to perform in the world.[51]

A favoured status was accorded those who had contributed socially by bearing children. Her family and society it was supposed would recompense her for the loss of her physical charms by surrounding her with respect and care in remuneration for services which she had rendered to them in the past. 'With the sweet consciousness of duty performed, she can now surround herself with a saintly halo of kind words. . . and pass onwards to the silence of eternal rest.'[52]

Thus, for the very dutiful woman, old age was sometimes seen as a golden age of senescence. If she had followed a sound life-style and not become chronically ill, the years after menopause could offer health and relaxation, a release from the periodic inconvenience of menstruation and a period of repose from the taxes and cares laid upon her by maternity. 'The post-menopausal period could thus become the Indian summer of a woman's life, a sabbath interlude of harmony and peace, to be followed by heaven.'[53] 'Thankful they have escaped the perils of childbearing and the tedious annoyances of a monthly restraint,' said Tilt, 'such women can enter a time of autumnal majesty and enjoy a vast improvement of health'.[54] Where premature infirmities, an unfavourable profession, or poor life-style habits had not hastened old age, women could preserve many of their earlier charms during this third age. Beauty, however, was no more said Walker, for 'form and shape have disappeared. . . sinkings and wrinkles are multiplied. . . the organs become rigid; and in some unhappy cases a beard protrudes'.[55]

Less homage was paid unmarried or childless older women, and less hope held out for their healthy old age. From a physiological standpoint, explained Currier, a sterile woman is a failure.[56] 'Persons who do not undertake the special functions of the sex are of secondary importance', said Cope, who thought them more likely to have led an aimless life.[57] According to Clouston, the repression of family life, motherhood and physiological altruism would always be a strain on the unmarried woman.[58] The non-reproductive woman not only threatened society and herself, she would also be prone to neurosis, ovarian insanity or old maid's mania.[59] The climacteric was a time when insanity was liable to develop in maiden ladies and extend into senescence, said Dr Hersman. 'Nature, just before the change of life, takes revenge for too severe repression of all manifestations of sex – this may take a turn similar to nymphomania.' Thus, he continued, 'we have the beginning and end of a very sad picture'.[60]

This was a particularly harsh indictment of the many spinsters who, for various reasons, had not borne children. Old age often brought severe economic and other difficulties to middle-class spinsters. Contemporary observers suggested that many governesses ended their days in lunatic asylums.[61] One in three spinsters over sixty in Victorian Britain needed poor relief and were forced into institutions. 'Spinsters in old age,' explains Anderson, 'were the residuum who failed to marry in a society in which the assumption was that all women should expect to marry.'[62] These attitudes were changing by the turn of the century as a number of new spinsters who were meaningfully employed or financially independent began reversing the traditional scorn for 'old maids', demonstrating that a single life-style could be a respectable option.[63] Such spinsters, rejecting marriage and motherhood, were seen by traditionalists as a threat to men, the family and the race. When, in old age, a number of them came to express regret for having rejected motherhood and to rue the barrenness of the career woman's triumph, male professionals were ready to compound that regret. G. Stanley Hall repeated popular medical observations by labelling those women who had chosen education or training instead of motherhood as 'functionally castrated' graduates and 'parturition phobiacs'.[64] The single woman, particularly if a member of a profession, was often branded in medical texts as a mannish maiden, an hermaphrodite no longer strictly female in sex.[65]

Medical theories for the ageing female

The menopause has characteristics which make the experience peculiarly vulnerable to the intervention of myth-makers . . . Whoever labels a woman's symptoms returns to her not her subjective experience but their own myth. . . . [Thus] the process of diagnosis is speech stolen and restored; through the myth restored to her, the woman's experience of her menopause is decided and controlled by the diagnostician.[66]

For late nineteenth-century American and English establishment physicians, perceived disorders of menopausal women, whether childless or not, and changing ways of viewing old age rendered the ageing woman a most appropriate candidate for medical attention. Constant monitoring and systematic treatment were increasingly seen to be required for the general sufferings of menopausal and ageing women and it was increasingly seen to be the duty of physicians to give considerable attention to such problems.[67] 'We must pay more attention to women at the time of the change and beyond,' said Dr. Humphrey after surveying the habits of old people in England, 'for we have been too much accustomed in the past to limit the work of development to the periods of adolescence and maturity.'[68]

Increased attention to medical management of the elderly was due partly to extensive medical discussion about the negative aspects of male senescence stimulated in an 1842 translation of Quetelet's French treatise on developmental stages. His work and that of pathologists in the Paris School of Medicine revealed specific diseases of old age, and suggested that senescence must be viewed as more than just a last gasp of energy before the vital force was finally spent. If disease was a discrete and inevitable condition of being old, then the entire stage of senescence became a perilous state of existence requiring close study and constant medical care. The old must therefore be treated differently from the young for they were now viewed as less likely to be productive, creative or agile as they aged.[69] Advanced old age, which had earlier been regarded as a manifestation of survival of the fittest was now denigrated as a condition of dependency and deterioration, and it was no longer seen to be natural for older people to participate in physically demanding activities. In terms of caring for the elderly, the physician was expected to assume the role of expert and the minutest detail of the senescent's routine became subject to medical approval.[70]

American and English physicians generally agreed with the French experts that the climacteric and senescence required considerable medical attention (and possibly a distinctive set of senile therapeutics), but they simultaneously retained a strong belief in old age as a depletion of vital energy about which very little could be done if it had already been spent. The notion that one could prolong life by conserving the 'vital principle' of the body had been popularized by, among others, Luigi Cornaro, an Italian Renaissance nobleman. By leading a temperate life, Cornaro wrote in his *Discourses*, the supply of life force could last for more than the time allotted by God (3 score and ten) to that allowed by Nature – 100 to 120 years. Cornaro's ideas were so popular that one English translation went through fifty editions during the eighteenth and nineteenth centuries.[71] The Cornaro theme flourished in the nineteenth century in D.H. Jacques, *'Physical Perfection': or, The Philosophy of Human Beauty; Showing How to Acquire and Retain Bodily Symmetry, Health and Vigour, Secure Long Life, and Avoid the Infirmities and Deformities of Age*, which included a chapter on longevity. 'The energy of life,' said Jacques, 'is in inverse ratio to its duration' and this notion tended to inform the late nineteenth-century physicians' daily interactions with the senescent.[72]

If some doctors questioned why athletes often lived longer than the very inactive despite having 'spent' so much energy or why the very young demonstrated less energy than those in early adulthood, such inconsistencies caused few establishment physicians to abandon the vital energy theory.[73] They continued to believe that weakness in old age resulted from the life energy having already been spent. 'Every living being has, from its birth, a limit of growth and development in all directions beyond which it cannot possibly go by any amount of forcing.'[74] Drained of energy, the senses dimmed, motor skills weakened, debilitation and disease inevitably followed. Thus the more wisely people spent their final portion of energy, the more likely they were to maintain a healthy balance between their body and the environment. It was the duty then, wrote Dr Van Oven:

> of all persons who have attained the climacteric age, carefully to avoid excesses and undue exertions, to watch at all times for the insidious approach of disorders; never to reject any slight ailment, but regard them as forerunners of more serious derangement, seek to repair the most trifling irregularities of function and give rest at once to any organ of the body which shows debility or fatigue.[75]

It was especially the duty of physicians to watch constantly over the regulation of these habits otherwise the last years became mere shadows of earlier productive years, often accompanied by body-wasting illness.

Establishment physicians used this reasoning in advising ageing females regardless of their current health, since having entered senescence their normal physiological condition had now become pathological. Although old women might be in perfect health, old age alone signified disability. Activities that had once been easily performed were now viewed as the potential cause of serious infirmities. Ageing women were perceived unquestionably to be invalids in need of constant care, lacking the necessary vital energy to participate in daily activities. Where life-style habits were discussed, physical activity, food, and occupation were all considered valid professional questions. Diet and exercise were particularly prominent among the medical therapies offered, in addition to widely used drugs such as mercury and opium. A correct regimen rendered the body less susceptible to senile illness, since overexertion could easily lead to cardiac arrest and a host of other life-threatening conditions. Ultimately, however, it was agreed that these could not be diverted. It was futile to attempt rejuvenation and return the anatomy and physiology of the elderly to its preclimacteric state.

Exercise prescriptions for the menopause and senescence

. . . along with fresh air, a certain amount of exercise, but not too much is needed.[76]

Advice about exercise for menopausal and ageing women more closely reflected the vital energy theory than the disease theories of the new clinicians, and hence followed similar lines of reasoning used by physicians for more youthful females. Menopause was invariably linked to menarche in nineteenth-century medical thought, the two events representing the stressful beginning and end of women's sexual activity. Precautions and rules laid down at menarche were considered equally profitable for women at the trying and delicate time of menopause. Indeed, commented Thorburn, the menopausal woman should be guarded like the young adolescent girl during puberty lest all manner of disease and discomfort strike.[77] Cautious exercise was recommended, along with avoiding excitement, severe mental or bodily effort and exhaustion. Menopausal women were advised against overtaxing their strength by continuous exertion at this stage of their life. 'Let every woman, and especially every mother, not squander the strength intended for personal preservation.'[78]

Rest was essential, with some hours of each day to be spent lying down, since medical authorities believed that the enormous energy expenditures during adolescence and the childbearing years were bound to have encroached upon the ageing woman's account and tired her considerably.[79] Her blood, for example, which was believed to be thinner than a man's to begin with, had been weakened consistently with each birth and at every menstrual period.[80]

Yet some exercise was useful at the change of life, insisted Dr Tilt. Gentle, regular and long-continued exercise in the cool of the day was considered beneficial. It relieved congestion of the internal organs, and caused the skin to perspire and the kidneys to excrete more urea. It reduced 'that redundant energy which, when unemployed, produces the fidgets, nervousness, and temper'. Long or quick walks were objectionable, however, 'for they aggravated uterine congestion, piles and varicose veins'. Driving was better, but horse-riding was debarred 'until after complete cessation of the menses, since it exacerbated bleeding'. The utility 'of exercise in favouring the menstrual flow sufficiently warrants the discontinuity of the practice while the change is in process, for then it is likely to cause flooding, piles and leucorrhea'.[81]

Indeed, at the age of forty to fifty and beyond, the need for appropriate exercise was seen to be the greatest.

> At that time, the circulation becomes defective, unless continually quickened by exercise; there is a tendency to passive congestion and functional derangements of various organs. . . The products of disintegrated food and tissue are not eliminated. Accumulating in the blood, they form the materies morbid, the matter on which death feeds.[82]

The combination of rest and gentle exercise for menopausal women would redirect the blood supply and activate the natural body tendencies to restore and prolong health and equilibrium.[83] Violent exercise, however, was sternly warned against. Severe muscular exertion could never compensate for the past expenditure of nervous energy.[84] If the elderly were to be allowed any outdoor sport it should include only slow, steady movements.[85] Exhausting walks were to be avoided as well.[86] Dr Madison Taylor recommended free, open-air exercise regulated with care and supervised with the same conscientiousness as other medical measures. He advised cautious, systematized and supervised physical training for the purposes of increasing elasticity in the tissues by active and passive stretchings and drill.[87] Dr Wainwright similarly felt that salvation for elderly women who had 'put on more flesh than is good for the health' lay in gentle bouts of muscular exercise. For such women, he quoted Wolfe regarding the appropriate regulation of exercise:

1. Exercise should be taken out of doors.
2. Exercise should not be dependent on the weather.
3. Exercise should not be taken after a meal or after long fasting.
4. One should not exercise to the point of weariness.
5. For those who are debilitated, they should not exercise but be passively exercised.[88]

However, most authorities agreed that such physical activity should take place quietly and within the family. Any attempt to re-enact energetic youth was to be discouraged because family needs should absorb all the energies of ageing women. Released from the responsibilities of childbearing, older women could continue to sacrifice themselves by assisting in the domestic affairs of their own or their children's homes.[89] Indeed, medical literature tended to assume that there would quite naturally be a metamorphosis transforming mothers into grandmothers, or 'second mothers'. Florence Nightingale's portrait in *Cassandra* of a dying woman's words illustrates how this sacrificial life was perceived by some to be not worth clinging to:

> Oh, if you knew how gladly I leave this life, how much more courage I feel to take the chance of another, than of anything I see before me in this, you would put on your wedding clothes instead of mourning for me.[90]

The male medical model of the female body

Mendeloff has argued that in developing health policy there is an argument that different periods of the life-span are valued differently. Elderly years are valued least. Infancy seems to get low ranking because parents' ties are just developing. The periods between all have some claim for special concern – indeed the prime years do seem to count for more. Once one's life-work has been accomplished, death is considered less objectionable.[91]

Late nineteenth-century male physicians would have concurred. Where women were concerned they believed that the prime years were of overwhelming importance for the future of a society seen by many to be disordered and declining. Women's prime years were their reproductive ones, especially the ten or twelve years following the establishment of menarche. The female constitution was sufficiently matured at twenty-one for marriage and childbearing.[92] Frances Willard surveyed eight of the most distinguished physicians in America and concluded that the best age for marriage was between eighteen and twenty-six.[93] A woman at twenty-five was at her best – physicians saw this as the most vigorous, active and useful part of her life. If a woman was not formed and healthy at twenty-five, she would never be so, said Clouston.[94] Preferably, a healthy woman at twenty-five was pregnant for the second or third time and could be expected to give birth to her last child around thirty-three years of age.[95] Aware of the loss of many mothers and children to disease and death, physicians recommended that women space their pregnancies carefully to maintain strength.[96] Dedicated to increasing the birth rate, the doctors agreed theoretically nevertheless that if more women collectively would marry and bear children, then individually they need not have so many so often.[97] At the same time, many establishment physicians worked to make abortion illegal and restrict women's access to information about birth control. Their desire to cope with the pattern of a declining birthrate among native-born white women and an increasing birthrate among working-class immigrant women, to protect their profession against the inroads of a new competitive element – educated women and to perpetuate a society increasingly threatened with massive social and economic change compelled the doctors to support scientific half facts and mythologies about healthy motherhood.

The medical model of the female body that male physicians developed for each stage of the life-span was allegedly decreed by nature, which granted health and an ordered society so long as women pursued their naturally ordained feminine role. Mind and body were inescapably opposed. The female body, needed to fulfil the feminine role, required scarce energy thus a woman could not be allowed to subscribe to much intellectual development. If women used their minds too much, overexerted their bodies or behaved in unfeminine ways then disease would surely follow. Reproduction would be threatened by any tampering with the delicate physiological balance of the female body and constitutional weakness passed on to the next generation.

Such explanations underlay the scientific discourse of many establishment medical men. Physical ill health mirrored social ill health, hence the aetiology of disease could be located in both social and physical disorders. Physical disorders emanated from disorders of the reproductive system, particularly at menarche and menopause. Social disorder resulted from non-compliance with the prescribed feminine role. Disease was the result of either or both, and prescriptions to alleviate it also related to both. Moderate exercise was prescribed to restore body-mind balance and to promote and maintain the right kind of healthy life-style. Competitive sport or over vigorous exercise created a physiological imbalance and was inappropriate socially except during childhood when growth and development did not compete with the reproductive system. In old age exercise was therapeutic rather than restorative. Having lost her reproductive capacity, the post-menopausal woman was physically useless to society and her social role lay in assisting her children and grandchildren within the home.

An understanding of the disease model which informed medical prescriptions for exercise explains, in part, why physicians considered women's reproductive structures and habits more important than the widespread and devastating diseases that took such a toll upon the population before the turn of the twentieth century. Some physicians with a special interest in public health pointed out that undue attention was paid to the reproductive system as a source of female disease. Dr Stephen Smith described his belief that many doctors used uterine disease as a lazy diagnosis for any and all of their patients' complaints.[98]

In most cases, however, physicians simply did not know or understand how to protect women from the ravages of disease and consequently 'pandered to worries about health rather than offering realistic remedies'.[99] Not until 1912, suggest Ehrenreich and English, did the average patient seeking help from the average doctor have more than a fifty-fifty chance of benefiting from the encounter.[100] However, by blaming women for their own ill health doctors could not be held responsible for either their own serious lack of medical knowledge about women's bodily functions or for their many ineffective practices. In stubbornly defending the veracity of their physiological model of disease many doctors were reluctant to accept new scientific findings about disease aetiology and retained strong professional conservatism. Morantz-Sanchez reminds us that the pronouncements about female nature by male physicians reveal less about those male physicians and their hostilities than about the cultural component of scientific assumptions and the social power exerted by those who are recognized interpreters of scientific theory. Evaluations of female health and exercise needs were informed less by empirical evidence than 'by cultural assumptions that had a particular non-medical use in ordering social and power relationships'.[101]

Yet middle-class women, young and old, relied increasingly upon physicians for advice and attempted to comply with life-style pre-scriptions despite the fact that female morbidity and mortality rates remained high. One's behaviour before the threats and realities of illness is necessarily rooted in the perception one has constructed of oneself and one's universe.[102] Many late nineteenth-century middle-class women accepted the analyses and prescriptions of the male medical establishment because they too believed that they were 'of no use without health'.[103] Foucault would explain that when a group (such as the American or British Medical Association in the late nineteenth century) establishes its political and economic hegemony, it is able to invest its words with power and thus impose order upon the unruly body. Exercise prescriptions were one attempt to impose order upon the female for the larger good.

Notes

1 Currier, *The Menopause*, p. 3.
2 As *Harper's Bazaar* put it in 1907, the women of the late nineteenth century had 'bloomed like flowers, fruited too generously and faded like an autumn garden'. *Harpers Bazaar*, 1907, pp. 810–811.
3 George Murray Humphry, MD, *Old Age: The Results of Information Received Respecting Nearly Nine Hundred Persons Who Had Attained the Age of Eighty Years Including Seventy-Four Centenarians*, Macmillan and Bowes, Cambridge, 1889, p. 5.
4 Patricia A. Kaufert, 'Myth and the menopause', *Sociology of Health and Illness*, IV, no. 2, July 1982, p. 145.
5 Peter N. Stearns, 'Old women: Some historical observations', *Journal of Family History*, V, no. 1, Spring 1980, pp. 44–57.
6 Judith Posner, 'It's all in your head: Feminist and medical models of menopause. (Strange bedfellows)', *Sex Roles*, V, no. 2, 1979, pp. 179–190; see also Kaufert, 'Myth and the menopause'; Marjorie C. Feinson, 'Where are the women in the history of aging?', *Social Science History*, IX, no. 4, Fall 1985, pp. 429–452; J. Roebuck, 'The invisible woman is a little old lady: The need for change in assumptions and paradigms', paper presented at the 37th Annual Meeting of the Gerontological Society of America, San Antonio, Texas, 1984.
7 Engelmann, 'The American girl of to-day', p. 10.
8 Jalland and Hooper, *Women from Birth to Death*, p. 282.
9 J. A. and Olive Banks, *Feminism and Family Planning in Victorian England*, Schocken Press, New York, 1964; See also Howard P. Chudacoff and Tamara K. Hareven, 'From the empty nest to family dissolution: Life course transition into old age', *Journal of Family History*, IV, no. 1, 1979, pp. 69–83.
10 J. W. Bell, M.D., 'A plea for the aged', *Journal of the American Medical Association*, XXXIII, no. 9, 1899, pp. 1136–1138.

11 Joan Arehart-Treichel, 'Life expectancy: The great 20th century leap', *Science News*, CXXI, 1982, pp. 186–188; Louis I. Dublin, Alfred J. Lotka and Mortimer Spiegelman, eds., *Length of Life: A Study of the Life Table*, The Ronald Press, New York, 1936, p. 41; The Abbott Table (1893–97) showed a life-span of 44·09 for males and 46·61 for females. The Glover Life Table (1900–02) estimated 46·07 for males and 49·42 for females. J. W. Glover, *United States Life Tables, 1890, 1901, 1901–10*, Bureau of the Census, Washington, D.C., 1921, pp. 132–143; G. C. Whipple, *State Sanitation*, Vol. 2, Harvard University Press, Cambridge, 1917, p. 300.

12 Smith, *The People's Health*, p. 316; Harrison, *Separate Spheres*, p. 64.

13 Dublin, Lotka and Spiegelman, *Length of Life*, p. 39.

14 Edward Shorter, *A History of Women's Bodies*, Basic Books, New York, 1982, p. 229; William Farr calculated in his vital statistics (1885) that five mothers died for every 1000 live births between 1847 and 1876. The actual rate of maternal death was undoubtedly higher and increased substantially after the fifth child. Jalland and Hooper, *Women from Birth to Death*, p. 118.

15 Frank I. Foster, M.D., *Handbook of Therapeutics*, D. Appleton & Co., New York, 1896; See also Smith, *The People's Health*.

16 Stearns, 'Old women', p. 44; See also Tilt, *The Change of Life*, Ch.1.

17 Smith-Rosenberg, 'Puberty to menopause', *Disorderly Conduct*, p. 191.

18 Paula Weideger, *Menstruation and Menopause: The Physiology and Psychology, the Myth and the Reality*, Alfred A. Knopf, Inc., New York, 1975, p. 198; Tilt, analyzing the histories of 1,082 women in England and France, found the average age of menopause to be forty-five years nine months. *The Change of Life*, pp. 23 and 97.

19 Pierce, *The People's Common Sense Medical Adviser*, p. 724.

20 Emily M. Nett, 'Midlife for women', Paper presented at the Canadian Sociology and Anthropology Meetings, Ottawa, June 1982, p. 7.

21 J. K. Shirk, M.D., *Female Hygiene and Female Disease*, Lancaster Publishing Co., Lancaster, PA, 1884, p. 132. One theory held that the ill health of menopause was due to the fact that blood, formerly lost at menstruation, now collected in the woman's body and caused physical disorder. Dr Edward Tilt explained that after the menopause, blood that once flowed out of the body at menstruation was turned into fat. Edward J. Tilt, M.D., *The Change of Life in Health and Disease*, 2nd ed., John Churchill, London, 1857, p. 54; Dr Pierce believed that the blood flowed to the head and caused mental excitability. Pierce, *The People's Common Sense Medical Adviser*.

22 Clouston, *The Hygiene of the Mind*, p. 230.

23 J. Braxton Hicks, 'The Croonian lectures on the difference between the sexes in regard to the aspect and treatment of disease', *British Medical Journal* (ii), April 21, 1877, pp. 475–476.

24 Humphry, *Old Age*, p. 13.

25 Walker, *Beauty in Women*, 1892, p. 205.

26 Tilt, *The Change of Life*, 4th ed., pp. 106–246; and 2nd edition, 1857, pp. 198 and 128–31.

27 Barnes, 'Lumleian lectures', pp. 586–587.

28 A. L. Galabin, *Diseases of Women*, 5th ed., London, 1893, pp. 489–491.

29 J. C. Webster, *Puberty and the Change of Life. A Book for Women*, London, 1892.

30 Tilt, *The Change of Life*, 1882, p. 101.

31 Napheys, *The Physical Life of Women*, pp. 273 and 277.

32 Pierce, *Common Sense*, p. 724.

33 W. Tyler Smith, 'The climacteric disease in women', *London Medical Journal*, I, July 1848, p. 601.

34 Currier, *The Menopause*, pp. 8–9.

35 Currier, *The Menopause*, pp. 12–13.

36 John Baldy, *An American Textbook of Gynaecology*, W. B. Saunders, Philadelphia, 1894, p. 84.

37 Tilt, *The Change of Life*, 4th ed., p. 11.

38 James Reed, 'Doctors, birth control and social values, 1830–1970', Morris J. Vogel and Charles E. Rosenberg, eds., *The Therapeutic Revolution: Essays in the Social History of Human Medicine*, University of Pennsylvania Press, Philadelphia, 1979; James C. Mohr, 'Patterns of abortion and the response of American physicians, 1790–1930', Judith Walzer Leavitt, ed., *Women and Health in America. Historical Readings*, The University of Wisconsin Press, Madison, WI, 1984.

39 Currier, *The Menopause*, p. 156.

40 J. H. Kellogg, *Ladies Guide in Health and Disease. Girlhood, Maidenhood, Wifehood, Motherhood*, Modern Medical Publishing Co., Battle Creek, Michigan, 1895, p. 372.

41 Prudence B. Saur, *Maternity: A Book for Every Wife and Mother*, L. P. Miller, Chicago, 1891; Austin, *Perils of American Womanhood*.

42 Tilt, *The Change of Life*, 4th ed, p. 14.

43 Hicks, 'Croonian Lectures', p. 475.

44 Skene, *Medical Gynecology*, p. 80.

45 Delaunay, 'Equality and inequality in sex', p. 190.

46 Lee Chambers-Schiller, 'The single woman: Family and vocation among nineteenth century reformers', Mary Kelley, ed., *Woman's Being, Woman's Place: Female Identity and Vocation in American History*, G. K. Hall & Co., Boston, 1977.

47 T. S. Clouston, *Clinical Lectures on Mental Discourse*, Henry C. Lee's Sons, Philadelphia, 1884, p. 388.

48 Hicks, 'Croonian lectures', p. 473.

49 Ehrenreich and English, *For Her Own Good*, p. 111. This theory was elaborated by Freud and Deutsch. Menopause was seen as the third edition of the infantile stage, the moment when the woman's service to the species ends. Biologically useless and permanently scarred, women became the dismissed servants of the race. Sigmund Freud, *Outline of Psychoanalysis*, Hogarth Press, London, 1949; Helene Deutsch, *The Psychology of Women*, Vol. 2., Grune and Straton, New York, 1945; Eric Erickson, 'Womanhood and the inner space', *Daedalus, Journal of the American Academy of Arts and Sciences*, Spring, 1964.

50 Stearns, *Old Women*, p. 46; Thomas R. Cole, *Past Meridian: Aging and the Northern Middle Class*, Unpublished Ph.D. diss., University of Rochester, 1980.

51 Augustus K. Gardner, *Conjugal Sins: Against the Laws of Life and Health and Their Effects Upon the Father, Mother and Child*, J. S. Redfield, New York, 1870,

pp. 150–151.

52 Napheys, *The Physical Life of Women*, p. 290.

53 Smith-Rosenberg, 'Puberty to menopause', p. 191; Eliza Farnham, *Woman and Her Era*, New York, 1864, p. 65.

54 Tilt, *The Change of Life*, pp. 102–3.

55 Walker, *Beauty in Women*, p. 163.

56 Currier, *The Menopause*, pp. 148 and 97.

57 Edward D. Cope, 'The relation of the sexes to government', *Popular Science Monthly*, XXXIII, October 1888, pp. 721–730.

58 Clouston, *Hygiene of the Mind*, pp. 209–210.

59 Forbes Winslow, *Mad Humanity: In Forms Apparent and Obscure*, C. A. Pearson Ltd., London, 1878, p. 228. The ovarian manic was sometimes alleged to develop immodest sexual appetites at menopause, for which unpleasant remedies such as injections of ice water into the rectum or vagina, or leeching of the labia and cervix were recommended. Smith, 'The climacteric disease', p. 607.

60 C. C. Hersman, M.D., 'Relation of uterine disease to some of the insanities', *Journal of the American Medical Association*, XXXIII, no. 2, September 16, 1899, p. 710; Frequencies of childlessness among native-born American middle-class women did rise in the latter part of the nineteenth century, but the reasons were extremely complex. However, even the strongest advocates of family limitation did not advocate childlessness and strong social pressure was exerted on women to fulfil the expectations of motherhood or count themselves a failure. Howard P. Chudacoff, 'The life course of women: Age and age consciousness, 1865–1915', *Journal of Family History*, V no. 3, Fall 1980, pp. 274–292; Peter Uhlenberg, 'A study of cohort life cycles: Cohorts of native-born Massachusetts women, 1830–1920', *Population Studies*, XXIII, 1974, pp. 407–420; Linda Gordon, *Voluntary Motherhood: The Beginnings of Feminist Birth Control Ideas in the United States*, Hartman and Banner, eds., *Clio's Consciousness Raised*.

61 Harriet Martineau, 'Female industry', *Edinburgh Review*, CIX, 1859, pp. 293–336.

62 Michael Anderson, 'The social position of spinsters in mid-Victorian Britain', *Journal of Family History*, IX, no. 4, Winter 1984, p. 392.

63 Ruth Freeman and Patricia Klaus, 'Blessed or not? The new spinster in England and the United States in the late nineteenth and early twentieth centuries', *Journal of Family History*, IX no. 4, Winter 1984, pp. 395–414.

64 Hall, *Adolescence*, 2, p. 634.

65 Smith-Rosenberg, 'Puberty to menopause'; Margaret A. Cleaves, M.D., *The Autobiography of a Neurasthene: As Told By One of Them and Recorded By ... Richard G. Badger*, The Gorham Press, Boston, 1910. Cleaves depicted herself as a mannish maiden, in her pursuit of a professional career; see also, S.P. White, 'Modern mannish maidens', *Blackwood Magazine*, CXLVII, 1890, p. 254.

66 Kaufert, 'Myth and the menopause', p. 148.

67 For a discussion of Doctors' attitudes towards the ageing, see Tilt, *The Change of Life*, 4th ed, and Charles D. Meigs, *Females and Their Diseases*, D.G. Brinton, Philadelphia, 1879.

68 Humphry, *Old Age*, p. 2.

69 L. A. Quetelet, *A Treatise on Man and the Development of His Faculties*, William and Robert Chambers, Edinburgh, 1842.

70 Tamara Hareven, 'The life course and aging in historical perspective', *Aging and Life Course Transitions: An Interdisciplinary Perspective*, Tamara K. Hareven and Kathleen J. Adams, eds., The Guilford Press, New York, 1982, p. 12; Carole Haber, *Beyond Sixty-Five. The Dilemma of Old Age in America's Past*, Cambridge University Press, Cambridge, 1983, p. 79; F. B. Smith also notes that an increasing part of the physician's wealth was underwritten by their attendance upon increased numbers of elderly patients and their chronic diseases, whose families could pay for those lengthy bedside vigils awaiting crises or death. *The People's Health*, p. 368.

71 Gerald A. Gruman, 'The rise and fall of prolongevity hygiene', *Bulletin of the History of Medicine*, XXXV no. 3, May–June 1961, pp. 221–229. On Cornaro's life and work, see William B. Walker, 'Luigi Cornaro, a Renaissance writer on personal hygiene', *Bulletin of the History of Medicine*, XXVIII, 1954, pp. 525–534; John Burdell, ed., *The Discourses and Letters of Luigi Cornaro, on a Sober and Temperate Life*, Fowler and Wells, New York, 1842.

72 D. H. Jacques, *'Physical Perfection': or, the Philosophy of Human Beauty; Showing How to Acquire and Retain Bodily Symmetry, Health and Vigor, Secure Long Life, and Avoid the Infirmities and Deformities of Old Age*, Fowler and Wells, New York, 1859, p. 207.

73 Haber, *Beyond Sixty-Five*, p. 66.

74 T. S. Clouston, 'Female education from a medical point of view', *Popular Science Monthly*, XXIV, December 1883, p. 215.

75 Bernard Van Oven, *On the Decline of Life in Health and Disease*, John Churchill & Sons, London, 1853.

76 Clouston, *Hygiene of the Mind*, p. 228.

77 J. Thorburn, *A Practical Treatise on the Diseases of Women*, London, 1885, pp. 192–193.

78 Napheys, *The Physical Life of Women*, p. 279; Pierce, *The People's Common Sense Medical Adviser*, p. 726.

79 Napheys, *The Physical Life of Women*, pp. 35–36.

80 Mitchell, *Doctor and Patient*.

81 Tilt, *The Change of Life*, 4th ed., p. 98 and 99.

82 Eugene Richards, 'The influence of exercise upon health', *Popular Science Monthly*, XXIX, July 1886, p. 333.

83 J. H. Kellogg, *Second Book on Physiology and Hygiene*, American Books, New York, 1894; Edwin Checkley, *A Natural Method of Physical Training: A Practical Description of the Checkley System of Physioculture*, W. C. Bryant, New York, 1890; D. H. Jacques, *How to Grow Handsome*, Fowler and Wells, New York, 1890, p. 31.

84 Clouston, *Hygiene of the Mind*, p. 277.

85 Wainwright, 'Exercise', p. 709.

86 Clouston, *Hygiene of the Mind*, p. 24.

87 J. Madison Taylor, M.D., 'The conservation of energy in those of advancing years', *Popular Science Monthly*, LXIV, April 1904, pp. 541–549.

88 Wainwright, 'Exercise', p. 707.

89 Taylor, *A Physician's Counsels*, pp. 93–94; For a discussion of the living arrangments of older women at this time, see Daniel Scott Smith, 'Life course, norms and the family system of older Americans in 1900', *Journal of Family History*, XIV, no. 3, Fall 1979, pp. 285–298. In 1900, over eighty per cent of widowed women with living children lived with one of them. Six in ten persons over sixty-four lived with a child; solitary residence was rarely practiced. Chudacoff and Hareven, 'From the family nest', p. 69.

90 Florence Nightingale, 'Cassandra', Ray Strachey, *The Cause. A Short History of the Women's Movement in Great Britain*, G. Bell & Sons, London, 1928, p. 417.

91 John Mendeloff, 'Measuring elusive benefits: On the value of health', *Journal of Health Politics, Policy and Law*, VIII no. 3, 1983, p. 563; It was not long ago that Wilson and Wilson talked about elderly women as representing the ghost of former womanhood. Robert A. Wilson and Thelma A. Wilson, 'The fate of the non-treated postmenopausal woman: a plea for the maintenance of adequate estrogen from puberty to the grave', *Journal of the American Geriatric Society*, XI, 1963, pp. 351–356.

92 E. H. Ruddock, *The Common Diseases of Women*, 6th ed., New York, 1888, pp. 83–84.

93 Frances Willard, *How to Win: A Book for Girls*, Funk and Wagnalls, London, 1889.

94 Clouston, 'Female education from a medical point of view', December 1883, p. 224.

95 Filene, *Him/Her/Self*, p. 11; Chudacoff provides data from Providence, Rhode Island, to show that the childbearing range in 1900 began at twenty-three to twenty-four and ended around thirty-four to thirty-seven. Chudacoff, 'Life course', pp. 274–292.

96 Ellis, *Determinants of Puritan Stock*.

97 Grant Allen, 'Plain words on the woman question', pp. 170–181.

98 Stephen Smith, *Doctors in Medicine: And Other Papers on Professional Subjects*, New York, 1892, p. 107.

99 Patricia Branca, *Silent Sisterhood. Middle Class Women in the Victorian Home*, Croom Helm, London, 1975, p. 66.

100 Ehrenreich and English, *Complaints and Disorders*, p. 33.

101 Morantz-Sanchez, *Sympathy and Science*, p. 208.

102 E. D. Pellegrino, 'Medicine, history and the ideas of man, medicine and society', *The Annals of the American Academy of Political and Social Sciences*, CCCXLVI, 1963, pp. 9–20.

103 William Edgar Darnall, 'The pubescent schoolgirl', *American Gynecological and Obstetrical Journal*, XVIII, June 1901, p. 490.

Part Two

Women's voices: female physicians and their views on health and exercise

4

Breaking the professional mould: women's struggle to enter the medical profession

> The inscription of incompatibility [of women and professional careers] is an inscription by governing men to legitimate the exclusion of women from professional power. The inscription of incompatibility masks the reality of exclusion.[1]

While nineteenth-century sexual ideology deterred most women from having a professional career, by mid-century numerous women in both England and the United States were becoming professionally involved in medicine with a particular view to improving the poor state of health of women and children. Middle-class women, these early female doctors argued, faced unique physiological problems throughout their life-course which could not be adequately or tastefully dealt with by male medical practioners.[2] Beset by ignorance of physiological facts and appropriate hygienic practices, such women were seen to be in dire need of an informed female support system, education in preventive health, and sensitive medical supervision by their own sex. In short, women physicians were increasingly seen as necessary to assist women in their important domestic role and to complement or compensate for traditional male medical practices. The purpose of the women's medical movement, said Elizabeth Blackwell, the first formally licensed female physician in England and America 'is for occupying positions which men cannot fully occupy and exercising an influence which men cannot wield at all'.[3]

The need for such an influence was borne out by an increasing number of gloomy reports from feminist hygiene experts and female doctors whose anxiety about female health, according to Ann Douglas Wood, was exacerbated by:

> an exaggerated but astute perception of the unconscious purposes underlying the attitudes and practises of doctors with women for patients. In their excited

view, current medical treatment was patently not science for which they professed respect, but a part of their male-dominated culture for which they had both fear and contempt.[4]

The poor state of health of many American and British middle-class women was only too clear to health reformers such as Catharine Beecher who, at mid-century, feared that 'ere long, there will be no healthy women in the country'.[5] Throughout the nineteenth century she and similarly-minded female health reformers argued that the regular male medical profession not only made little effort to remove the causes of female disease but also, in part, contributed to it by rendering middle-class women helpless victims as a result of unnecessary, ineffective and morally questionable practices.[6] In England Elizabeth Garrett Anderson argued that although many women were not healthy, the extent of female ill health was over exaggerated by male doctors.[7] By 1895 Mary Putnam Jacobi was attributing an economic factor to male medical enthusiasm for illuminating female disease. 'It is considered natural and almost laudable to break down under all conceivable varieties of strain', she wrote. 'Constantly considering their nerves, urged to consider them by well-intentioned, short-sighted advisers, [women] pretty soon became nothing but a bundle of nerves.'[8]

Feminist Charlotte Perkins Gilman also objected to what she perceived as the tyranny of male medical control over female wellbeing. American men, she complained, had 'bred a race of women weak enough to be handed about like invalids; or mentally weak enough to pretend they are and to like it'.[9] She recounted in numerous literary works her bitter experiences with male medical practices along with her advocacy of preventive health measures, especially physical activity as a means of emancipation. Gilman, along with many other feminists, shrewdly realized that women themselves best understood the reasons for their ill health and the kind of daily habits which would lead to wellbeing through healthy life-styles.

To many feminist minds male establishment physicians stood accused of using professional authority to repress women and curtail their activities by exaggerating, prolonging and even encouraging their ailments, real or imaginary. Masculine dominance over women, therefore, could be avoided if women paid greater attention to their personal health and sought the assistance when needed of a female physician who understood women's bodies and needs. Gilman herself turned to physician Mary Putnam Jacobi for treatment of her depressions, after finding little solace from male experts. 'I found her the most patient physician I had ever known, and the most perceptive. She seemed to enter into the mind of the sufferer and know what was going on there, and I have carried with me, and always shall, the deepest . . . feelings for that broad mind.'[10] Jacobi's willingness to treat Gilman as an equal partner in prescribing a cure, explains Morantz, contrasted directly with the authoritarian Dr S. Weir Mitchell's rest cure for nervous women and emphasized the pervasive belief that women physicians could somehow empathize and deal more competently with female health concerns.[11]

Feminist campaigner Josephine Butler experienced the same relief as Gilman in consulting English physician Elizabeth Garrett in 1868. Having consulted nine doctors in three countries about her apparent heart condition, Butler finally consulted a woman physician.

> I was able to tell her so much more than I ever could or would tell to any man. . . Oh, if men knew what women have to endure and how every good woman has prayed for the coming of a change. . . . How would any modest man endure to put himself in the hands of a woman medically as women have to do in the hands of men? . . . I pray to God that many Miss Garrett's may arise.[12]

Arguments advanced in favour of women doctors

> Women are naturally inclined and fitted for medical practice. I maintain that not only is there nothing strange or unnatural in the idea that women are fit physicians for women and men for men; but, on the contrary, that it is only custom and habit which blind society to the extreme strangeness or incongruity of any other notion.[13]

The initiation of women into the medical profession was both a response to spreading dissatisfaction with regular physicians and a logical outcome to the mid-nineteenth-century feminist and popular health reform movements which emphasized special female qualities for ministering to the health and fitness needs of women and children.

At mid-century the medical profession was in disarray on both sides of the Atlantic. Turbulent professional developments in England, especially overcrowding, led to the inauguration of the British Medical Association in 1853. Its efforts concentrated on centralizing and consolidating professional power through a medical register of doctors.[14] The 1858 Medical Act was a concrete recognition of the desperate need to create more uniform standards of qualification and practice by improving medical education and regulating recruitment. Despite this Act, English doctors disagreed about even the most basic diagnoses and treatment, let alone how to regulate relationships among themselves.[15]

The *Lancet* lamented at the time that 'medicine is not looked upon as the profession of a gentleman'.[16] Novelists regularly portrayed doctors as ignorant, coarse and grasping.

In America there was little uniform training or licensing, and sporadic efforts to regulate the profession were ineffective.[17] Few medical schools required more than two years' attendance and even fewer provided clinical experience.[18] Medical education was largely an apprentice system and a profusion of proprietary schools with extremely low admission requirements had sprung up. Most physicians lacked formal medical degrees.[19] Henry Bigelow, writing scornfully of Harvard Medical School students, reported that 'more than half of them can barely write'.[20] One important consequence of the lack of well-trained physicians was that a number of medical sects composed of irregularly trained doctors filled the vacuum and competed intensely for patients. Concerned with the potential loss of patients, regular doctors complained in a leading article in the *Lancet* in 1857 that:

> such persons [irregulars and quacks] exist in numbers which would surprise those less conversant with the state of the case than ourselves. Hanging about the suburbs of town, infesting its central parts and acting ostensibly as druggists, these people absorb much money and destroy many lives and much health.[21]

Across the Atlantic, homeopaths, hydropaths, Thomsonians, Grahamites and others sold their varied expertise to a public clamouring for relief from disease, and regular 'allopathic' physicians established the American Medical Association in 1847 to try to limit the irregulars' ability to practise medicine.[22] Regular doctors became increasingly vocal in their desire to defend public health against the irregulars, 'an enemy more subtle than disease' who could 'never do honour to the profession'.[23] Indeed, some observers discerned greater emphasis on the struggle to restrict professional registration than on efforts to improve a medical education which Mary Putnam Jacobi described as 'rudimentary . . . The intrinsic tests were so shifting and unreliable, the standard of attainments so low, that it was proportionately necessary to protect the dignity of the profession by external, superficial, and arbitrary safeguards.'[24]

Public denunciation of the 'heroic' measures used by regular doctors was also growing. Common practises such as bloodletting, purges and cauterization (Currier called doctors who used such measures 'bleeders, pukers, purgers')[25] killed as often as they cured and generated increasing criticism for their painful ineffectiveness.[26] The time had passed, said Ann Preston (future Dean of the Woman's Medical College of Pennsylvania) when 'the licensed graduate whose lancet is sprung for every headache and heartache that he may meet can obtain public confidence'.[27] Early Victorian novels painted horrifying pictures of mid-century English male medical practices. In *Recommended to Mercy*, 'Dr Langton was a practitioner of the good old school; physiking and phlebotomizing, cauterizing and torturing after the manner of his predecessors.' Frequent bloodletting was often supplemented by harsher measures. 'In vain, they tried their remedies: their ice to his head, their cooling medicines, their blisters to his feet.'[28] Ignorance, poor training and excessive practices thus combined to generate a widespread loss of medical prestige and so strengthened the mid-nineteenth-century popular health reform movements along with the varied efforts of women to become more involved in preventive medicine.[29]

Early feminists and health reformers had already played a critical role in transforming public attitudes towards sickness and death by arguing that men and women should take more responsibility for their own health.[30] In seeking to obtain the solution to women's health problems by providing them with more accurate information about their own physiology, middle-class women, who made up the health reformers' primary constituency, placed a new emphasis on health and the body. Furthermore, they contributed by directing the reformist mind to the physical conditions of women's life and to health and educational reform in general.[31] The sentiment grew that 'the health of the body and the uses made of it decided whether nations or societies would rise or fall'.[32] Feminists and health reformers increasingly relied upon science and hygiene as ideological tools to promote female advancement and to counter the outrages they believed were being inflicted upon women by traditional medical practices.

Only by laying claim to scientific authority did female reformers believe that they could rescue women from the twin evils of physiological ignorance and heroic medicine. They were sure that these were largely responsible for the terrible decay of female health. Only through a commitment to preventive hygiene did they see a way to improve women's domestic and social condition. Preventive hygiene based upon scientific principles involved, among other things, the educated use of pure air, loose clothing and exercise. Its practice, female reformers believed, led to a perfect balance of mind and body that would only subsequently be disturbed by lack of symmetry, excess and disease. Thus obedience to balanced hygienic rules could prevent physical and social degeneration. If the will could learn to rule the body's natural forces, disease would never appear and the body could be relied upon as the principal instrument of social control.[33] It was this belief, clearly articulated by such female health reformers as Mary Gove Nichols, Catharine Beecher and Harriet Hunt, that inspired the actions of many first-generation nineteenth-century women doctors. They realized that 'only healthy, vigorous women could meet the challenges thrust upon them by a society in transition'.[34] Elizabeth Garrett Anderson, lecturing to the London Association of Schoolmistresses in 1868, declared that 'health is to be regarded as a means and a power rather than as an end in itself, and what is wanted from the body is that it should become a strong and willing slave, instead of a tyrannical and capricious master'.[35] Elizabeth Blackwell also extolled the need to rule one's body: 'bodies that can move in dignity, in grace, in airy lightness or conscious strength, bodies erect and firm, energetic and active bodies that are truly sovereign in their presence, are expressions of a sovereign nature'.[36]

For women to take more control over their bodies, to believe that they could play a greater role in determining their own future, they needed instruction in preventive hygiene. Women doctors seemed particularly suitable to do that. Shocked by the realization that male doctors were unable to deal adequately with female disease, and determined to improve the health knowledge and practices of American women, Harriett K. Hunt sought to become the first woman doctor by apprenticing herself to Thomsonian physicians and then establishing her own eclectic practice in Boston. Although very successful in practice, her attempts to seek formal training and recognition were rejected twice by the Harvard Medical College in 1847 and 1851. 'No woman of true delicacy,' claimed a resolution of Harvard students in response to her application, 'would be willing to attend medical lectures with men. And they, in turn, would be unwilling to mix with any woman who 'unsexed' herself.'[37] Nonetheless, Hunt continued her medical practice while supporting feminist demands for trained female doctors who could specialize in preventive hygiene.[38] It was clear, she lectured, that the female physician must be preventive. 'She must look upon life through sanitary channels and she must use her natural abilities to concentrate upon those aspects of health care for women and children that male doctors could not provide.'[39]

Mary Putnam Jacobi also emphasized prevention through the promotion of information about health. In 1874, she informed the First

Woman's Congress that the existence of women doctors would have:

> an immense influence in dissipating the stupid prejudices which had for so long concealed from women the general physiological knowledge which was most important for them to know. The study of the mechanism of the human body is not mere dirty work, but one of the most sublime occupations; [the] mysteries are not sacred but embarrassing masses of ignorance waiting to be dispelled.[40]

Although women needed information about their bodies, it was felt that Victorian sensibilities had prevented them from discussing their bodily symptoms freely with male doctors. There was also a general concern to protect the female from potential male abuse. Elizabeth Blackwell always used her concern for the potential compromise of a woman's modesty by male physicians to show how much women doctors were needed. She remembered in 1860 how many middle-class women had confided to her their shame and anger at their rough handling by male accoucheurs.[41] Indeed she was persuaded to enter medicine by a friend who, dying of a uterine disorder, confessed that her suffering might have been alleviated had she not been too embarrassed to report her symptoms to a male doctor.[42] Pioneer doctor Sophia Jex-Blake declared that she was amazed how women could go to men for uterine treatment. She argued that many did not, claiming considerable suffering among women too pure-minded to expose certain ailments to male doctors.[43] Josephine Butler was one of many reformers who ardently crusaded against the male doctor's infringement of female privacy and liberty. 'Every woman,' she insisted, 'has a right to protect the secrets of her own person.'[44]

Women doctors, early supporters supposed, would encourage women patients to expose their bodies more willingly, thereby revealing a host of diseases hitherto hidden to male doctors.[45] This would hasten their cure and develop an understanding of appropriate prevention techniques. Female physicians would treat their patients as sisters, showing womanly sympathy with their special physiological organization. Josephine Lowell echoed popular female sentiment that 'a woman can know a woman as a man cannot'.[46] This was especially important in delicate sexual matters. It seemed self-evident, Sophia Jex-Blake pointed out, that a woman's most natural adviser would be one of her own sex, who could appreciate more fully than any medical man her state, both of mind and body.[47] Elizabeth Garrett Anderson noted in 1871 that increasingly her patients were women from all over London who, for matters of delicacy, wished to be treated solely by women for gynaecological conditions.[48]

Women physicians were believed to be especially important for guiding and protecting the sexuality of young girls.

> The skilled and sympathetic woman physician, rather than the man, should accompany young girls through their school and college life . . . she will have constantly present to her an adequate conception of the ideal or normal life of women . . . moreover, her assistance will serve to avoid and alleviate much needless suffering.[49]

Educated medical women, said Dr Eliza Mosher, 'touch humanity in a manner different from men; by virtue of their womanhood, their interest in children, in girls and young women, both moral and otherwise in homes and in society'.[50]

Many pioneering women doctors in both England and America emphasized that these maternal, nurturant and counselling qualities specially qualified women to be doctors. Indeed, if there was a dominant point of view among women doctors in the nineteenth and early twentieth centuries, says Morantz, 'it was that women belonged in the medical profession by virtue of their natural gifts as healers and nurturers'.[51] Mary Putnam Jacobi urged the training of women doctors not so much because she believed their strength and intelligence equalled those of men, but because 'the special capacities of women as a class for dealing with sick persons are so great'.[52] Elizabeth Blackwell, usually considered the first formally trained woman doctor in America and the first to receive an English licence to practise, saw her womanhood as a weapon against the masculine medical world and expected female physicians to become the professional allies of wives and mothers everywhere.[53] To Blackwell, women physicians were merely different kinds of mothers who simply carried their maternal instincts into medicine. The true physician, she said, 'must possess the essential qualities of maternity'. As spiritual mothers of the race women physicians could be 'more truly incarnations of the grand maternal life than those who [were] technically mothers in the lower physical sense'.[54]

The female struggle to enter the nineteenth-century medical profession was spurred on by the argument that women's natural nurturing talents could form a 'connecting link' between the female domestic life and the newly emerging scientific medical world. If medical training was necessary to provide support for scientific motherhood, then medical knowledge would assist women in becoming better mothers and making society more homelike.[55] That argument rendered male physicians particularly vulnerable to the female incursion into medicine after mid-century, 'for if women were to enter any profession, their special talent for nurturing seemed to dictate a career in medicine'.[56] There was no line of practical work outside domestic life, Elizabeth Blackwell explained, so eminently suitable for women as the legitimate study and practice of medicine.[57] An aggrandizing male medical profession intent on safeguarding its own interests should be required to demonstrate that women's domestic and maternal nature, far from being an asset to medicine, was an unbeatable liability.[58]

The efforts of the nineteenth-century male medical profession on both sides of the Atlantic to prevent aspiring female doctors from entering training institutions, medical societies and hospitals by demonstrating women's physical and emotional unsuitability for the doctor's role shaped the attitudes and practices of the first female physicians. Aspects of the debate which attempted to restrain female professional advancement, and the strategies women developed to overcome establishment hurdles are essential in reaching an understanding of the doctor-patient relationships developed among women and the types of therapeutic advice (including exercise prescriptions) proposed by those women who managed to become regular doctors. Because they often possessed or had pressed upon them a strong sense of femaleness, and because of the harsh pressures brought to bear upon early female medical aspirants to prove their competence and stamina, one might expect from them less inclination to attribute female ill health to allegedly inherent defects in the female physiology and a less general anxiety over managing female energy for the reproductive process.[59] In preventive health matters there was in the female medical discourse a greater enthusiasm for promoting female health, vigour, physical mobility and commitment to the practice of a somewhat different kind of medicine than that advocated by their male counterparts – one that was less technocratic and interventionist, milder, and more reliant upon nature.[60] Women physicians, says Morantz-Sanchez, 'sincerely believed that they would behave differently from men and that they had their own special contributions to make to society'.[61]

Male medical objections to women doctors

History, physiology and the general judgment of society unite in the negative of woman's fitness for the medical office.[62]

The male medical establishment, fearing economic competition in an overcrowded and depressed profession, initially blocked entrance for women into regular medical schools and refused admission to medical societies to women with training in irregular medical colleges.[63] Fear of female competition for patients in the second half of the nineteenth century also surfaced, no doubt because a large proportion of physicians' clients were women, and women physicians, claiming a special affinity for dealing with female disorders, were perceived to be competing for the growing and lucrative market in obstetrics and gynaecology. The obstetrical business was 'one of the essential branches of income to a majority of well-established practitioners' and inroads made by female physicians were a cause of serious concern.[64] 'Are they to enter into hard and public competition with us . . . no longer keepers at home,' commented a doctor in *The Lancet* in 1862.[65] Another claimed that a 'body of female doctors attending women would displace an equivalent number of male doctors or diminish their incomes.'[66] The *Boston Medical and Surgical Journal* ruefully quoted a Scottish doctor:

> An' when the leddies git degrees,
> Depen' upon't there's nocht'll please
> Till they hae got oor chairs an' fees,
> An there's an end o' you an' me.[67]

Concerned with their own survival, male physicians were hardly in a mood to welcome on board a group of women whose potential number could sink the already foundering ship.[68]

The male medical objections centered upon the belief that women were both physically and emotionally unsuitable for medical practice. A resolution passed by the Philadelphia County Medical Society stated:

> The physiological peculiarities of women, even in single life, and the disorders consequent on them, cannot fail frequently to interfere with the regular discharge of their duties as physicians in constant attendance on the sick. . . .The members of this society, therefore, cannot offer any encouragement to women becoming practitioners of medicine.[69]

Added to the claim that medical training and the work of a physician were incompatible with the duties of women to bear children and run households, there were arguments to show that women would be hardened and defeminized by the disagreeable and laborious aspects of medical education. Only a man could brave the 'revolting' scenes of childbirth, quoted *The Lancet*. Women pursuing a medical career would unsex their sisterhood because 'any woman who is logical, philosophical, and scientific departs from the normal woman in her physical as well as her mental characteristics'.[70] Put bluntly, Dr Bennett explained, women were 'sexually, constitutionally and mentally unfitted for the hard and incessant toil of medical practice'.[71]

Beginning in the late 1860s and early 1870s, however, skilful biological arguments were developed and widely disseminated to bar women from medicine. In America Dr Horatio Storer first raised the issue of the 'periodical infirmity' of women physicians he observed while working as head surgeon in the New England Hospital for Women and Children. Since women were susceptible to the influence of their reproductive system, he argued, and 'subject to recurrent waves of mental and physical instability caused by menstruation, they could not be trusted to furnish medical assistance consistently and scientifically'.[72] As monthly cripples, he thought women more in need of medical aid than able to furnish it.[73] Storer was clearly prejudiced, since he had quarrelled with those women physicians who administered the hospital about restrictions they had placed on his high-risk surgery from which many of his patients had died. None the less his criticisms carried weight.

Dr Edward Clarke took up Storer's theme, claiming that although women had the right to practise, they unfortunately lacked the capability. Let them try a fifty-year experiment, he allowed, even though he doubted they would ever become successful practitioners.[74] His early pronouncements engendered little consternation among an increasingly successful group of female physicians. But when he expanded his initial thoughts in *Sex in Education; or, A Fair Chance for Girls*, the male medical case concerning the negative relationship between the intellectual education and the physiology of women was fully elaborated. From arguing initially against the specific dangers of medical education, Clarke expanded his thesis to include the baneful physiological results of all female education after puberty. A girl could healthily study only four hours a day (two thirds that of boys) and should take at least three days off every fourth week. Girls and women, he declared, needed a 'special and appropriate education that shall produce a just and harmonious development of every part', and medical training was not part of that.[75]

Several female physicians and feminists published reactions to Clarke, demonstrating the unscientific and misogynous nature of his argument.[76] Dr Clarke's book seems to have 'found a chance at the girls rather than a chance for them', said Julia Ward Howe in a reply to *Sex in Education*:

121

. . . All could wish that he had not played his sex-symphony so harshly, so loudly or in so public a manner . . . The notion that you cannot feed a woman's brain without starving her body might better be recaste to show that if more attention is given to physical education, body and mind become capable of more sustained effort. Some instances of remarkable robustness in women have been the result of a physical education identical with that usually given to boys. We are thus left in doubt whether the book was written for men or for women.[77]

Women would not believe Clarke, said Elizabeth Stuart Phelps, 'simply because they know better . . . Every healthy woman physician knows better,' she insisted, 'and it is only the woman physician, after all, whose judgement can ever approach the ultimate uses of the physicist's testimony to these questions.'[78]

Among the female physicians who responded, Mary Putnam Jacobi in particular challenged Clarke's thesis by examining the relationship between menstruation, rest and female disabilities. She explained that 'the singular avidity with which the press and the public have seized upon the theme discussed in Dr Clarke's work. . . is a proof that this appeals to many interests besides those of scientific truth'. Indeed, she continued, 'his arguments are not accepted because they are demonstrable, but enlisted because they are useful'. In regard to the periodical functions, 'a mysterious interest has always been attached. . . From the Mosaic law to Raciborski, from the denunciation of the schoolmen to the rhapsodies of Michelet, they have been invoked in every theory on the nature of women; that is in every theory on the organization of society.'[79]

In a prize-winning article (the Boylston Medical prize was selected with the author's name removed), Jacobi demonstrated empirically that there was nothing in menstruation that particularly necessitated periodic rest for most women. Proper physical exercise along with good nutrition, she suggested, would prevent menstrual pain, and certainly mental activity was not dangerous to women's health.[80] Allowing that menstruation could deplete female energy stores, she nevertheless insisted that women had the health and strength to combine reproductive development and higher education. Many other studies by women physicians followed, including one demonstrating the good health of practising female physicians and their triumph over menstruation.[81]

Despite such a scholarly defence, as the century wore on male doctors continued to demonstrate their anxiety over the growth of female power and influence in medicine and to argue the serious consequences attendant upon women involved in professional endeavours. Dr Nathan Allen, a prominent Massachusetts physician, suggested that higher education caused women to become nervous and lose their capacity to nurse their infants. 'In consequence of the great neglect of physical exercise and the continuous application to study, together with various other influences, large numbers of our American women have altogether an undue prominence of the nervous temperament.'[82] Similarly Dr S. Weir Mitchell, the eminent Philadelphia neurologist, wrote scathingly in 1873 of the destruction caused by women pursuing professional studies. 'She is not fairly up to what Nature asks from her as wife and mother. How will she sustain herself under the pressures of these yet more exacting duties which nowadays she is eager to share with man?'[83] Dr N.S. Davis of Chicago wrote in the same vein. Abundant evidence, he said, showed that 'there are two channels of expenditure of physiological force in woman – the terrible strain of higher and professional education . . . and the expense of being properly trained for motherhood'.[84]

Not surprisingly, male anxieties over the biological difficulties of female doctors were not extended to female nurses who maintained constant vigilation of the sick while remaining docile and submissive to the physician in charge. Sophia Jex-Blake made much of this point in England, where the training of women doctors proceeded more slowly than in America. Although Elizabeth Blackwell had obtained a licence to practise in England in 1859, this opportunity had been immediately closed to other women.[85] Seeking another route, Elizabeth Garrett Anderson sought unsuccessfully the opportunity for medical training and licensing at the Apothecaries Hall in 1865. Sophia Jex-Blake tried without success to force the University of Edinburgh to allow her to complete her medical training and eventually obtained her medical degree from the University of Bern in Switzerland. In a court case against male administrators at the University of Edinburgh, she argued that women were both naturally inclined and fitted for medical practice:

> and if this be so, I do not know who has the right to say that they shall not be allowed to make their work scientific when they desire it, but shall be limited to merely the mechanical details and wearisome routine of nursing, while to men is reserved all intelligent knowledge of disease, and all study of the laws by which health may be preserved or restored.[86]

Women were fit physicians for women and men for men, she argued. History showed just how competent women had been in these affairs until the recent expropriation of all aspects of medicine by men. As to female capacity for medical work, she noted:

> It has always struck me as a curious inconsistency that while almost everybody applauds and respects Miss Nightingale and her followers for their brave disregard of conventionalities on behalf of suffering humanity, and while hardly anyone would pretend that there was any want of feminine delicacy in their going among the foulest sights and most painful scenes to succour, not their own sex, but the other, many people yet profess to be shocked when other women desire to fit themselves to take the medical care of those of their sisters who would gladly welcome their aid. Where is the real difference?[87]

The British medical establishment knew where the difference lay. An article in *The Lancet* articulated the precise difference between woman as doctor and woman as nurse.

> In the economy of nature . . . the ministry of women is one of help and sympathy. The essential principle, the keynote of her work in the world is aid; to sustain, succour, revive and even sometimes shelter man in the struggle and duty of life, is her peculiar function. The moment she affects the first or leading role in any vocation, she is out of place. . . awkward, unfit and untrustworthy.[88]

In any case, continued the article, 'if women undertake the duties of physicians, we shall presently feel the want of nurses. . .'. Reacting to suggestions that women should enter medicine, the Medical Council of Great Britain declared that 'the study and practice of medicine and surgery, instead of affording a field of exertion well fitted for women, does, on the contrary, present special difficulties which cannot be disregarded'.[89] In other words, women doctors were unfit for strenuous toil and night visits but quite capable of doing so as nurses, which was their legitimate province.

British male medical rhetoric increasingly reflected the same anxieties as those articulated by Dr Edward Clarke of Harvard about the entry of women into the medical profession. Although Ehrenreich and English note that the virulence of the American sexist opposition to women had no real parallel in Europe, this may have been partly due to the fact that far fewer British women aspired to medical careers at this time.[90] However, even though Clarke had focused particularly upon the damaging effects of higher education on American girls and women, his arguments were soon applied with equal vigour to English women. A leading contributor was Dr Henry Maudsley of University College London, who reformulated Clarke's thesis on the deleterious effect of higher education upon women, especially those seeking medical training. In 'Sex in mind and education', Maudsley explained to his public that:

> It will have to be considered whether women can scorn delights and live laborious days of intellectual exercise and production, without injury to their functions as the conceivers, mothers and nurses of children. For it would be an ill thing. . . that we got the advantages of a quantity of female intellectual work at the price of a puny, enfeebled and sickly race . . . Is it well too for them to contend on equal terms with men for the goal of man's ambition?[91]

Elizabeth Garrett Anderson replied the following month in the *Fortnightly Review*. Most of the women who had contended with men in pursuit of professional goals, she remarked, 'have had no chance of being any the worse for being allowed to do so on equal terms. They have had all the benefit of being heavily handicapped'. She was convinced that 'it is a great exaggeration to imply that women of average health are incapacitated from serious work by the facts of their organization. Among poor women . . . the daily work goes on without intermission and, as a rule, without ill effects.' Challenging the thesis that intellectual activity undermined the health of normal girls, she considered that intense physical activity could be far more damaging. She believed the health of American women inferior to that of English women because of the lack of exercise, overheated houses, higher education at too early an age, and the dangers of co-education. Garrett Anderson admitted that this could be used as an argument to slow down but not to prohibit women's professional development. As a trained and practising physician, however, she was proof that English women could study extensively, and she reminded her male medical colleagues of the attention paid by many English schools to the health and ongoing strength of their female pupils. 'We can speak of the conditions under which English girls work, and we are able to say distinctly that on many vital points they are just those which Dr Clarke and the other American doctors urge as desirable.'[92] This was the case at Roedean, for example, where the school's prospectus announced that 'special pains will be taken to guard against overwork, and from two to three hours daily will be allotted to out-door exercise and games'.[93]

Undeterred by such claims, Dr T.S. Clouston consolidated Maudsley's attack on the dangers of 'the present tendency to over-educate the female sex'.[94] In a lecture series at Edinburgh, Clouston criticized educators for disregarding the needs of the female constitution. The female organism was more delicate than that of men, he claimed. The machine was less tough, it broke down at slighter causes and needed more careful medical management. It was not fitted for the regular grind kept up by men.[95] It had neither the strength nor the regularity. Therefore any process of education which abused the female machine necessarily stunted the women and robbed the world. Dr Withers Moore, President of the British Medical Association, cemented the argument in an 1886 address:

> growing girls are not rich enough to bear the expense of being trained for motherhood and also that of being trained for competition with men in the severer exercises of the intellect. Women should be protected from the rude battle of life by the work and labor of men. . . It is not good for the human race that women should be freed from the restraints which law and custom have imposed upon them, and should receive an education intended to prepare them for the exercise of brain-power in competition with men . . . Bacon, for want of a mother would not be born.[96]

Despite the fervent arguments of Drs Storer, Clarke, Clouston, Maudsley, Withers Moore and other well-known medical men, none presented convincing statistical evidence. 'We have not the facts to do so', admitted Clouston, who then went on to provide casual observations as undeniable testimony.[97] Claiming it to be obvious that each sex had an appropriate and exclusive place and work, establishment physicians repeated the refrain whenever they wanted to prevent women from becoming doctors. Their arguments were sometimes effective. Studying to become a doctor at the Women's Medical College in Philadelphia, Jane Addams left after the first year admitting physical exhaustion. According to Sarah Blaisdell, Addams lost physical vigour, having 'taxed it . . . very severely both in study and in doing for others'. She had depleted her 'original stock' of vigour and was eventually forced into Mitchell's hospital for nervous disorders. He was, in fact, the second doctor to order her to rest her mind and body from her medical studies, and she never did become a doctor.[98]

Notes

1 Swindells, *Victorian Writing and Working Women*, p. 21.
2 Martha H. Verbrugge, 'The Social Meaning of Personal Health: The Ladies Physiological Institute of Boston and Vicinity in the 1850's', in Susan Reverby and David Rosner, eds., *Health Care in America. Essays in Social History*, Temple University Press, Philadelphia, 1979, pp. 45–66.
3 Elizabeth Blackwell, 'The influence of women in the profession of medicine', Elizabeth Blackwell, ed., *Essays in Medical Sociology*, 1902, reprint, Arno Press, New York, 1972, II, p. 28.
4 Ann Douglas Wood, 'The fashionable diseases', p. 41.

5 Catharine E. Beecher, *Letters to the People on Health and Happiness*, 1855, reprinted., Arno Press, New York, 1972, p. 9.

6 Beecher, *Letters to the People*, pp. 115–138.

7 Elizabeth Garrett Anderson, quoted in Ehrenreich and English, *Complaints and Disorders*, p. 25.

8 Mary Putnam Jacobi quoted in Ehrenreich and English, *Complaints and Disorders*, p. 19.

9 Charlotte Perkins Gilman, *Women and Economics: A Study of the Economic Relation Between Men and Women as a Factor in Social Evolution*, Harper and Row, New York, 1966, 1st pub., 1898.

10 Gilman's reminiscences about Mary Putnam Jacobi are noted in Alumnae Transactions, Women's Medical College of Pennsylvania, 1907, p. 66.

11 Morantz-Sanchez, *Sympathy and Science*, p. 214.

12 Janet Horowitz Murray, *Strong-Minded Women and Other Lost Voices from Nineteenth-Century England*, Pantheon Books, New York, 1982, p. 317; Josephine Butler to Albert Rutson, 22 February 1868, *Josephine Butler Papers*, Fawcett Collection, City of London Polytechnic.

13 Sophia Jex-Blake, M.D., *Medical Women. A Thesis and a History*, 1886, reprint ed., Source Book Press, New York, 1970, pp. 6–7.

14 Swindells, *Victorian Writing*, p. 27.

15 Hilary Marland, ed., *Medicine and Society in Wakefield and Huddersfield 1780–1870*, Cambridge University Press, Cambridge, 1987, pp. 266 and 302.

16 *The Lancet*, 2 October 1858, p. 358; See Smith, *The People's Health*, p. 376.

17 Speert, *Obstetrics and Gynecology in America*, p. 77.

18 J. Marion Sims, *The Story of My Life*, New York, 1884; William G. Rothstein, *American Physicians in the Nineteenth Century: From Sects to Science*, Johns Hopkins University Press, Baltimore, 1972; John S. Haller, Jr. *American Medicine in Transition, 1840–1910*, University of Michigan Press, Urbana, 1981; Richard H. Shryock, *Medicine and Society in America, 1660–1860*, New York, 1960; Patricia Vertinsky, 'Body shapes: The role of the medical establishment in informing female exercise and physical education in nineteenth century North America', in Mangan and Park, eds., *From 'Fair Sex' to Feminism*, p. 265.

19 Mary Roth Walsh, 'The rediscovery of the need for a feminist medical education', *Harvard Educational Review*, XLIX, no. 4, November 1979, p. 448.

20 Henry Bigelow, quoted in G. H. Brieger, *Medical America in the Nineteenth Century*, The Johns Hopkins University Press, Baltimore, 1972.

21 'Quackery in the manufacturing districts', *The Lancet*, II, 1857, p. 326; In the UK see 'Fringe Medical Practice', in Marland, *Medicine and Society*, pp. 205–245; See also Smith, *The People's Health*.

22 For a discussion of the struggle between regulars and irregulars, see, for example, Harris Livermore Coulter, 'Political and Social Aspects of Nineteenth Century Medicine in the United States', unpublished Ph.D. thesis, Columbia University, 1969. Briefly, Thompsonians taught that disease was the result of an excess of cold in the body; hot baths and herbs were the main remedies. Grahamites promoted health through hygienic measures, vegetarianism, whole-wheat flour and abstinence from alcohol. Hydropathy included the use of therapeutic baths and drinking waters. Osteopathy was a system of therapy using body massage and spinal manipulation.

Homeopathy advocated the administration of minute quantities of drugs that would produce symptoms similar to those of the disease being treated.

23 Proceedings of the Michigan Medical Association, 1850, pp. 17–18 and 14.
24 Mary Putnam Jacobi, 'Women in medicine', in Annie Nathan Meyer, ed., *Woman's Work in America*, Henry Holt & Company, New York, 1891, p. 149.
25 Currier, *The Menopause*, p. 49.
26 Vertinsky, 'Body shapes', p. 264; Leach, *True Love*, p. 22.
27 Ann Preston, Thesis, 'General Diagnosis', Medical College of Pennsylvania Archives, 1851.
28 Matilda Houston, *Recommended to Mercy*, I, London, 1862, p. 43; Mrs Henry Wood, *Mildred Arkell*, III, London, 1865, p. 305, in Myron F. Brightfield, 'The medical profession in early Victorian England, as depicted in the novels of the period, 1840–1870', *Bulletin of the History of Medicine*, XXXV, no. 3., May–June 1961, pp. 221–229.
29 Although women had traditionally been involved in midwifery, by the 1820s, male physicians had managed to close the door on training opportunities for women with the argument that they were too delicate, too moral and unable to use the new mechanical techniques for birthing appropriately. The gradual professionalization of medicine allowed male physicians to break the midwife's traditional hold on the occupation. The prestige of the profession eventually allowed physicians to make claims to superior competence as childbirth attendants and co-opt the developing medical technology and knowledge applicable to childbirth. In the process they redefined the nature and care of childbirth to suit their own professional needs. This was especially so in the United States where physicians were particularly assiduous in marking out their territory and there was less of a tradition of respected professional midwives. Datha Clapper Brack, 'Displaced – the midwife by the male physician', Hubbard, Henifin and Fried, eds., *Biological Woman: The Convenient Myth*, pp. 208–209. See also Walter Channing, *Remarks on the Employment of Females as Practitioners in Midwifery, by a Physician*. Boston, 1820, and Walsh, *Doctors Wanted*. As Mary Putnam Jacobi pointed out, women had practiced freely in medicine as long as the practice of medicine was free, and decided upon by a natural taste for dealing with the sick. Mary Putnam Jacobi, 'Shall women practice medicine?', *North American Review*, CXXXIV, January 1882, pp. 52–75.
30 Regina Markell Morantz, Cynthia Stodola Pomerleau and Carol Hansen Fenichel, eds., *In Her Own Words. Oral Histories of Women Physicians*, Greenwood Press, Westport, CN, 1982, p. 14.
31 Regina Markell Morantz, 'Making women modern: Middle class women and health reform in nineteenth century America', *Journal of Social History*, X, no. 4, Summer 1977, pp. 490–507; Verbrugge, *Able-Bodied Womanhood*, p. 8; Kathleen E. McCrone, 'Play up! Play up! and play the game,' Sport at the late Victorian girls' public schools', Mangan and Park, eds., *Fair Sex*, p. 122.
32 Leach, *True Love and Perfect Union*, pp. 19 and 21.
33 Leach, *True Love*, p. 26.
34 Morantz, 'Making women modern', p. 495; See also Verbrugge, *Able-Bodied Womanhood*, p. 19.
35 E.G. Anderson, 'Miscellanea, Physical Training of Girls', *Englishwoman's*

Journal, October 1868, p. 151.

36 Elizabeth Blackwell, 'Extracts from the laws of life, with special reference to the physical education of girls', *English woman's Journal*, I, 1858, pp. 189–190.

37 *Boston Evening Transcript*, 3 January, 1851.

38 Walsh, *Doctors wanted*, p. 32.

39 Jacobi, 'Women in medicine', Meyer, *Women's Work*; Harriet Hunt, *Proceedings of the Women's Rights Convention*, October 1851, Boston, 1852.

40 Mary Putnam Jacobi, 'Social aspects of the re-admission of women into the medical profession', paper and letters presented to the First Women's Congress of the American Association for the Advancement of Women, New York, 1874, p. 173; Mary Putnam Jacobi, 'Shall women practice medicine', *North American Review*, CXXXIV, Jan 1882, p. 57.

41 Ingleby Scott, 'Dr. Elizabeth Blackwell', *Once a Week*, June 16, 1860, p. 577.

42 Margaret Forster, *Significant Sisters. The Grassroots of Active Feminism, 1839–1939*, Secker and Warburg, London, 1984, p. 63.

43 Margaret Todd, *The Life of Sophia Jex-Blake*, Macmillan and Co. Ltd., London, 1918, p. 247; Sophia Jex-Blake, *Medical Women*, p. 50.

44 Josephine Butler, Parliamentary Papers, 1882, HMSO, London, p. 340; Brian Harrison, 'Women's health and the women's movement in Britain: 1840–1940', Webster, ed., *Biology, Medicine and Society*, p. 45.

45 They had remained hidden because of an entrenched proscription against examining women's bodies. 'He is but the panderer of vice… and an unchaste man, who ruthlessly insists upon a vaginal taxis in all cases of women's disease', said Dr Charles D. Meigs of Philadelphia. Meigs, *Females and Their Diseases*. Since respect for women's modesty often precluded the physician's inspection of her genitalia, much was obviously overlooked.

46 Josephine Lowell, 'Open letter', *The Century Magazine*, XLI, no. 1, February 1891, p. 634.

47 Jex-Blake, *Medical Women*, p. 49; Jacobi, 'Women in medicine', p. 427.

48 Jo Manton, *Elizabeth Garrett Anderson*, Methuen & Co. Ltd., London, 1965, p. 226.

49 M. Carey Thomas, *The Century Magazine*, XLI, no. 1, February 1891, p. 637.

50 Eliza Mosher, M.D., 'The value of organization – what it has done for women', *Women's Medical Journal*, XXVI, 1916, p. 3.

51 Morantz-Sanchez, *Sympathy and Science*, p. 4.

52 Jacobi, 'Women in medicine', p. 177; See also Rosalind Rosenberg, *Beyond Separate Spheres. Intellectual Roots of Modern Feminism*, Yale University Press, New Haven, CT, 1982, p. 17.

53 Elizabeth and Emily Blackwell, *Medicine as a Profession for Women*, Tinson, New York, 1860, pp. 15–19.

54 Elizabeth Blackwell, 'Opening of winter session of London School of Medicine for women in 1889', in Forster, *Significant Sisters*, p. 57; Blackwell, 'The influence of women', *Essays in Medical Sociology*, p. 21.

55 Regina Markell Morantz, 'The connecting link: The case for the woman doctor in 19th century America', Leavitt and Numbers, eds., *Sickness and Health in America*, p. 167; See also Kathryn Kish Sklar, *Catharine Beecher: A Study in American Domesticity*, Yale University Press, New Haven, 1973.

56 Walsh, *Doctors wanted*, p. 107; See also Burstyn, 'Education and sex'.

57 Dorothy Clarke Wilson, *Lone Woman. The Story of Elizabeth Blackwell, The First Woman Doctor*, Little, Brown & Co., Boston, 1970, p. 367.

58 Walsh, *Doctors wanted*, p. 108.

59 Virginia Drachman, 'Women doctors and the women's medical movement: Feminism and medicine, 1850–1895', Ph.D. diss., State University of New York at Buffalo, 1976.

60 Morantz and Zschoche, 'Professionalism, feminism, and gender roles', p. 570.

61 Morantz-Sanchez, *Sympathy and Science*, p. 60.

62 Theoph. Parvin, Prof. *Diseases of Women*, quoted in Jacobi, 'Women in Medicine', *Woman's Work*, p. 143.

63 Richard H. Shryock, 'Women in American medicine', *Journal of the American Medical Association*, V, 1950, p. 375.

64 Editorial, *Boston Medical and Surgical Journal*, LXXVIII, 1862, p. 106.

65 *The Lancet*, II, 1862, p. 123.

66 'Reply to Sophia Jex-Blake's address at St George's Hall', *The Lancet*, I, 1872, p. 618.

67 *Boston Medical and Surgical Journal*, LXXXIX, 1873, p. 23.

68 Walsh, *Doctors wanted*, p. 134; The entire question of economic competition in medicine merits further study, notes Walsh, though a beginning has been made by Lloyd C. Taylor, Jr., *The Medical Profession and Social Reform, 1885–1945*, St. Martin's Press, New York, 1974.

69 Pamphlet entitled *Preamble and Resolution of the Philadelphia County Medical Society upon the Status of Women Physicians*, Stuchey, Philadelphia, 1867.

70 *The Lancet*, 9 January, 1858, p. 44; *The Lancet*, II, 1869, p. 321.

71 A. Hughes Bennett, M.D., *The Lancet*, I, 1870, p. 887.

72 Horatio Robinson Storer, *Boston Medical and Surgical Journal*, LXXV, 1866, pp. 191–192.

73 Walsh, *Doctors wanted*, p. 113.

74 Edward Clarke, M.D., *Boston Medical and Surgical Journal*, 1869, pp. 345–356.

75 Clarke, *Sex in Education*, pp. 159 and 140.

76 Julia Ward Howe, ed., *Sex and Education, A Reply to Dr. Clarke's Sex in Education*, 1874, reprint ed., Arno Press, New York, 1972; Duffey, *No Sex in Education*, J. M. Stoddart, Philadelphia, 1874; George Fisk and Anna Manning Comfort, *Women's Education and Women's Health: Chiefly in Reply to 'Sex in Education'*, Syracuse, NY, 1874; Anna C. Brackett, ed., *The Education of American Girls*, G.P. Putnam's Sons, New York, 1874; Dr Clarke's evidence was apparently limited to six cases that had come to his attention; see Mabel Newcomer, *A Century of Higher Education for American Women*, Harper, New York, 1959, p. 29.

77 Howe, *Sex and Education*, pp. 6 and 29.

78 Elizabeth Stuart Phelps, quoted in Howe, ed., *Sex and Education*, p. 130.

79 Mary Putnam Jacobi, 'Mental action and physical health', in Brackett, *The Education of American Girls*, 1874, pp. 258, 260.

80 Jacobi, *The Question of Rest*.

81 Emily F. Pope, Emma L. Call, and C. Augusta Pope, *The Practice of Medicine by Women in the United States*, Wright and Potter, Boston, 1881; Walsh has identified 145 scientific articles by women physicians between 1872 and 1890

dealing with female health, menstruation and related difficulties. Mary Roth Walsh, in Hubbard, Henifin and Fried, *Biological Woman*, p. 259.

82 Nathan Allen, quoted in Edward W. Ellsworth, *Liberators of the Female Mind; The Shirreff Sisters, Educational Reform and the Women's Movement*, Greenwood Press, Westport, CT, 1979, p. 54.

83 Weir Mitchell, *Wear and Tear*, p. 57.

84 S. Davis, MD, quoted in Lucy M. Hall, 'Higher education of women and the family', *Popular Science Monthly*, XXX, March 1887, p. 612.

85 Horn explains that Blackwell decided to become a physician at a propitious moment. When she began to apply to medical school in 1845, the profession was expanding yet had not developed barriers to discriminate against women. She was able to slip through, catching the profession off guard. Her pioneering steps, however, hardly opened the doors to women in the profession. Margo Horn, 'Sisters worthy of respect: Family dynamics and women's roles in the Blackwell family', *Journal of Family History*, VIII, no. 4, Winter 1983, pp. 367, 382.

86 Jex-Blake, *Medical Women*, pp. 68 and 6.

87 Jex-Blake, *Medical Women*, p. 40.

88 *The Lancet*, 17 August, 1878, p. 314.

89 W.H. Davenport Adams, *Woman's Work and Worth in Girlhood, Maidenhood and Wifehood*, John Hogg, London, 1880, p. 473.

90 Barbara Ehrenreich and Deirdre English, *Witches, Midwives and Nurses*, The Feminist Press, Suny, NY, 1973, p. 28; Sophia Jex-Blake underscored that fact that the protracted fight for access to the profession in England had slowed down. Despite the fact that an 1875 Act of Parliament had permitted universities to confer degrees on women and another had forbidden the Royal College of Surgeons to exclude them, extraordinary difficulties were constantly encountered by women seeking medical training and work in hospitals. By contrast, she said, 'if we turn to America we find that medical women are numbered, not by tens but by hundreds, and that their practice … is of the most extensive kind.' Jex-Blake, *Medical Women*, p. 246.

91 Henry Maudsley, 'Sex in mind and education', *Fortnightly Review*, 1874, p. 479.

92 Garrett Anderson, 'Sex in Mind', pp. 583 and 591.

93 Atkinson, 'Fitness, feminism and schooling', Delamont and Duffin, *The Nineteenth-Century Woman*, p. 110.

94 Clouston, 'Female education from a medical point of view', Dec. 1883, p. 228.

95 Clouston, 'Female education from a medical point of view', Jan. 1884, p. 322.

96 Withers Moore, MD, quoted in Lucy M. Hall, 'Higher education of women', p. 612.

97 Clouston, 'Female education', Jan. 1884, p. 334.

98 G. J. Barker-Benfield, ' "Mother as emancipator", the meaning of Jane Addams' sickness and cure', *Journal of Family History*, IV, no. 4, Winter 1979, p. 404; Blaisdell to Addams, 24 December 1881, Correspondence, Swarthmore College Peace Collection.

5

Female physicians:
professional goals
and exercise prescriptions

The professional orientation of female doctors

As the nineteenth century progressed, women increasingly ignored the warnings of medical men by seeking and winning medical training wherever they could. Kept out of medical schools, they organized their own. Denied access to hospitals, they set up training hospitals specifically for women. Often barred from the club-like world of male medical societies, they organized their own female medical societies – the formation of the New England Hospital Medical Society in 1878 ushered in the era of the professional association of women physicians.[1] In 1880, 2,423 women physicians were identified in America – 3 per cent of all medical professionals. In 1890 there were 4,557 female physicians.[2] In 1893 a national network of women physicians in America followed the founding of the *Woman's Medical Journal*, and by the century's end there were over 7,000 women serving as physicians.[3] Women, said James Bryce, 'had made their way into most of the professions more largely than in Europe'.[4] Partly because there was less provision for women's education in England, the numbers there were considerably smaller. There were eight women doctors in 1871, eleven in 1879, twenty-five in 1881, seventy-three in 1889, 101 in 1891, 264 in 1895 and 495 in 1911 (less than 2 per cent of the total).[5]

While not all women doctors approached professional objectives from a single perspective, some seeing medicine as a professional and scientific pursuit with others viewing medicine primarily as a social mission, their stance on female health and exercise was quite similar. Daniel Scott Smith has labelled the dominant perspective of the early pioneer women doctors 'domestic feminism', a perspective which reinforced the belief that exercise and other hygienic habits had an important contribution to make to healthy motherhood and efficient homemakers.[6] Jill Conway has also shown how women reformers of the late nineteenth century often regarded themselves as social missionaries but were unable (or unwilling) to step aside from the controlling power of stereotypes of the female temperament. Lacking a clear class consciousness, they expected their own sex 'to be agents of social change because of the unique qualities with which they believed the feminine temperament was endowed'.[7] Thus many became examples of a Victorian type of female sage, unquestioningly accepting traditional views of female physicality and mental capacity and portraying women as civilizing and moralizing forces in society. Their rejection of Victorian economic and bourgeois values was rarely accompanied by a questioning of Victorian sexual stereotypes. Such women moved into professional life by claiming they were expanding the domestic sphere rather than leaving it, hence becoming specialists in co-operation – professional housekeepers, as it were.

Women who entered public life espousing the ideology of maternal and domestic values often gave up maternity themselves, accepting the popular view that public work and maternity were incompatible. Elizabeth Blackwell and Lucy Sewall typified women physicians playing the role of social rather than biological mothers.[8] They both subscribed to the traditional image of a community-oriented physician, claiming an altruistic commitment to the welfare of others, even at the expense of her own.[9] 'My whole life is devoted unreservedly to the service of my sex,' said Elizabeth Blackwell,

> the study and practice of medicine is . . . but one means to a great end, for which my very soul yearns with intensest passionate emotion . . . for which I would offer up my life with triumphant thanksgiving, if martyrdom could secure that glorious end: the true ennoblement of woman, the full harmonious development of her unknown nature, and the consequent redemption of the whole human race . . .[10]

Elizabeth Garrett Anderson also claimed to be dedicated to medicine as a social mission, though she married and had children. Like Blackwell, she represented many early women doctors who viewed social reform and the public health issues of women and children as their absorbing concern. By encouraging women doctors to focus upon preventive rather than curative medicine they prompted women physicians to view the health needs of women and girls, as they became wives and mothers, as their particular province. Elizabeth Blackwell claimed throughout her career that women physicians differed from men because they could use their motherly qualities and intuition to improve female health.[11] 'Sanitation,' she agreed with Florence Nightingale, 'is the supreme goal of medicine.'[12] Captured by the appeal of focusing on improving their fellow women's health and making society more homelike, a stream of women sought to emulate her example by seeking entry into medical schools throughout Europe and North America and obtaining formal licence to practise.

A smaller number of women approached medicine with less messianic zeal to become scientific experts. In spite of being told repeatedly that woman's mission was not to pursue science and that women were incapable of rational thinking,[13] many nineteenth-century women doctors, chief among them Mary Putnam Jacobi, viewed medicine as a scientific profession rather than a social mission. Jacobi chose medicine out of interest in chemistry and love for scientific rationalism, seeing 'scientific research as an absolute good because it added to the fund of human knowledge'.[14] She travelled to Paris and l'Ecole de Médecine to pursue advanced studies in medical science, determined to bring more rigorous methods to an American system she saw as lax and unscientific. Upon her return, one of her aims in joining the staff of the Women's Medical College of the New York Infirmary was to stimulate scientific spirit among women medical students and to pursue experimental work herself. The medical students, she noted, 'must learn how to observe, to experiment, to think', for the chief task of a women physician is the creation of a scientific spirit.[15] Soon accepted by her male colleagues as a first-rate scientist and physician, she became the first woman admitted to the New York Academy of Medicine. Pursuing similar professional goals to her mainstream male colleagues, she established her excellence in spite rather than because of being a woman. Women physicians, she cautioned, should see themselves as physicians first, and if they had special qualities it was because they were deliberately acquired rather than innate. Far from specializing only in the health problems of women and children, she felt that women physicians should profess a wide range of medical specialities to establish a broad professional presence in the profession, not remain 'dawdling on the threshold to forever remind [themselves] and everyone else that [they had] just come in'.[16]

While Blackwell and those like her sought to promote the female doctor's unique contribution to her own sex, Jacobi and, later, dedicated women such as Florence Sabin worked to minimize differences between male and female physicians.[17] Despite their different professional orientations, however, in matters of female health and exercise their practical recommendations were often remarkably similar. The importance of exercise to healthy womanhood was commonly acknowledged whether the main goal was emancipation or heightening reproductive efficiency. The scientific proficiency displayed by an increasing number of female doctors at the end of the nineteenth century and into the twentieth showed that most women were not physically disabled by either academic study or by menstruation and menopause. Accumulating evidence showed that women could work long and hard in many arenas without physical or mental penalty. Yet overall, having established both their own capacity and the potential of other women, many female doctors still subscribed to views of exercise which reflected those of their male establishment colleagues. Despite rhetoric to the contrary and a strong challenge to the menstrual disability theory, the exercise prescriptions of early female doctors bore a striking resemblance to male medical therapeutics, showing the widespread and general acceptance of the popular pseudo-scientific theories of the era which informed beliefs about exercise. They differed only in the seriousness which they attached to improving family hygiene and female health and the special attention that many of them paid to female exercise needs. In this sense, says Morantz, female medical educators with a scientific bent differed little from female moral reformers and social feminists who professed a home-based ideology.[18] The following studies of selected women doctors and their written views on female health and exercise convey more unanimity than uniqueness, except for the most militant feminists and the most ardent reactionaries.[19]

Female physicians, physical culture and exercise prescriptions: the early pioneers

Elizabeth Blackwell

Although many women doctors wrote about the benefits of exercise, including the dangers of overexertion, a trio of early pioneer physicians were particularly influential in illuminating the relationship between physical activity and the socially desired healthy robustness in women. 'We should ponder the question,' said Elizabeth Blackwell in 1852, 'whether in our modern days we have not lost much stout virtue, with the failure of our bodily powers. . . What would not our delicate ladies

. . . give for that vigorous life . . . full of energetic activity . . . and pursue every occupation of the day, with the power of robust health?' 'Exercise,' she added, 'is the grand necessity which everything else should aid.'[20]

Elizabeth Blackwell, the first regular woman doctor in both America and England, wrote several treatises on female physical education and the desirability of uninterrupted health as a national heritage.[21] 'The necessity of exercise during the growth of the body,' she said, 'sufficiently indicates the prominent place which exercise should occupy in our systems of education.'[22]

The domestic feminism of Elizabeth Blackwell was clear in her lectures entitled *Laws of Life, with Special Reference to the Physical Education of Girls*.[23] These lectures, which focused upon female health and physical education for girls, were written in New York and first delivered to a group of Quaker women who gave her a start in practical medical life by producing her first much needed women patients.[24] One of these patients prevailed upon George Putnam, the publisher, to bring out a paper-bound brochure on the *Laws of Life*, and this found its way to England where it was read and commended by John Ruskin.[25] When she came to England to register under the 1858 Medical Act, Blackwell gave the series of lectures at the Marylebone Literary Institution where they were well received.[26]

Blackwell's message was that sheltered and pampered city girls would be fulfilled only by improving their physical potential. Urging health reform, she advocated:

> the tearing off of swaddling clothes, the encouragement of climbing, running, riding, dancing and free play in childhood; freedom from strangling corsets . . .; training in skills which would give her a worthwhile goal in life, prevent a too early marriage often resulting in invalidism, [and] courses in all schools and colleges in science and sanitation.[27]

Such an 'entire neglect of all provision for the exercise of city children', she noted, demanded serious consideration. 'Not only do we entirely neglect to call the motor nerves into proper action, but the whole effect of school and indoor life is directly calculated to exalt the undue susceptibility of the sensitive nature.' In England, she suggested, the neglect of female physical training was bad enough, but in the United States it was even worse due to 'the madness of American customs' and 'the folly of its educational system'. English girls thus had an advantage over Americans in having more home education, more fresh air, more parks and fields, simpler food, more riding and archery, a more

extended period of education, later marriages and no central heating![28]
The first care for the young girl was to develop health and strength:

> We need muscles that are strong and prompt to do our will, that can run and
> walk indoors and out of doors and convey us from place to place as duty or
> pleasure calls us . . . We need strong arms that can cradle a healthy child, . . .
> backs that will not break under the burden of household cares, a frame that is
> not exhausted and weakened by the round of daily duties.[29]

Girls should care for their bodies, she continued, so that they could be
ideal vessels for motherhood, unlike 'the poor over-driven hacks in our
omnibuses'. Sufficient exercise should be taken outside, she said, for a
proper and healthy development of the body. Nor was there a hurry to
press girls to become physically mature. Delay, she believed, would be
fortuitous, for it was important to avoid premature activity of the powers
appropriate to the next stage. Once puberty arrived, a girl had to deal
with the transformation to a potential mother and at this time there were
four laws of life that she should follow: The first law, which was the
foundation of all, was the law of exercise. Movement and existence, she
explained, were identical, or at least inseparable. Thus:

1. She should exercise regularly.
2. She should live in an orderly fashion.
3. She should try to blend the life of the soul and the body.
4. She should always try to put her body to proper use.[30]

By the time the female adolescent was sixteen or seventeen, with the
right training she would have acquired a strong and perfectly obedient
body ready for childbearing. Between twenty and twenty-five the body
attained its full vigour, so marriages before this age should be
discouraged. During pregnancy she was exhorted to follow similar
hygienic laws, including a regimen of periodic exercise with attention to
regular habits, cold bathing, plain food and loose clothing.[31]

'If the health of the mother breaks down,' Blackwell explained later in
The Religion of Health, 'family happiness is destroyed and the welfare of
the nation [is] imperilled both in the present and the future.'[32] Not only
was it imperative that a mother obey the laws of health, it was her duty to
secure the right health conditions for her children. 'Think of this, O
Mothers!' she exhorted. 'It is in your power to render them [your
daughters] healthy and strong in body, and the mothers, in their turn, of
a stronger race than ours. Do not continue in the fatal error of our age,
forcing the intellect and neglecting the development of the body.'[33] To
assist English women improve their living habits, Blackwell helped

establish the National Health Society whose motto was 'Prevention is better than cure'.[34]

Medical men, said Blackwell, had an excellent opportunity for educating women in sanitary knowledge because of their authority, yet they rarely took advantage of this since their training in male medical schools was so deficient in hygienic matters. Lucy Hall agreed with her, complaining that:

> There is something almost ludicrous in the spectacle of a physician, educated and professedly observing, passing over without a word about the death-dealing follies which are making invalids of tens of thousands of women all about him, while he lifts his voice in dismal croaking over the awful prospect which looms before his jaundiced eyes of a time when more women shall be educated. . . He might have spared one thought for that doomed multitude, shut off forever from honourable motherhood. . .[35]

Educators too, Blackwell remarked, could better use their time in the health education of youth. Any course of studies laid down for either children or adolescents, she suggested, should not just protect them from harm but do them physical good for their future tasks. Plenty of outdoor exercise and direct training in precision, agility and strength were needed. Blackwell further suggested that scientific gymnastic training such as the famous system designed in Sweden by Ling would best meet the needs of developing youth. Advocating the Ling system, she said 'we need a rational system of gymnastic training, not to super-sede country rambles and the healthful society of natural objects, but to form the basis of a sound education, to ensure the perfect development of the body'. All active sports such as riding, dancing, swimming and archery were also encouraged and short periods of mental application were to be consistently terminated by direct physical activity.[36] 'Further-more,' she continued, 'nature would never again present so valuable an opportunity of remodelling the constitution', and women physicians were particularly appropriate for this task:

> A doctor of . . . preventive medicine who shall become acquainted with the constitution of each student and determine how far exercise must be modified to meet individual peculiarities, is an indispensable member of the faculty of any college that undertakes to educate in Health. With this observation and caution, modern gymnastics and exercise in various forms will become an invaluable part of education.[37]

Blackwell revised the *Laws of Life* for publication in England upon her visit there in 1858, when she placed her name on the Medical Register of the United Kingdom.[38] She would have remained in England but for personal financial difficulties. 'I am convinced that England is the place where we should work to best advantage . . . so greatly does England want just our experience', she wrote to Lady Byron.[39] Before she returned to New York, however, she developed a lengthy correspondence with Elizabeth Garrett who, inspired by her success at becoming a registered doctor, was attempting to gain admission to medical school in England and carry on Blackwell's work. Garrett had also been strongly influenced by Sarah Emily Davies, one of the founders of Girton College, Cambridge. When Blackwell in 1869 finally returned to England, her country 'by birth, choice, permanent home and last resting place', the campaign to allow women to become doctors was well under way and Dr Elizabeth Garrett had been practising medicine for four years.[40]

Elizabeth Garrett Anderson

Like Blackwell, Elizabeth Garrett believed that women had not only a particular gift for medicine but had a responsibility for improving the health of women and children for their domestic responsibilities.[41] In an inaugural address at the London School of Medicine in 1877 Garrett spoke of her belief that it 'is almost certain that our special experience as women will help in the practice of medicine'.

> First, no young man in England knows how debilitating it is to live a life of dullness and inactivity; secondly, women doctors will hopefully be less resigned to chronic ill health in women and more determined to promote their good health.[42]

Garrett's views on physical education for girls and women were first articulated at a speech delivered to the London Association of Schoolmistresses in 1868. Physical training, she pointed out, 'necessarily included all that related to the care of health, as well as to the development of strength and grace'. 'Exercise [was] to be varied, frequent, and never fatiguing. Walks to be taken briskly in small parties . . . Ten minutes' quick dancing, as waltzing and galloping every evening.' Gymnastics, she suggested, should be conducted with speed and agility as an aim rather than strength. Musical gymnastics were particularly suitable because they added pleasure to the routine of exercising. As for games, croquet afforded insufficient exercise while battledore and tennis were more vigorous. Most important was the question of rest in relation to exercise. Both were to be thorough, especially for fast-growing girls, who should lie down for a few minutes after gymnastics, then rest long and easy at night.[43] Garrett repeated some of these themes at an 1870 London School Board candidates' meeting to which she had been invited. Asked if she considered physical training and especially swimming necessary for girls, she declared her belief that 'physical education was especially necessary for girls and swimming so useful she had practised herself for many years to perfect the art'.[44] In subsequent School Board meetings she also insisted that children needed light and air, and washrooms and space to play, and throughout her career she continued to press for games for girls. The idea of female collegiate life was fairly new, she admitted, but women needed better education as wives and mothers. 'Women are not harmed by regular and steady work,' she insisted. 'On the contrary, many of the most miserable cases of nerve weaknesses in women are due to the want of it.'[45]

In May 1872 Elizabeth Garrett Anderson, by now married to Skelton Anderson, began a series of lectures for women on anatomy and physiology, followed by an extensive reply to Dr Henry Maudsley's well-publicized attack on women's higher education. Garrett Anderson, who, in fact, shared Maudsley's basic premises concerning the importance of sexual differences, demanded to know if menstruation was really such an incapacitating affliction. After all, she pointed out, reproductive organs were formed in girls at birth and not suddenly at adolescence. Analogous changes took place in the constitution and organization of young men, she noted, which, when added to the many ways that boys further taxed their strength, rendered them, rather than young women, at risk from intellectual study. Women were handicapped by social rather than physiological reasons. Given the daily work demanded of working-class women, she suggested, 'the assertion that, as a rule, girls are unable to go on with an ordinary amount of quiet exercise or mental work during these periods seems to us to be entirely contradicted by experience'. Furthermore, she continued, 'a life at a good day-school, with time for fresh air and exercise, is healthier than sitting over the fire with a novel at home'.[46]

As Elizabeth Garrett Anderson settled into her own family life, she also became Dean and later President of the London School of Medicine for Women, and the only woman member of the British Medical Association from 1872 to 1893. Even in the twilight of her career Garrett Anderson wrote about a healthy way of life for women from puberty to menopause. At puberty, she reminded, girls need a healthy, active life with much open-air exercise, plenty of good food and plenty of occupation. Of the climacteric she wrote:

in natural menopause there is a beneficient absence of haste. . . .; physiological compensation is established and in many cases the woman is in better health after the menopause than she was before it. She has paid her tax to humanity and she is now free from calls of that kind on her strength and activity.[47]

Mary Putnam Jacobi

While Elizabeth Garrett Anderson countered Dr Maudsley's attack on higher education for English women, Mary Putnam Jacobi provided convincing scientific evidence in the United States to refute male medical establishment claims that too much mental and physical exertion was debilitating the reproductive vigor of American middle-class women.

Jacobi's intellect was ably demonstrated in the research she developed for Harvard's Boylston Medical Prize in response to the question, 'Do women require mental and bodily rest during menstruation, and to what extent?' She had already examined the question in 'Mental action and physical health' where she suggested that common sense and good hygiene could allow girls to study without ruining their health.[48] Pointing to the poor health of girls observed by Dr Edward Clarke, she suggested that competition, close confinement, long hours and unhealthy sedentary habits may have been more responsible for their problems than the exertion of mastering school textbooks. The single manoeuvre of 'confining girls to a sofa and a novel for a week in every four', she argued, could not possibly cure all the ailments of Clarke's female patients.[49] Furthermore, Jacobi pointed to statistics from various parts of the world confirming the hard work performed by working-class and other women without provision for rest during menstruation. The English textile industries, for example, employed almost half a million women in 1871, while in the United States the 1870 census showed that a sixth of the female population over the age of ten worked in industry. It was, she noted,

> impossible to exclude young girls from manufactures, our industry has need of the labour of women and women are in imperative need of the salaries afforded by wholesale industry . . . Existing regulations are little prepared to yield to nature her inexorable demand for rest during one week out of every four in the adult life of women. . . If it be said, it is necessary that women rest during menstruation, we must ask, necessary for what purpose? The preservation of life? Evidently not, since the most superficial observation shows thousands of women of all races and ages engaged in work of various degrees of severity without attempting to secure repose at the menstrual epoch[50]

The research project she developed for the Boylston Prize approached the question pragmatically. 'How,' she asked, 'did women who rested during menstruation feel compared to those who did not?' Did the working capacity of a woman diminish during menstruation, leading to inferior work? If women who did not rest were liable to disease, then the rested ones should be revealed to be the ones in better overall health. To test this hypothesis, she sent out, to a wide variety of women, 1,000 questionnaires containing sixteen questions asking about the type of menstrual difficulties experienced, the amount of walking typically accomplished during this time, the general level of health and the type of mental activity offered at school or higher education. She also systematically collected physiological data from six subjects for periods up to three months: pulse rates, temperature, urea excretion and muscular strength as measured by a hand dynamometer.

Two hundred and eighty-six women returned questionnaires. A third of them (ninety-four women) stated they suffered no pain during menstruation or deterioration of general health. Few of this group rested more than an hour a day during menstruation. Eighty-four per cent of the spinsters, however, suffered pain versus 11 per cent of the married women, causing Jacobi to suspect an often noted connection between celibacy and discomfort. Their pain must be due, she concluded, to their depression at a failure to achieve a married state which caused a depletion of nutrition to the nerve centres and hence pain during menstruation.

Rest, reasoned Jacobi, did not appear to be necessary for normally menstruating women, and mental activity was not dangerous:

> There is nothing in the nature of menstruation to imply the necessity, or even the desirability of rest, for women whose nutrition is really normal. . . The menstrual flow is the least important part of the menstrual process, and arguments for rest drawn from the complexity of the physiological phenomena involved in this should logically demand rest for women during at least twenty days out of the twenty-eight or thirty. In other words, should consign them to the inactivity of a Turkish harem.[51]

What was connected to menstrual disability, she concluded, was lack of exercise, poor study habits, celibacy, childlessness and frivolous social activities. Jacobi also developed a convincing argument that women often possessed a high degree of vitality as a result of maternity rather than being drained by it. 'It is not usually recognized to what an extent the organic vigour of women is naturally destined to be increased by child-bearing.'[52]

Jacobi's research was a brilliant medical attack on the myth that menstruation debilitated women and the most impressive single physiological statement in favour of co-education written by a feminist.[53] The study stimulated her interest in the relationship of educational methods to health and mental development. Systematic exercise as part of the educative process was even more necessary for girls than boys, she explained, since boys were so much more likely to get it spontaneously. She viewed as an encouraging sign the developing partnership between the public educator and the physician joining hands and becoming counsellors. School gymnastics, she believed, should be subject to direct medical supervision and should take place in the high school for between twenty-five and forty-five minutes a week.[54]

With the birth of her own children her interest shifted to primary education and a sharp criticism of the methods used to keep 'unfortunate young victims in uninterrupted session through three full hours in succession'. Declaring 'if there is a more direct method of raising a nation of invalids and idiots, I am not acquainted with it', she advocated shorter school hours and abundant physical culture for children in their early years of education.[55] In this regard she was in complete agreement with an increasing number of female medical colleagues who were being hired by educational institutions at all levels to supervise the health and hygiene of girls and young women. Indeed, in addition to private practice, women doctors were increasingly involved in founding and managing large urban hospitals and dispensaries for women and children, in caring for female prisoners and patients in insane asylums, and in teaching at female colleges and some state universities.[56]

Female physicians in educational institutions

Not only hygiene but physical education to develop the bodies of growing girls was taking the place of polite and effeminate delicacy, and there were not wanting medical women to study and teach medical gymnastics and corrective exercises to children and young people.[57]

Just as many early women doctors came to the medical profession through schoolteaching, teaching hygiene courses to women became a significant professional activity for women doctors in the late nineteenth and early twentieth centuries.[58] Initially, women developing private practices found such lectures a useful way in which to earn money and gather female clients. Health and hygiene instruction including detailed exercise prescriptions, for example, was a large part of the work accomplished by female physicians hired to work in health spas and the popular water-cure establishments of irregular doctors.

It was in the women's schools and colleges, however, and later in the state universities, that women physicians such as Eliza Mosher, Lucy M. Hall and Clelia Duel Mosher became significant instructors in female health, hygiene and physical culture. One consequence of the dire warnings by male physicians about the potential health hazards faced by women students was that, rather than barring them from their institutions, educators sought better means of monitoring the health of their female adolescent charges. Hiring a resident female physician served the purpose of monitoring the health of women students and supervising their hygienic affairs, as well as providing instruction in health and physical culture.[59] Sara Burstall from Manchester commented particularly upon the increasing number of supervisory women physicians in American educational institutions in her survey of American educational practices. 'It appears that there is, in America, a very close relation between the medical profession and physical education. Medical women are in charge of this department in all the chief women's colleges.'[60] Similarly, Burstall described the development in England of a close relationship between physical training and medical inspection. The doctor and the gymnastics mistress were the main experts and controllers of the physical and mental aspects of girls' lives.[61]

Dr Alice T. Hall, for example, Professor of Physical Training, Lecturer in Human Anatomy and Physiology, and director of the gymnasium at the Women's College of Baltimore (later Goucher College), claimed her college to be the first to rank the Department of Physical Education equally with other departments, requiring female students to complete an hour of physical activity per day throughout the four years of working for a degree. Hall studied briefly with Dr Dudley Sargent before visiting physical training centres in Germany and Sweden. Deciding 'that the Swedish system was the one that could be used to the greatest advantage in America', she modelled her Baltimore programme on that of the Royal Central Gymnastic Institute at Stockholm and hired a graduate as the first gymnasium assistant. She also was assisted by Edward M. Hartwell, physician and pioneer physical educator, who helped her to obtain a set of machines for massage and Swedish gymnastics as well as in planning her exercise programme for college women.[62] Her department became a model for many other colleges and universities.[63]

Eliza M. Mosher

Eliza Mosher, who became an exemplar of resident female physicians in higher educational institutions, considered herself a third-generation pioneer doctor with as single-minded a dedication to medicine and as deep an interest in female health and physical education as the earlier pioneer Elizabeth Blackwell.[64] She was one of the first females to enter and graduate from the University of Michigan Medical School, but even before this she had spent a year as clinical assistant to Lucy Sewall, 'one of the best educated physicians in Boston', at the New England Hospital for Women and Children.[65] Following graduation, Mosher, with Lucy Hall as partner, set up a private practice concentrated particularly upon preventive medicine for young girls who were overdoing, under-eating and needed 'a good overhauling – life, habits and all'.[66] She continued to develop her interest in female health and hygiene at her next post as first woman physician and then superintendent at the State Reformatory Prison for Women at Sherbon, Massachusetts. Not only did she supervise the health of women prisoners, she also developed special activity programmes through which self-control and self-respect might be developed.[67] In 1896 she was persuaded by the president of the University of Michigan to become the first woman faculty member at the University of Michigan, Dean of Women and Professor of Hygiene in the Literary Department (the Dean of Medicine refusing to appoint a woman to his faculty).[68] As resident physician to women and director of physical education, she took her role as teacher of hygiene very seriously and developed a broad-based physical education programme for women.[69] She taught personal hygiene, physical culture, home economics and public health, systematically weighed and measured all her female charges, supervised their behaviour and devised corrective exercises for them.

Numerical analyses of body size and strength, as well as postural analyses, were stressed increasingly by medical personnel as a way scientifically to manage the body and standardize levels of health.[70] Using a record-keeping system developed by her companion Lucy Hall, Mosher personally supervised and recorded every aspect of her students' growth, development and appearance. Particularly interested in postural analysis, she founded the American Posture League, invented a special kindergarten chair and wrote about the relationship of posture to health and exercise.[71]

Mosher's attitude toward health and physical culture was typical of many female physicians who became resident physicians and directors of physical education at educational institutions towards the end of the nineteenth century. Her determination to demonstrate that female college students could enjoy better health than the average woman was matched only by the zeal with which she supervised the exercise programmes of her charges. As one student noted, 'she marched us around like a regiment of soldiers. It was useless to say one word against physical education. Dr Mosher called anyone who didn't like it just plain lazy.'[72] Writing about health and physical culture in *Health and happiness, a message to girls* and 'The Health of American Women', Mosher demanded that women use their bodies to their fullest capacity and pay particular attention to:

1. Wholesome and nutritious food taken at regular intervals.
2. Pure air during the whole twenty-four hours.
3. Undisturbed and sufficient sleep.
4. A suitable amount of exercise out of doors and in the gymnasium.
5. Absence of undue worry and hurry.
6. A healthful mode of dress.
7. Congenial employment and temperance in all things.[73]

Instilling these laws in her female students at the University of Michigan and other institutions where she worked would, she was sure, help dispel the myth that higher education disabled women's health. Supported by the careful records kept by Lucy Hall, she was able to claim that 'women college graduates enjoy[ed] a sum total of twenty per cent better health than the average woman'.[74]

Like Mary Putnam Jacobi and others, Eliza Mosher and Lucy Hall challenged Clarke, Clouston and Withers Moore whose arguments they claimed lacked reliable data. It was true, admitted Hall, that the birth rate among middle-class New Englanders was falling, but the relationship of this phenomenon to the higher education of women could not be substantiated. 'All this much-talked-of physiological expenditure is a myth. Strength comes with use.'[75] Longitudinal surveys of the health status and physical development of school and college girls confirmed that fears of widespread disability resulting from intellectual study were groundless.[76] Unbalanced training was the real problem, not brain strain, indolence and purposeless drift rather than mental and physical education. Worst of all fates was to have a feeble underdeveloped physique unable to pursue the noble plan of motherhood.

Women could study and achieve motherhood, claimed these female college physicians, and, with the right kind of physical education, improve their maternal capacity. Despite her views on social feminism, Mosher, like many of her colleagues, viewed the physical training of college women as the grand route to motherhood, 'the highest and holiest crown of womanhood'.[77] It would be a great economic loss to the state, she said, if 'through ill health or physical disability, women [were] unable to bear and properly rear children'.[78] Her commitment in her work, therefore, was to a form of scientific motherhood in which the advantages accruing from preserving the health of college women could be recouped by society in the form of more efficient households and better babies. Indeed, throughout a long and influential career, including twenty years as the senior editor of the *Medical Women's Journal* and time spent organizing the Medical Women's National Association, Mosher, while demonstrating educated women's fitness and ability to function in a modern world, always highlighted maternity as central to the female role.[79]

Clelia Duel Mosher

Clelia Duel Mosher, a Johns Hopkins graduate, cousin of Eliza Mosher and medical adviser to women students at Stanford University, also understood the important role of women physicians in advocating and supervising the physical culture of women students. She was particularly assiduous in designing and documenting extensive tests and measurements of the growth and development of college women, artfully using statistics to publicize the facts concerning female health and strength.[80] Just one generation of better conditions and improved exercise had significantly altered girls' physical development, she claimed, hence physical differences were clearly not as permanent as had been assumed. 'The need for truth with regard to women's physical limitations,' she wrote, 'has become imperative.'[81]

Pointing out again that the traditional view of women being incapacitated by monthly periods increased the idea of impaired efficiency, Mosher followed Mary Putnam Jacobi in approaching scientifically the question of potential menstrual disability.[82] Based on the study of more than 2,000 women during 12,000 menstrual periods conducted over thirty years, along with diary notes and laboratory observations, Mosher concluded that menstrual pain stemmed from uterine congestion and as a counter suggested specialized exercise rather than rest.[83] Her findings supported Leta Stetter Hollingworth's careful study of the mental and motor abilities of twenty-three women during menstruation which showed that performance was not impaired by menstruation and that physical suffering was in all likelihood due more to suggestion than physiological problems. Doctors had exaggerated the effects of periodicity, said Hollingworth, partly because 'normal women do not come under the care and observation of physicians'. 'Men to whom it would never have occurred to write authoritatively on any other subject,' she declared, 'regarding which they possessed no reliable or expert knowledge, have not hesitated to make the most positive statements regarding the mental and motor abilities of women as related to functional periodicity.'[84] Thus women had been persuaded to believe that the difficulties of the few could be expected by all.

The first step in the physical regeneration of women, claimed Mosher, lay in altering their mental attitudes about bodily functions. First, every girl should be taught that menstruation was not a bad time and that incapacity was unnecessary because 'the effect upon the mind of constantly anticipated misery can scarcely be measured'.[85] Nor should women regard menopause with apprehension:

> Instead of morbid unhappiness, the climacteric or change of life should produce . . . no more than a mild regret that the period of youth and potential motherhood is over, and should be naturally welcomed as release from the inconvenience attendant upon menstruation.[86]

In short, those who were busy and useful were those who avoided disease and premature old age. Being a woman was no reason for not being perfectly well, and physical fitness was important not only for each individual but for the nation and the race. College education with its emphasis on athletics could enhance the health and strength of the 'new woman'. 'This splendid modern woman, approaching the old Greek ideal of physical perfection' would be 'the mother of finer sons and daughters, the promise of a stronger race.' Nor was the achievement to be restricted to college women.

> In the municipal playgrounds, swimming pools, gymnasia and girl scout activities, woman today has such an opportunity as was never before given. It rests alone with her whether she rejects it, clinging to the old idea of physical weakness and dependence, or with open mind takes the opportunity of testing the richness of physical perfection and the fullness of life which comes in its train, making of herself a better citizen, a better wife, a better mother.[87]

By examining the reaction of female doctors working to improve the health of girls through exercise in schools and colleges on both sides of the Atlantic, Paul Atkinson shows how the introduction of physical training allowed the female body to be treated 'as a field for cultural intervention rather than as a passive field of naturally determined processes [and suffering]'. Rather than rejecting establishment medical concepts, female doctors merely modified them and, by using strict physical training in conjunction with medical inspection to mould women who could be fit for a male world, these women doctors 'created an especially strong form of discipline and control over young ladies' bodies'.[88]

Women doctors and eugenics: renewed anxieties in the early twentieth century

We may outrun
By violent swiftness, that which we run at,
And lose by over-running.[89]

Despite Clelia Duel Mosher's promise of new physical freedoms for the early-twentieth-century woman, doctors increasingly emphasized that the purposes for pursuing health and fitness should be focused more rather than less upon honing the female reproductive system. In the early twentieth century the race suicide theory combined with an increasing emphasis upon the heredity laws focused medical minds upon women's bodies with a new intensity. Women were reminded of their responsibility to future generations and asked to commit themselves with renewed fervour to developing strong and healthy bodies. Since mental and moral traits were still believed to be transmissible through the Lamarckian mechanism, the desire was to strive ever more diligently for the Greek ideal – a sound mind in a sound body. This meant, said Dr Mary Wood Allen, that 'each girl's health is a matter of national and racial importance'.[90] The urgency of the mission made the efficient management of the body more crucial. A fit and energy conserving woman could reproduce more effectively, and although women doctors were convinced that moderate exercise enhanced physical efficiency, many of them worried that unnecessary energy waste would prevent the fulfilment of traditional womanly duties.

Eugenics was plainly evident in many writings about female health, exercise and sport by women physicians on both sides of the Atlantic in the early twentieth century. In addition to increased anxieties about a falling birthrate among middle-class women, there were revelations about low physical-fitness levels in many young military recruits, and nervous predictions about the spread of inferior genetic stock through the indiscriminate breeding of immigrant hordes.[91] The low health standards of Boer War recruits caused an outcry in Britain and produced a national inquiry into physical deterioration. In the city of Manchester, for example, 8,000 out of 11,000 volunteers were rejected as unfit for military service.[92]

Women especially were blamed for neglecting their maternal obligations. The Committee on Physical Deterioration struck by the British Government claimed that 'there is no lack of evidence of increasing carelessness and deficient sense of responsibility among the younger women of the present day'.[93] Work outside the home, too much sport, too much idle leisure, too much education and too little training were all blamed for retarding racial progress.[94] The demise of the race was predicted if women continued to neglect their familial duties, overexert themselves in unnatural domains or lead sedentary urban lives which induced physical debility.[95]

Eugenicist Karl Pearson had no doubt that the trend towards female emancipation was the main problem. We must first settle, he said, 'what is the physical capacity of woman, [and] what would be the effect of her emancipation on her function of race-reproduction before we can talk about her rights'.[96] Maternity, he suggested, should be considered an essential social activity not to be impaired by individual intellectual development.[97] The dangers of overeducation in relation to the ability to mother were reformulated with increasing vigour. Pearson, echoing Herbert Spencer's earlier remarks, explained that 'if child-bearing women must be intellectually handicapped, then the penalty to be paid for race predominance is the subjection of women'.[98] In America G. Stanley Hall agreed with Dr Nathan Allen's earlier concern that women's education was an important reason for the immigrant population outnumbering the indigenous American stock of New England.[99] He restated the dangers vividly in his voluminous writings on youth and adolescence. 'The more scholastic the education of women, the fewer children and the harder, more dangerous and more dreaded is parturition.'[100] The destiny of the race, twentieth-century eugenicists held, rested with women who were responsible for maintaining good, healthy stock for the future.[101] To this end, any necessary sacrifice of self-development was to be demanded by society.[102]

Along with the dangers of overeducation and excessive intellectual stimulation came new fears (tied to the old energy balance theories) that a woman's health and childbearing capacity might be damaged by excessive physical activity, especially during adolescence. So a new line of defence was drawn up, explains McCrone.

> Just as it had been maintained that women who attempted to compete with men academically and professionally would put their femininity and reproductivity at risk, so it began to be argued that muscular fatigue was no remedy for mental exhaustion and would have similar dreadful effects . . . Strenuous games . . . drained energy from vital organs, thus damaging women's bodies irreparably and threatening the survival of the race.[103]

This uneasy feeling was apparent in the discourse of a number of female doctors as well as both male and female leading educators. Sara Burstall was not alone in worrying in 1907 that 'the pendulum has probably swung too far in the direction of over-exertion'.[104] Dr Jane Walker warned that girls and women were making a fetish of exercise and causing harm to their bodies.[105] Of the women doctors who were strongly influenced by eugenicist ideas (and who elaborated upon the perceived health risks of athletics and vigorous exercise), none was so voluble as Arabella Kenealy, a British doctor whose books and articles were disseminated widely on both sides of the Atlantic.

Arabella Kenealy

Discussing 'Woman as an athlete' in 1899, Kenealy warned that women would not accomplish their womanly duties if they insisted upon engaging in vigorous physical activity and competitive sport. 'It is not wished . . . to discredit the exercise essential to the building up of healthy bodies, and of maintaining the balance, mental, emotional and physical. Only the forced athletics which destroy this balance are condemned.' Nature, she continued, 'groaned for the muscle-energy wasted by excessive sport'. Too active women were squandering the birthright of 'the babies':

> The old system for girls of air and exercise inadequate to development and health was wrong, but for my part I am inclined to doubt if it was really so pernicious in its physiological results or so subversive of domestic happiness and the welfare of the race as is the present system which sets our mothers bicycling all day and dancing all night and our grandmothers playing golf.[106]

More than the conservation of energy was at stake, however. Kenealy, in the shadow of Freud, wrote that it was abnormal for females to possess strength and stature and a virile mentality. Indeed, females could gain such attributes only at the cost of the masculinity of their future sons. 'A woman who wins golf and hockey matches may be said

. . . to energize her muscles with the potential manhood of possible sons . . . with their potential existence indeed, since over-strenuous pursuits [could] sterilize women as regards male offspring.' In other words, muscular women produced weakling males.[107]

The new importance attributed to the special circumstances of adolescence was also apparent in Kenealy's writings where she underscored the differences in female physical behaviour which followed puberty. 'From having been a strong, young, active, boy-like creature, now . . . the girl loses physical activity and strength. A phase of invalidation sets in. Instinctively, she no longer runs and romps . . . She becomes a complex of disabilities.' What happened, said Kenealy, was that 'nature suddenly locked the door upon her differentiating and escaping energies in order that these might be conserved and knit into organization'. Thus her transition to womanhood was one 'almost entirely of adaptation, physiological and psychical to the functions of wifehood and child-bearing'. Her intelligence at eighteen was less keen than it had been at twelve. Her physical energy, however, fitted her to be 'mother of the Child – the blossom of the Race'. In sum:

> Woman is 'une malade' because, throughout the more than thirty years of her potential maturity she suffers periodically those which, biologically speaking, are minor childbirths . . . Nature exacts from her this recurring toll to Life and to the Race, not only to preserve in healthful and efficient function the power and mechanism of actual child bearing but . . . perpetually to recruit her emotional womanhood and wifehood.[108]

Kenealy was particularly worried that girls were becoming over-strained by such strenuous exertions as hard drill, cricket, hockey and football, which she considered would develop masculine muscles where feminine muscles should be, and make girls 'Amazons of the playing fields'. 'To the characteristic sterile and bold glint of the young woman of strenuous pursuits,' she complained 'could be added the mule-look of conscious immodesty, all stripping her of reserve and dignity alike.' Kenealy blamed overstrenuous, middle-aged feminists for providing an inappropriate role model for younger women, who could ill afford to have shrunken breasts, narrow pelvises and immature or defective reproductive organs. Furthermore, she noted, heart diseases had increased by 50 per cent since sports and athletics had become a cult. Forced athletics was ruining the health and attitudes of early twentieth-century women.

> The spectacle of young women, with set jaws, eyes strained tensely on a ball, a fierce battle-look gripping their features, their hands clutching at some or

other instrument, their arms engaged in striking and beating, their legs disposed in coarse ungainly attitudes, is an object-lesson in all that is ugly in action and unwomanly in mode.

The need, said Kenealy, was for women to direct vital power into making a splendid race. For the sake of the nation women should be 'house-proud, home-abiding, faithful wives and admirable mothers'.[109]

Elizabeth Sloan-Chesser

It has become a platitude to say that over-exercise must be avoided. But it cannot be too frequently repeated that whilst moderate exercise will improve the vitality and the health of every organ in the body, exercise carried to the point of fatigue and strain may do irreparable harm.[110]

Despite her own success in becoming a medical doctor and her claims in support of female emancipation, Dr Elizabeth Sloan-Chesser joined Kenealy in extolling the sacrifice demanded by motherhood and in envisioning a eugenic ideal in which the home was the cradle of the race, with the production of a great race 'the Empire's first line of defence'.[111] Any woman disagreeing with this social mandate, suggested Sloan-Chesser, must be abnormal.[112]

Sloan-Chesser wrote extensively (if less hysterically than Kenealy) about health and exercise for girls and women, and particularly reflected the new emphasis upon efficiency and good citizenship. Without good health, she explained, a woman was a less useful member of society, a less capable worker and a less efficient mother. Indeed, if she became ill, it was probably her own fault! She criticized the female tendency to neglect muscular exercise after the school years. Every woman should spend part of her day practising some physical culture. The best sort, she explained, should serve a useful purpose. Domestic work, from sweeping and dusting to making beds, was very useful if done methodically and energetically with the windows open. Walking was ideal exercise. For the sedentary, fifteen minutes of simple exercise night and morning combined with a daily walk in the fresh air provided the minimum exercise required to keep a woman in health.[113]

Sloan-Chesser believed that both physical culture and manual training should play a larger role at school in order to lay the foundation of efficient home-makers. She recommended that young girls of six and seven be first allowed to romp and play in the open air like young barbarians before being restrained as they matured. At adolescence the strain of growth and educational pressure began to take their toll, thus work and play had to be carefully regulated. Sloan-Chesser felt that at this time physical training and hygiene education became critically important, and that the adolescent girl should be trained to pay attention to her body but restrained from giving out more energy in study than she could afford. Her health was, after all, 'more precious than knowledge'.[114]

The type and amount of sport and physical culture employed had to be measured carefully. It was more dangerous for girls to overstrain themselves than for boys but no girl could develop physically on the best lines without playing some games. Running and jumping could be practised in moderation. Swimming was desirable, cycling appropriate if the saddle was well positioned and speed and distance regulated. Hockey was suspect because it overtired girls. Cricket was a first-rate game for girls and lawn tennis and fencing (for girls over twelve) were also favoured. To these could be added calisthenics in the form of Swedish drill and dancing.

Chesser completed her prescriptions for female physical culture with five health hints which epitomized medical attitudes towards female sport and exercise in the early twentieth century and which have proved enduring.

1. Regulation – many people injure themselves by going in for too strenuous exercise.
2. Over-fatigue – excessive exercise will injure the nervous system and may cripple the heart.
3. Rest – periods of rest should always be taken after games or physical exertion for recuperation and repair.
4. Diet – during training, diet should be regulated.
5. Clothing – girls should wear short, well-cut skirts with a proper sports blouse or jersey.[115]

The fear that excessive athletics and gymnastics would harm both individual and race thus coloured the exercise prescriptions of Elizabeth Sloan-Chesser, Arabella Kenealy and other influential women doctors such as Mary Scharlieb. Overindulging in games, the latter claimed, would produce a 'neuter' girl disinclined to maternity.[116] Where exercise was concerned, balance was the key, 'for no human being ought to live a one-sided life . . . The ideal woman is neither the girl who spends her life playing games, riding horses or training dogs, nor is she the girl who spends her day in uninterrupted study.' Once a young woman's education was complete, a female medical adviser could ensure that she was physically fit for the obligations of married life and that prospective marriage partners were fit for 'the production of healthy children for the service of the state'.[117]

Angenette Parry

This is peculiarly the age of the athletic girl.[118]

In the United States Angenette Parry, a graduate of the Women's Medical College of the New York Infirmary, summarized contemporary medical thinking on the relation of athletics to female reproductive life at a 1911 New York Academy of Medicine meeting. Though it is difficult to define athletics, she wrote, 'it behooves us . . . to get an all around conception of the facts of the case so that where harm is being done we may sound the warning'. While it would be folly to limit the athletic activities which could mean the salvation of women from childhood to old age, she continued, it was important for physicians to direct and control the situation so that:

> our growing girls . . . shall have all the joy and exhilaration of increasing out-of-door life . . . the whole woman invigorated by intelligent athletic activities, quickened circulation, improved appetite, a better balanced nervous system, and a saner outlook on life and its responsibilities . . . In this athletic age, we must face the responsibility of intelligently advising women young and old along athletic lines.[119]

Surveying the opinions of obstetricians, college physicians, and directors of physical training concerning the effect of athletics upon female reproductive functioning, Parry concluded that menstrual wellbeing was enhanced by moderate physical activity, although girls could injure themselves seriously by immoderate sport and intercollegiate contests. (There was unanimous agreement concerning the nervous physical strain of the latter.) In the case of childbirth, most of Parry's respondents believed labour to be favoured by moderate athletics, although a number claimed that excessive exercise hindered labour.

> A woman who has had wise, graduated physical training up to what may be called moderate athletics . . . is in the best possible shape for easy, uncomplicated labour, rapid convalescence, with the ability to nourish her own child generously . . . The children of such mothers should . . . be of the best quality as to health and vigour.

In addition to labour difficulties, uterine displacements were often blamed upon strenuous competitive games, violent activity and heavy lifting. The important thing, medical authorities agreed, was that women needed appropriate muscular training, and if they would not do 'normal, manual work', i.e., housework, then the next best thing was athletics.

The physician would decide what constituted 'moderate' athletics and then supervise girls and women throughout their schooling and childbearing years. Each girl would then have

> the advantage of a thorough grounding in the physiological facts essential to her highest physical development. She should be fully aware of the inevitable penalties to be paid for carelessness, recklessness and exercise too violent or stimulating for her individual organization. She should understand clearly what she may and may not do during the menstrual period.

It was essential, said Parry, that the female medical profession do its full duty in advising and training 'our splendid army of American girls into the highest type of physical perfection possible for womanhood and motherhood'.[120]

The impact of female physicians upon women's health and prescriptions for exercise

If there was any party line among the first and second generation of women doctors it was that women had a right to good health and a responsibility to maintain that health in order to be a better mother. Many early pioneers dedicated their energies to the practice of a social medicine that sought to improve women's health and strength. Exercise prescriptions formed an increasingly important part of the good hygiene they recommended so assiduously for girls and women. Their dedication to a special mission meant that many of the early female physicians did not marry, fearful perhaps that they could not 'serve two masters' while living 'by and for the people'.[121]

Yet, notes Burstyn, 'the historian finds it difficult to ascertain whether these women perceived themselves to be part of a movement to redefine the roles of all women, or merely as opening new options for others as deviant as themselves'.[122] Certainly the massive amount of data collected on the health of women students demonstrates the female physicians' enthusiasm for monitoring and promoting female health, and the variety of sports and physical activities which blossomed at women's schools and colleges on both sides of the Atlantic is evidence of their efforts in support of healthful activity during this era .[123] However, in collecting data and going to such lengths to refute male medical charges about female incapacity for higher education, professional work and strenuous physical activity the female doctors may have hindered their original thinking.[124] While establishing the utility of exercise during the critical periods of a woman's life, most women physicians nevertheless subscribed conscientiously to the notion that female physical exercise should be moderate and noncompetitive, and that it should develop fitness for motherhood rather than strength for independence. The legitimate function of athletic exercise was the promotion of physical fitness for a better womanhood.[125]

Although Dr Arabella Kenealy's anti-feminist diatribes against women's sports and athletics represented the conservative end of the continuum (Dyhouse calls it 'a hysterical pitch'), they were supported quite widely.[126] Despite the clear-minded, independent thinking of scientist-physicians such as Mary Putnam Jacobi,[127] most of the pioneer women doctors had a sense of social mission which saw women primarily as reproductive agents and housewives and thereby matched the views of the male medical establishment. The exercise prescriptions delivered by women doctors often mirrored those of their conservative male counterparts, assimilating notions of improving women's health through hygienic practices and moderate physical exercise.

Harrison questions whether or not we can demonstrate any impact of female physicians upon women's health during this period. In England, he suggests, there were too few of them to make a difference, although their activities might have been valuable as a restraint (real or perceived) upon the anti-feminism of so many male doctors.[128] Both in Britain and in the United States the professional status of women doctors was too insecure to support vigorous dissent from prevailing, conservative attitudes toward women and their bodies. Many women doctors were as reticent as their male colleagues in discussing female physiological facts. Elizabeth Garrett Anderson doubted whether sexual matters could be discussed with propriety except in professional journals.[129] Although Elizabeth Blackwell eventually spoke and wrote freely about sexual matters, believing women should be assisted in overcoming their ignorance and anxieties, she could not find a publisher for her *Counsel to Parents on the Moral Education of Their Children*.[130] She eventually published the work herself. The twentieth century was well underway before Christine Murrell publicly challenged the notion that man was the physiological norm and woman the deviation.[131] By then a sharp retrenchment in medical school admission quotas for women was in process, stimulated in America by Flexner's report on the reform of medical training and a new hardening of attitudes against women at work on both sides of the Atlantic.[132]

The fact that female physicians continued to be concerned with the question of female modesty (indeed, this was one of the most forceful arguments put forward by feminists and female physicians in defence of medical training for women) suggests that many of them fully accepted the very notion of Victorian delicacy and decorum so strongly endorsed by men and which contributed to keeping women enclosed in their separate sphere.[133] The women doctor's public contempt for the frivolous behaviour and poor health habits of many middle-class women often exceeded male medical establishment criticisms of the fashionable dress, sedentary behaviour and giddy social lives of women patients. 'One of the most difficult things to prescribe is a daily walk,' commented a female physician in the *Woman's Medical Journal* of 1893. 'To induce a patient to get out and walk is an almost utter impossibility. She will look at you in a hopeless, helpless sort of way and ask where she shall go, whither she shall wend her steps.'[134]

Above all, many pioneer women doctors emphasized their 'femaleness' and their special qualities of female nurturance rather than focusing upon furthering women's intellectual and physical capacity and scientific curiosity. As Dr Ann Preston remarked, 'the relative intellectual ability of the sexes is altogether an irrelevant question'.[135] What was remarkable of the thinking of these women, explains Morantz, was the degree to which their own attitudes mirrored those of their male colleagues. These professional women, she suggests, were prisoners of their time and culture, 'hampered by the limitations of and contradictions in their own ideology'.[136]

This is hardly surprising given that professions are by nature exclusionary and that once inside the pale, women physicians became subject to the professional's need to defend conservative medical theories and a shared professional perspective. This perspective ennobled motherhood and provided support for those therapeutic practices, including exercise prescriptions, thought professionally appropriate to return health, strength and purpose to women for their appointed role.

Medical culture has a powerful socialization process which tends to exact conformity as the price of participation.[137] Harrison concludes that 'far from transforming the ideas and methods of the medical profession, the American and British woman doctor seems to have accommodated herself quickly to the ethos of her male-dominated profession'.[138] Success depended partly on accepting the male model, and it can be argued that once women became doctors they became as one with men as a professional body, whatever individual capacities they retained for different action.[139] Perhaps it is these individual capacities, the actual practices and prescriptions personally tailored to the daily needs of all kinds of women, which ultimately could tell us most about late-nineteenth-century middle-class women and their physical needs and capabilities. Certainly, while many female doctors came to share essentially the same scientific and professional standards and practised medicine in fundamentally the same ways as male doctors, the importance of female culture to individual women doctors must be recognized. Many women doctors strove to preserve their distinctive femaleness even as they embraced new professional values.[140] Such women were very much both women and doctors when it came to prescribing exercise for girls and women.

In the early years of the twentieth century the success of women doctors in any medical sphere was cast in doubt as increasing anxieties over co-education (especially women's success in that domain), over-crowding in the medical profession and the Eugenics Movement helped restrict opportunities for women. Mary Putnam Jacobi noted insightfully of women doctors that 'failure could be pardoned them, but . . . success could not'.[141] She realized that the success of women physicians depended largely upon their adoption of male curricula, clinical standards and procedures. Critics of female education, however, argued that it had been a mistake to unsex women by allowing them to be educated like men.[142] The strident anti-feminist ideology which flourished in the early twentieth century renewed with fervour the argument that motherhood and housekeeping, not the professions and especially not the medical profession, were the legitimate careers of women.

No one articulated this position more clearly than the psychologist G. Stanley Hall, who in 1908 was invited to address the graduating class of the Boston College of Physicians and Surgeons. His speech, notes Walsh, 'was unequivocally hostile to the aspiring woman doctor as he reiterated the old stereotypes of feminine hysteria and menstrual disability'.[143] As one measure of the power that these traditional stereotypes held over the popular mind and the way in which they were used by the male medical establishment and other experts of the body, the first half of the twentieth century became 'an era of stagnation and even regression for women in medicine'.[144] This situation was inevitably reflected in popular middle-class attitudes towards women's bodies and the perceived boundaries of desirable female exercise and sport.

Notes

1 Kate Campbell Hurt Mead, M.D., *Medical Women of America, A Short History of the Pioneer Medical Women of America and a Few of Their Colleagues in England*, Froben Press, New York, 1933, p. 43.

2 Cora Bagley Marrett, 'On the evolution of women's medical societies', *Bulletin of the History of Medicine*, LIII, no. 3, Fall 1979, p. 435.

3 Clelia Mosher claimed there were 7,387. Clelia Duel Mosher, M.D., *Woman's Physical Freedom*, (2nd ed.), The Women's Press, New York, 1923, (1st edition, 1915), p. 10; Ruth J. Abram, ed., *Send us a Lady Physician, Women Doctors in America, 1835–1920*, W. W. Norton, New York, 1985, p. 57.

4 James Bryce, 'The American Commonwealth II', Ernest Earnest, *The American Eve in Fact and Fiction, 1775–1914*, University of Illinois Press, Urbana, IL., 1974, pp. 589–90.

5 Census of Great Britain, Parliamentary Papers, Cd 7018, lxxvii, 1913, p. 552; Harrison, 'Women's health and the women's movement', Webster, ed., *Biology, Medicine and Society*, p. 51; Ellsworth lists 477 English women doctors in 1911, of whom 382 were married, p. 293; Smith quotes *The Physician and Surgeon, General Practitioner*, as noting the numbers for 1901 as 212, and for 1911, 477. Smith, *The People's Health*, p. 382; Mary Putnam Jacobi explained that the difference in numbers of women physicians in England and the United States was due to the fact that in America the admission of women to medicine was effected in response to a popular demand whereas in Europe it came from above, from the deliberations of small groups of highly cultivated people. Thus in Europe, 'women have had the education but not the patients, and in America they have had the patients and not the education.' Mary Putnam Jacobi, on the opening of the Johns Hopkins Medical School to Women, *Century Magazine*, CDXI, 1, February 1891, p. 634.

6 Daniel Scott Smith, 'Family limitation, sexual control and domestic feminism in Victorian America', Hartman and Banner, eds., *Clio's Consciousness*.

7 Jill Conway, 'Women reformers and American culture, 1870–1930', *Journal of Social History*, V, no. 2, Winter 1971–72, p. 166.

8 Alhough Elizabeth Blackwell never married (nor indeed did any of her sisters), she never expressed criticism of marriage or rejected the institution outright. She replaced notions of marriage with a profound sense of social mission and applied all her talents to her medical career. Horn, 'Sisters worthy of respect', p. 367.

9 Mary B. Mahowald, 'Sex-role stereotypes in medicine', *Hypatia*, II, no. 2, Summer 1987, pp. 21–38.

10 Elizabeth Blackwell, quoted in Elizabeth Cady Stanton *et al.*, eds., *History of Woman Suffrage*, 6 vols., Fowler and Wells, New York, 1881–1922, Vol. 1, pp. 90–91.

11 Forster, *Significant Sisters*, p. 57.

12 Elizabeth Blackwell, *Pioneer Work in Opening the Medical Profession to Women*, Longmans, Green & Co., London, 1895, p. 176.

13 See the discussion in W. W. Parker, M.D. 'Woman's place in the Christian

world and superior morally, inferior mentally to man not qualified for medicine or law the contrariety and harmony of the sexes', *Transactions of the Medical Society of the State of Virginia*, 1892, pp. 86–107.

14 Regina Markell Morantz, 'Feminism, professionalism and germs: The thought of Mary Putnam Jacobi and Elizabeth Blackwell', *American Quarterly*, XXXIV, no. 5, Winter 1982, p. 467.

15 Rhoda Truax, *The Doctors Jacobi*, Little, Brown & Co., Boston, 1952, pp. 131–132; Mary Putnam Jacobi, 'Specialism in Medicine', Victor Robinson, *Pathfinders in Medicine*, Medical Life Press, New York, 1929, p. 358.

16 Jacobi, quoted in Morantz, 'Feminism, professionalism and germs', p.473; Jacobi, 'Annual Address Delivered at the Commencement of the Woman's Medical College of the New York Infirmary, May 30, 1883', *Archives of Medicine*, X, 1883, pp. 59–71.

17 Morantz-Sanchez comments that this central theme in the story of women in medicine, the tension between 'feminism' and 'morality' on the one hand and 'professionalism' and 'science' on the other, has plagued women physicians up to the present day. Morantz, 'Feminism, professionalism and germs', p. 472.

18 Morantz, Pomerleau and Fenichel, eds., *In Her Own Words*, pp. 20 and 21.

19 Although this is not a comprehensive overview of women doctors, I have tried to select those who are representative of the professional orientations that have been discussed, of the different environments in which they practised, and of medical women's attitudes towards women and exercise on both sides of the Atlantic from the mid-nineteenth century to the first decades of the twentieth century. Generalizations about the experiences of women physicians are possible, Morantz-Sanchez suggests, at least on the basis of impressionistic evidence. *Sympathy and Science*, p. 92.

20 Blackwell, *Extracts from the Laws of Life*, pp. 189–190.

21 Actually a woman disguising herself as a man and calling herself James Barry had secured a diploma in medicine from the University of Edinburgh in 1812 and pursued a distinguished career as a military doctor until her death. Esther Pohl Lovejoy, *Women Doctors of the World*, The Macmillan Co., New York, 1957, p. 130.

22 Elizabeth Blackwell, M.D., *Lectures on the Laws of Life with Special Reference to the Physical Education of Girls*, 2nd edition, Sampson Low, Son and Marston, London 1871, p. 94.

23 Elizabeth Blackwell, M.D., *Laws of Life with Special Reference to the Physical Education of Girls*, G. P. Putnam, New York, 1852.

24 Blackwell, *Pioneer Work in Opening the Medical Profession*, p. 194.

25 Rachel Baker, *The First Woman Doctor: The Story of Elizabeth Blackwell, M.D.*, George G. Harrap & Co. Ltd., London, 1946, p. 131.

26 Smith, *The People's Health*, p. 381.

27 Wilson, *Lone Woman*, p. 285.

28 Blackwell, *Laws of Life*, 1871, pp. 126, 137, 168 and 164.

29 Blackwell, *Laws of Life*, 1871, p. 102.

30 Blackwell, *Laws of Life*, 1871, p.35.

31 Nancy Ann Sahli, 'Elizabeth Blackwell: A biography', Ph.D. diss., University of Pennsylvania, 1974, p. 123.

32 Elizabeth Blackwell, 'The religion of health', Lecture delivered at St. George's Hall, London, Feb. 9, 1871 in Blackwell, *Essays in Medical Sociology*, Vol 1, p. 229.

33 Blackwell, *Laws of Life*, 1871, p. 31.

34 Mary St. J. Fancourt, *They Dared to be Doctors; Elizabeth Blackwell, Elizabeth Garrett Anderson*, Longmans Green and Co., London, 1966, p. 127.

35 Lucy M. Hall, 'Higher education of women', pp. 614–615.

36 Blackwell, *Laws of Life*, 1871, pp. 143, 171 and 174.

37 Blackwell, *Laws of Life*, 1871, p. 247.

38 Blackwell, *Lectures on The Laws of Life*, 1858, published again in 1871.

39 Blackwell, *Opening the Medical Profession*, p. 227.

40 Lovejoy, *Women Doctors*, p. 132.

41 Banned from British medical schools, Garrett eventually obtained a licence to practice from the Apothecaries Hall and then had to obtain her degree in Paris. Although the battle for admission to medical school was won later by Sophia Jex-Blake, it was not until 1876 that teaching hospitals were persuaded to accept women students.

42 Elizabeth Garrett Anderson, Inaugural Address, London School of Medicine, October 1, 1877, quoted in Davenport Adams, *Woman's Work and Worth*, p. 475.

43 Elizabeth Garrett, M.D., 'Miscellanea', *Englishwoman's Journal*, 12 October 1868, pp. 151–152.

44 Elizabeth Garrett, *The Times*, 12 Nov. 1870.

45 Garrett Anderson quoted in Barbara Stephen, *Emily Davies and Girton College*, Constable, London 1927, p. 257–8.

46 Garrett Anderson, 'Sex in mind', p. 593.

47 Elizabeth Garrett Anderson, 'Puberty' and 'Menopause', D. Chalmers Watson, ed., *Encyclopaedia Medica*, Green and Sons, London, 15 vols., 1899–1910.

48 Mary Putnam Jacobi, M.D., 'Mental action and physical health', Brackett, ed., *The Education of American Girls*, 1893, pp. 255–306.

49 Jacobi, 'Mental action', p. 297.

50 Mary Putnam Jacobi, 'Social aspects of the readmission of women into the medical profession', paper presented to the First Woman's Congress of the Association for the Advancement of Women, New York, 1874, p. 169.

51 Jacobi, *The Question of Rest*, p. 19.

52 Jacobi, 'Shall women practice medicine?', pp. 52–75.

53 Leach, *True Love and Perfect Union*, p. 155.

54 Jacobi, 'Mental action', p. 303; Mary Putnam Jacobi, quoted by Laura Liebhardt, M.D. 'Our schoolgirl', *Woman's Medical Journal*, 1, no. 2, 1893, p. 212.

55 Truax, *The Doctors Jacobi*, p. 208.

56 Showalter, in *The Female Malady* describes how female writer Louisa Lowe campaigned in England in the 1870s and 80s against the lunacy laws and was the first to suggest the placement of women doctors in female lunatic asylums. 'Except as occasional consultants,' she suggested 'the less men doctors have to do with female lunatics the better.' Louisa Lowe, *The Bastilles of England; or, The Lunacy Laws at Work*, Crookenden, London, 1883, p. 137.

57 Mead, *Medical Women of America*, p. 59.
58 Elizabeth Blackwell was one of many women who initially earned their living as school teachers. Anna Howard Shaw wrote vividly of her early struggles for an education and her years as a 'schoolmarm' in order to support her family and pay for her studies to become an M.D. at Boston University. Anna Howard Shaw, M.D., *One Story of a Pioneer*, Harper and Bros., New York, 1915; Morantz-Sanchez, *Sympathy and Science*, p. 151.
59 In England, too, as Gathorne-Hardy has pointed out, if one of the most potent arguments against girls receiving a decent education was that they were too weak, then, as well as proving they were not, now schools and colleges could take pains to make them stronger. This attitude was at the root of most of the early games activities at girls' schools and colleges. Jonathan Gathorne-Hardy, *The Public School Phenomenon, 1597–1977*, London, 1977, pp. 168–170. See also McCrone, 'Play up, Play up, and play the game', *Fair Sex*, p. 104.
60 Burstall, *The Education of Girls*, p. 149.
61 Atkinson, 'Fitness, feminism and schooling', *The Nineteenth-Century Woman*, p. 110; Sara Burstall, 'Medical inspection', in Sara Burstall and M. A. Douglas, eds., *Public Schools for Girls*, Longmans, London, 1911, pp. 220–225. In practice, Dorothy Ainsworth recorded, a gymnastics teacher was usually hired to do the actual teaching of physical education, although as long as systems of gymnastics were based upon medical diagnoses, a resident female physician was thought absolutely essential to oversee the health and hygiene of college students. Dorothy S. Ainsworth. *The History of Physical Education in Colleges for Women*, A.S. Barnes and Co., New York, 1930, pp. 61–70.
62 Roberta J. Park, 'Edward M. Hartwell and Physical Training at The Johns Hopkins University, 1879–1980', *Journal of Sport History*, XIV, Spring 1987, p. 116.
63 Alice T. Hall, quoted in E. Hitchcock, 'Some principles regarded as essential in the direction of the department of physical education and hygiene', Isabel C. Barrow, ed., *Report of the Discussions and Papers of the Physical Training Conference*, George H. Ellis, Boston, 1899, p. 60. See also Park, 'Sport, gender and society', *Fair Sex*, p. 80; The Swedish system of Per Henrik Ling took its place in American and British schools and colleges, following or adding to the German gymnastics system, the new gymnastics of Dio Lewis and the systems of Delsarte and Sargent. The system became firmly established in both Britain and the United States and was very closely linked to medical supervision and monitoring of students. Paul Atkinson, 'The feminist physique: Physical education and the medicalization of women's education', Mangan and Park, *Fair Sex*, p. 48. See also Peter C. McIntosh, *Physical Education in England Since 1800*, G. Bell and Sons, London, 1952, pp. 129–131.
64 'A woman who stuck it out', *Literary Digest*, LXXXV, 4, April 1925, pp. 64–70. Mosher emulated Elizabeth Blackwell in other ways too, by not marrying and by adopting a child and approximating traditional family life with a female companion, Lucy Hall, who was also a doctor. Florence Hazzard, 'Heart of the oak', typescript biography of Eliza Mosher in the Eliza Mosher

MSS, Michigan Historical Collections, p. 15; This relationship, speculates Morantz-Sanchez was not intense, and appeared to be more of a mentor-novitiate partnership than a passionate attachment. *Science and Sympathy*, p. 133.

65 Hazzard, 'Heart of the Oak', p. 10.

66 22 May, 1887, Eliza Mosher MSS, Michigan Historical Collections.

67 Dr. Eliza M. Mosher. 'Memorial', *Bulletin of the Medical Women's National Association*, 23 January, 1929, pp. 6–13.

68 Dorothy McGuigan, *A Dangerous Experiment, One Hundred Years of Women at the University of Michigan*, University of Michigan Press, Ann Arbor, 1970, p. 47.

69 Morantz, Pomerleau and Fenichel, eds., *In Her Own Words*, p. 20.

70 Dudley Sargent led the field in developing anthropometric measures for the purpose of standardizing health and his system was used in schools and colleges around the country. Dudley A. Sargent, 'The Physical Development of Women', *Scribner's Magazine*, 5 Feb, 1889, pp. 172–185; *Handbook of Developing Exercises*, Rand, Avery, Boston, 1882.

71 Eliza M. Mosher. *Proceedings of the American Association for the Advancement of Physical Education*, 1892, Press of the Springfield Printing and Binding Co., Springfield, Mass, 1893, pp. 116–133; Also discussed in Jessie Hubbell Bancroft, 'Eliza M. Mosher, M.D.', *Medical Woman's Journal*, XXXII, 5 May 1925, pp. 122–129.

72 McGuigan, *Dangerous Experiment*, p. 64.

73 Bancroft, 'Eliza M. Mosher, M.D.', p. 128; Elizabeth M. Mosher, 'The health of American women', Benjamin Austin, ed., *Woman; Her Character, Culture and Calling*, Book and Bible House, Brantford, 1888, p. 245. One cannot help noticing the similarity of these health rules to those proclaimed by current health experts as the right road to health, wellness and long life. See for example, a discussion of longevity's lucky seven in Breslow and Somers, 'The lifetime health-monitoring program, a practical approach to preventive medicine', *New England Journal of Medicine*, CCXCVI, March 1977.

74 Lucy M. Hall, 'Higher education of women', p. 615; Lucy M. Hall, M.D., 'Physical training of girls', *Popular Science Monthly*, XXVI, February 1885, p. 496.

75 Hall, 'Higher education', pp. 614 and 615.

76 See for example, Jane Frances Dove, 'Cultivation of the body', in Dorothy Beale, Lucy Soulsby and Jane Frances Dove, *Work and Play in Girls Schools*, London, 1898, p. 416; *Health Statistics of Female College Graduates*, Massachusetts Bureau of Labor Statistics, Boston, 1885; Mrs. Henry Sidgwick, *Health Statistics of Women Students of Cambridge and Oxford and of Their Sisters*, Cambridge, 1890; Willystine Goodsell, *The Education of Women: Its Social Background and Its Problems*, New York, 1923.

77 Eliza M. Mosher, 'The health of American women', p. 240.

78 Eliza M. Mosher, 'The better preparation of our women for maternity', *Women's Medical Journal*, XII, Sept. 1902, p. 8.

79 Bancroft, 'Eliza M. Mosher, M.D.', pp. 122–29.

80 For example, longitudinal records of her students' height over a thirty-year period showed that college freshmen had gained 15 inches in height. Clelia

Duel Mosher, 'Some of the causal factors in the increased height of college women', *Journal of the American Medical Association*, LXXXI, August 1923, pp. 528–535.

81 Duel Mosher, *Woman's Physical Freedom*, p. 17.

82 Duel Mosher, 'Normal menstruation', p. 178.

83 Duel Mosher, 'A physiologic treatment of congestive dysmenorrhea and kindred disorders associated with the menstrual function', *American Medical Association*, 25 April 1914; 'Functional periodicity in women and some modifying factors', *California Journal of Medicine*, January–February 1911, pp. 1, 4 and 6; Mosher, *Physical Freedom*, p. 19.

84 Hollingworth, *Functional Periodicity*, pp. 95 and 97.

85 Mosher, quoted in Hollingworth, *Functional Periodicity*, p. 10.

86 Mosher, *Physical Freedom*, p. 47.

87 Mosher, *Physical Freedom*, pp. 80 and 87.

88 Atkinson, 'Feminist physique', *Fair Sex*, p. 54.

89 Shakespeare, quoted in Arabella Kenealy, *Feminism and Sex Extinction*, p. 126.

90 Mary Wood Allen, *What Every Woman Ought to Know*, The Vir Publishing Company, Philadelphia, 1913, p. 220.

91 Elizabeth Sloan-Chesser, M.D., *Woman, Marriage and Motherhood*, Methuen & Co. Ltd., London, 1913, p. 201; Havelock Ellis, *The Task of Social Hygiene*, London, pp. 148–149; The birthrate had been declining steadily in England in the last two or three decades of the 19th century, stimulating much debate about national efficiency. G. F. McCleary, *The Maternity and Child Welfare Movement*, London, 1935, p. 5; M. Hewitt, *Wives and Mothers in Victorian Industry*, London, 1958; See also Dyhouse, 'Good wives and little mothers', pp. 21–35; Anna Davin, 'Imperialism and motherhood', *History Workshop*, V, Spring 1978, p. 10; Similarly, in America census returns in Massachusetts showed a drop in the birth rate among native Americans. Nathan Allen, 'The normal standard of women for propagation', *American Journal of Obstetrics*, IX, April 1876, pp. 1–39; Ellis, *Determinants of Puritan Stock*.

92 Carol Dyhouse, 'Social Darwinistic ideas and the development of women's education in England, 1888–1920', *History of Education*, V, no. 1, 1976, pp. 46–47.

93 *Report of the Inter-Departmental Committee on Physical Deterioration*, Vol I, London, HMSO, 1904, p. xxxii.

94 Alice Ravenhill, 'Eugenic ideals for motherhood', *Eugenics Review*, I, 1909–10; C. W. Saleeby, *Parenthood and Race Culture*, Mitchell Kennerley, London, 1909; William Whetham and Catherine Whetham, *The Family and the Nation*, Longmans and Green, London, 1909, and *Heredity and Society*, Longmans and Green, London, 1912; Catherine Whetham, *The Upbringing of Daughter*, Longmans and Green, London, 1917.

95 Edwin A. Ross, 'The causes of racial superiority', *Annals of the American Academy of Political and Social Sciences*, XVIII, 1901, pp. 85–86.

96 Karl Pearson, 'The woman question', *The Ethic of Free Thought*, London, 1888, p. 371.

97 Karl Pearson, 'Woman and labour', *Fortnightly Review*, May 1894, p. 576.

98 Pearson, 'The woman question', p. 372; Herbert Spencer in *The Principles of*

Biology, Vol. II, New York. D. Appleton, 1867, pp. 485–486.

99 Nathan Allen, 'Physical degeneracy', *Journal of Psychological Medicine*, IV, 1889, pp. 725–764.

100 G. Stanley Hall, *Youth: Its Education, Regimen and Hygiene*, New York, 1906, p. 280.

101 Havelock Ellis, *The Task of Social Hygiene*, London, 1912, p. 6; Saleeby, *Woman and Womanhood*, p. 6.

102 Duffin has shown how, when twentieth-century feminists were seen to present a challenge to the prevailing definition of women's place and social function, their place in the natural order was affirmed all the more strongly. The biological and medical arguments became more explicitly formulated, and the boundaries were more sharply drawn. Lorna Duffin, 'The conspicuous consumptive: Woman as an invalid', Delamont and Duffin, eds., *Nineteenth-Century Woman*, p. 128.

103 McCrone, 'Play up', *Fair Sex*, p. 116.

104 Burstall, 1911, *English High Schools for Girls*, p. 98.

105 Jane Walker, 'Athletics for girls', *Women Workers: The Papers Read at the Conference Held at Tunbridge Wells, 1906*, P.S. King, London, 1906, p. 100.

106 Arabella Kenealy, 'Woman as athlete', *Nineteenth Century*, XLV, 1896, p. 642.

107 Arabella Kenealy, *Feminism and Sex Extinction*, T. Fisher Unwin Ltd., London, 1920, p. 278.

108 Kenealy, *Sex Extinction*, pp. 110, 111, 114, 119, 120.

109 Kenealy, *Sex Extinction*, pp. 128, 135–7, 139, 278.

110 Elizabeth Sloan-Chesser, M.D., *Physiology and Hygiene for Girls' Schools*, G. Bell & Sons Ltd., London, 1914, p. 155.

111 Sloan-Chesser, *Woman, Marriage and Motherhood*, p. 273; Elizabeth Sloan-Chesser, M.D., *Perfect Health for Women and Children*, Methuen & Co. Ltd., London, 1912, p. 54.

112 Sloan-Chesser, *Woman, Marriage and Motherhood*, p. 269.

113 Sloan-Chesser, *Perfect Health*, pp. 3, 15.

114 Sloan-Chesser, *Perfect Health*, p. 98.

115 Sloan-Chesser, *Physiology and Hygiene*, pp. 156, 126.

116 Mary Scharlieb, M.D., 'Adolescent girlhood under modern conditions, with special reference to motherhood', *Eugenics Review*, I, April 1909 – January 1910, p. 179.

117 Mary Scharlieb, M.D., *The Seven Ages of Woman: A Consideration of the Successive Phases of a Woman's Life*, Cassell and Co., London, 1915, pp. 30, 52 and 69.

118 Angenette Parry, 'The relation of athletics to the reproductive life of women', *American Journal of Obstetrics and Diseases of Women and Children*, LXVI, no. 3, September 1912, p. 342.

119 Parry, 'The relation of athletics', pp. 342 and 346.

120 Parry, 'Athletics', pp. 346, 351–2, 356, 357.

121 Gertrude Baillie, 'Should professional women marry?', *Women's Medical Journal*, II, February 1894.

122 Joan N. Burstyn, *Victorian Education and the Ideal of Womanhood*, Croom Helm, London, 1980, p. 147.

Female physicians

123 Mary Roth Walsh, 'The quirls of a woman's brain', in Hubbard, Henifin and Fried, eds., *Biological Woman*, pp. 241–264; see also, Brackett, 1874, *The Education of American Girls*.
124 Burstyn, *Victorian Education*, p. 151.
125 Christine M. Murrell, *Womanhood and Health*, Mills and Boon Ltd., London, 1923, p. 112.
126 Dyhouse, 'Social Darwinistic ideas', p. 43.
127 Mary Putnam Jacobi wrote 128 articles for medical journals and magazines and nine books. Kate Campbell Hurd-Mead, *Medical Women of America*, Froeben Press, New York, 1933, p. 77.
128 Harrison, 'Women's health and the women's movement', pp. 53–54.
129 Garrett Anderson, quoted in Harrison, 'Women's Health', p. 21.
130 Elizabeth Blackwell, *Counsel to Parents on the Moral Education of Their Children*, F.J. Parsons, Hastings, 1878.
131 Murrell, *Womanhood*, p. 89.
132 Walsh, 'Quirls', p. 259.
133 Morantz, 'The lady and her physician', in *Clio's Consciousness*, p. 48.
134 Editorial comment on 'the exercise question', *Woman's Medical Journal*, 1, no. 12, 1893, p. 237.
135 Ann Preston, *Valedictory Address*, A. K. Terrlinus, Philadelphia, 1858, p. 8.
136 Morantz, Pomerleau and Fenichel, eds., *In Her Own Words*, pp. 5 and 25.
137 Martin, *The Woman in the Body*, p. 13.
138 Harrison, 'Women's health', p. 55.
139 Delamont, in Delamont and Duffin, *The Nineteenth-Century Woman*, p. 52; Forster, *Significant Sisters*, p. 89.
140 Virginia D. Drachman, *Hospital with a Heart. Women Doctors and the Paradox of Separatism at the New England Hospital, 1862–1969*, Cornell University Press, Ithaca, NY, 1984, p. 13.
141 Jacobi, 'Women in medicine', *Woman's Work in America*, p. 196.
142 Grant Allen, 'Plain words on the woman question', p. 452.
143 Walsh, *Doctors wanted*, p. 203.
144 Walsh, *Doctors wanted*, p. 237; Virginia Drachman cautions that it is also important to realize the impact of the transformation of American medicine on the lives of women doctors in the early twentieth century, as well as the effects of discrimination and professionalism. Most of the literature on this transformation, she notes, has paid little attention to women doctors. Drachman, *Hospital With a Heart*, p. 12.

Part Three

**Radical views on
medical wisdom
and physical culture**

6

Escape from freedom:
G. Stanley Hall's totalitarian views
on female health
and physical education

> Missionaries, whether of philosophy or of religion, rarely make rapid way, unless their preachings fall in with the prepossessions of the multitude of shallow thinkers.[1]

The turn of the century brought with it a renewal, and indeed an expansion, of the biological deterministic views which had been used to circumscribe the movement of women for most of the previous century. Rather than ushering in a new era of emancipation for women, the early 1900s were, in a number of ways, characterized by a regression to the more extreme notions of female inferiority and sex differences that had distinguished the 1860s and 70s. The trend was a direct reflection of the Darwinian-based eugenics movement that increasingly affected medical and popular thinking.

Eugenics, says Haller, became 'a sort of secular religion for many who dreamed of a society in which each child might be born endowed with vigorous health and an able mind'.[2] A better civilization would develop should the fit be encouraged and the unfit discouraged from propagating, and various theories were propounded to fashion this ideal. One approach was to let the unfit die out by leaving them alone and providing no medical assistance or charity. Others attempted to promote selective-breeding policies. Middle-class women, especially, were exhorted to become more productive; to turn their interests away from higher education, professional aspirations and thoughts of suffrage and economic independence, and to rededicate their energies to the serious business of scientific motherhood. Female emancipation, they were told by respectable physicians, scientists and social workers, threatened family integrity and social stability. The demise of the family would spell disaster at the national level. In America Theodore Roosevelt termed the threat 'race-suicide'.[3]

Despite its deterministic and pessimistic implications, eugenics was very much part of the Progressive movement. It began as a scientific reform in an age of reforms and was closely associated with the rise of psychology and pedagogy, sciences which were beginning to play a dominant role in the formulation of social theories and the shaping of social thought at this time. Prominent psychologists, such as G. Stanley Hall, an ardent eugenicist, played a leading role in defining the social reality of the time, promoting education as a tool of social control in much the same way as the medical authorities of the previous era had utilized medical advice and prescriptions to introduce and perpetuate their pseudo-scientific theories. While Hall joined doctors, politicians and other experts in linking the declining birth rate among the better classes to the indifferent health and lack of maternal dedication among many middle-class women, his answer to the problem of female invalidism was far broader than the advice and prescriptions of the medical profession.

Hall's vast, complicated and optimistic scheme was to create the right conditions, through socialization and the educational process, to assist evolutionary progress and thus elevate society to a superstate. Woman's role was a limited but extremely crucial one in this endeavour. With the understanding that body always took primacy over mind, women were to be assisted in improving their health and vigour through a national programme of physical training. This would lay the basis of a careful policy of selective breeding. Thus the reformative potential of physical education would become a potent means of regulating women's reproductive power in a patriarchal society bent upon evolutionary advance.

Through the voluminous discourse of fourteen books and 350 published papers, Granville Stanley Hall, professional educator, trailblazer of American psychology and father of the child-study movement, popularized a social and educational philosophy based upon a genetic psychology which gave to women 'reverent exemption from sex competition and reconsecrate[d] her to the higher responsibilities of the human race' – those of wifehood and motherhood.[4] Although Bleier claims that the ultimate effectiveness of movements and programmes can only be weakened if they rely upon theories of biological determinism,[5] Hall's romantic articulation of the rightness of nature and its implications for the developmental and educational needs of girls and women (especially their physical development) has made a lasting impact upon educational thought and practice and hence upon Western society as a whole.[6] Ideas which gave more importance to the hygienic and moral functions of physical and health education for girls than to intellectual training, critical thinking or a competitive outlook, and which de-emphasized and discouraged co-educational activity, vigorous athletic pursuits and highly organized games for adolescent girls were stamped indelibly into currency in the late nineteenth and early twentieth centuries.[7]

In an address to the National Educational Association in 1903, G. Stanley Hall reiterated establishment medical opinion that women were in danger from over-brain-work since it affected 'that part of her organism which is sacred to heredity'. In his speech he characteristically interpreted female emancipation as freedom from masculine ideals rather than freedom to share them.[8] Such an escape for females from the 'illusory' freedoms promised by higher education and professional training represented, to the influential Hall, a cause worth working for. Women, he insisted, had a procreative function in society and should dedicate themselves singlemindedly to the ideal of being the very best of what they were destined to be. Women were 'the light and the hope of the world', their only duty to promote family integrity and to breed freely.[9] National supremacy, he noted, would 'ultimately go to that country that is most fecund [for] . . . the nation that breeds best, be it Mongol, Slav, Teuton or Saxon, will rule the world in the future'.[10]

The elevation of female physicality and the deprecation of female intellectualism was fundamental to Hall's social philosophy. In his view, academic study instilled an aversion to the maternity for which a woman's body and soul were made. 'For every woman the ideal, in fact, the only full life, was marriage and motherhood – whatever interfered with that life was unethical and a sin against both the race and the highest destiny of the individual woman.'[11] Indeed, he claimed, without maternity, a woman could have no rest or peace. Her formal education, therefore, as well as her early childhood socialization must support nature in fitting her for this task and make her the 'fittest possible instrument for racial improvement'.[12]

A central theme in Hall's work was the development and explication of methods of control and educational techniques based upon scientific developmental principles. As scientific discourse about the physical requirements of the body expands, reminds Foucault, the human body is brought increasingly within the orbit of state or professional power. Within this orbit, power is exerted through a combination of disciplinary techniques and regulatory methods.[13] For Hall, neither the physician (who only knew how to address the body) nor the minister (who was obsessed with notions of supernatural intervention) had sufficient expertise to elaborate these techniques. Only the trained and experienced psychologist, imbued with genetic sense and understanding the importance of health and muscle culture, could guide the physical development and education of the female towards 'the constraint and joy of pure obligation'. Such guidance would assist her to become 'the conduit through which 'mansoul' might some day become a 'superman' in a 'superstate'.[14]

To pursue his dream of promoting progressive evolutionary advance, Hall believed that the tasks of the psychologist, the scientist and the pedagogist must all converge on learning 'first to know, and then to control' the conditions of female development. Indeed, Hall's respect for physiological development was such that he looked to it to define both the goals of education and the conditions of learning.[15]

Toward a science of human development: first to know . . .

Central to Hall's concerns for understanding and guiding the physical development and education of girls were his theories on human development. These were based upon a unique and comprehensive integration of the literature from the philosophical and natural sciences with developmental psychology.[16] Essentially, he reshaped certain aspects of popular beliefs about children and youth by combining them with new ideas in science (especially evolutionary theory) and with large scale observation of and gathering data on contemporary children's growth and habits. Hall collected his information about children through multitudinous questionnaires distributed to mothers, teachers and administrators, and by collecting and organizing sets of data concerning children's activities. Between 1894 and 1915 he and his students distributed 194 questionnaires on child-study topics. In consequence he developed a persuasive picture of adolescence and youth culture which captured the public's imagination and had a strong impact upon educational and medical theory and practice in the early years of the twentieth century on both sides of the Atlantic.[17]

In some respects Hall's image of the adolescent years has retained a long-lasting currency, imprinting itself upon educational thought and practice, particularly in physical and health education. On the other hand, his ability to tolerate only one approach to understanding reality eventually rendered his aristocratic, racist and sexist social philosophy unacceptable to many and showed his prophetic visions of educating a super-race to be anti-intellectual and anti-rational. Curti claimed that Hall's ideas simply reflected the dominant ideologies within his own society and his unconscious subservience to the existing social system.[18] Karier, however, suggests that he might better be viewed as a prophet of the twentieth century's totalitarian man. 'He not only sensed the truly reactionary longings of an alienated man, but also intuitively grasped the kind of symbols which could satisfy those longings, and in doing so, he seemed to touch the future.'[19]

Hall's dream of a super-state rested upon beliefs about selective breeding and genetic psychology which he articulated in a scientific theory of human development. He adopted the essential features of genetic psychology from Darwin's *On the Origin of Species* (1859) and *The Descent of Man* (1871) in which the theory was propounded that natural selection is the creative force of evolution, building 'adaptation in stages by preserving, generation after generation, the favourable part of a random spectrum of variation'.[20] Darwin had not, of course, initially subscribed to a progressionist aspect of the evolutionary scheme or to a rigidly determined pattern of evolutionary stages, seeing evolution rather as a complex and tangled web of relationships, its direction haphazard and open-ended.[21] His view of the process was flexible and hazy enough, however, that he was eventually persuaded to incorporate the Lamarckian doctrine into his formulations of evolutionary theory. According to Lamarck, acquired characteristics could be transmitted to future generations through reproduction and thus, through the mechanism of inheritance of acquired characteristics, social behaviour had the potential of becoming a major factor in the human evolutionary scheme.[22] Lamarckianism came to play an important role in Darwin's work 'as mounting attacks against the principle of natural selection forced him to retreat somewhat from his earlier formulations of evolutionary theory'.[23]

This notion of unilinear social evolution supplied Hall in the 1890s with the needed link between social and intellectual progress and organic mental evolution whereby the law of exercise facilitated physical and mental evolutionary progress. Indeed, Hall's Lamarckianism had its most systematic formulation in the 'recapitulation' theory of mental development.[24] In extending Haeckel's biogenetic law and Spencer's ideas to the realm of the mind, Hall assumed that the developing individual human mind retraced, in its major outlines, the mental history of the race in the same way that the development of the human embryo (ontogeny) recapitulated the physical evolutionary history (phylogeny) of its ancestors.[25] Hall believed that if he studied in detail the habits of children and then compared this data with anthropological information about primitive people, he would be able to reconstruct and thus understand man's ancestral mental history.[26]

The origin of instinct was a critical question in the Lamarckian notion for it was important to be able to assume that habits could become organized as instincts before transmission. Instincts, said Charles Ellwood, future president of the American Sociological Society, evolved through 'certain coordinations of nerve cells and muscle fibres which tend to discharge in one way rather than another, and which make personal and social development tend to take one direction rather than another'.[27] Thus instincts came to be viewed as the gradual and internalized products of habitual behaviour which, most importantly, were modifiable through appropriate mechanisms for adaptation. To Hall, the modern mind was a mass of instincts which had been acquired from primitive man and which manifested themselves at various stages of the child's development. 'Instincts,' he asserted, 'feelings, emotions, and sentiments are vastly older and more determining than the intellect . . . Moreover, they are basically right.'[28] Despite the rediscovery of Mendelian genetics in 1900,[29] these beliefs held remarkable staying power for at least the next twenty years since it was difficult for social Darwinists such as Hall to reject a comforting doctrine which guaranteed progress through accumulated individual effort. Education and gradual character development could thus become long-term instruments for the improvement of mankind.[30]

Hall's boundless belief in the educational implications of both Lamarckianism and the theory of recapitulation pressed him to attempt to discover the optimal developmental moments for the introduction of new hereditary characteristics. 'Historicism, as it were, entered the psyche, bringing in its train the problem of judging among relative values and problematic directions of growth.'[31] His empirical investigations and theoretical suppositions led him first to articulate five basic principles which underlay the science of all human development and then apply them to the special conditions of female development.[32] Hall used these basic principles as a platform for explaining the particular significance of adolescence to female development, function and racial progress.

i) *Adolescence is the staging point for evolutionary advance*
Hall believed that adolescence was the only point of departure for the

superanthroid that man or woman was to become. If he could some-how co-ordinate the characteristics of childhood and youth with the development of the race, he felt he would be able to establish criteria by which to diagnose and measure arrest and retardation in the individual and the race.[33] He was persuaded by anthropologist Lewis Henry Morgan that the development of mankind could be viewed as passing through three stages from savagery to barbarism to civilization and through three corresponding stages of social organization: collectivism, individualism and then collectivism again.[34] In applying these stages to development, Hall felt that all children should be viewed as young and selfish barbarians until they reached the adolescent years which signalled a second birth and a new susceptibility to cultural influences.[35]

The adolescent stage, then, was a critical time of intervention, a plastic stage and a time of storm and stress which was infinitely malleable and responsive to the call of the future.[36]

ii) *Nature is right*
Since individual growth entailed a complete retracing of the steps of species evolution, Hall insisted that there should be no interference in the child's natural development and that the continued operation of ancient instincts during childhood should be unfettered until adoles-cence. Nature alone could lift the child to the stage of civilization at early adolescence which would complete the journey of recapitulation.[37]

iii) *Each stage of development requires catharsis*
The notion that each stage of growth was distinct, unique and inviolable and required full expression complemented the nature-is-right prin-ciple.[38] Catharsis 'required that an uncivilized trait characteristic of early racial history should be fully practised in childhood to prevent its occur-rence in adult years'.[39] There was to be no repression of psychic instincts, or full development could not take place at each stage.[40] The most critical period of life was adolescence, however, since civilization depended upon the completion of these uncertain final stages.

iv) *Physical growth is more developmentally significant than cognitive growth*
Surveying Darwin's picture of evolutionary development, Hall con-sidered the power of the intellect to be a relatively late development. It seemed clear to him, therefore, that healthy physical and emotional growth took precedence over cognitive development and that the latter

177

must often be retarded since only a small elite showed intellectual promise.[41] Man, he agreed with Schopenhauer, was at best one third intellect and two thirds will, and muscles were the true organs of the will.[42] 'Rational muscle culture', the development of health and a strong body must, therefore, take precedence over accumulation of knowledge.[43] 'The apple of intelligence,' he warned, 'must not be plucked at too great a cost of health, for muscles come before mind, will before intelligence, and sound ideas rest on a motor basis.'[44] A far better motto than Cicero's *vivere est cognitari* was *vivere est velle*.[45]

v) *Growth occurs unevenly in stages and nascent periods*
According to Hall's understanding of the recapitulation principle, physical growth occurred rhythmically in stages with ripening periods. A child or pre-adolescent remained on a growth plateau while passing through each of the ancestral forms and then experienced an accelerated spurt between stages. Hall called these transitions 'nascent' periods at which recapitulatory momentum and developmental energy peaked. The major difficulty, of course, was to establish the correct moment of these nascent benchmarks in order to guard and nurture their development.[46] Furthermore, since he claimed that each part of the body possessed a unique racial history, nascent periods or the age curve of growth had to be established for them too. Only then could the parent or teacher know 'to what degree to stimulate each part in its stage of most and least rapid growth, and how to apportion training of mind and body'.[47]

Hall observed, however, that adolescence was a 'nascent period of now or never', a critical time of muscle growth fraught with danger and environmental and emotional pressures – a time more than any other requiring 'protection, physical care, [and] moral and intellectual guidance'.[48]

The special conditions of female development

The ideological screen through which Hall viewed evolutionary human development particularly coloured his understanding of female growth and function and how this affected educational policy and the correct nurturing of girls.

Evolutionary progress, Hall believed, had accentuated the differences between the sexes.

In savagery, women and men are more alike in their physical structure, and in their occupations, but with real progress the sexes diverge and draw apart, and the diversities always present are multiplied and accentuated.[49]

Sexual divergence, Hall agreed with Darwin, began with the lowly protozoa and steadily increased as the superior physical and mental abilities of the human male became established through sexual and natural selection. As a result women were less completely evolved than men, their physical and mental characteristics more childlike than adult.[50] Herbert Spencer further refined Darwin's argument to explain that a woman's earlier evolutionary arrest must have been due to the demands of maternity which diverted needed energy for mental and physical growth to the reproductive process.[51] 'If we read biology and the history of the race aright, the perfection of woman cannot be the perfection of man,' said Miss Findlay in support of such views, since 'the two perfections differ too much in function to be comparable'.[52]

The notion of function was a key to post-Darwinian evolutionary arguments concerning female development. Since biology must have fitted the sexes to their respective social functions, sex roles must be biologically prescribed. Nature, reminded Herbert Spencer, had fitted women to be childrearers, and men to be workers in the public domain, and had equipped them differently, physically and mentally, for these roles:

That men and women are mentally alike is as untrue as that they are alike bodily . . . To suppose that along with the unlikeness between their parental activities there do not go unlikeness of mental faculties is to suppose that here alone in all Nature there is no adjustment of special powers to special functions.[53]

Within the special functions of the female, therefore, lay the key to her special growth and development and the agenda for her particular educational needs. Through evolutionary history women had become physically weaker and, in Lamarckian fashion, maternal duties had fostered (and been emphasized as instincts by repetition) their emotional development at the expense of their intellectual growth. This explained how the female brain had been marred by disuse and why emotional traits had become deeply engrained in women. 'She better than man,' said Hall, 'represents the feelings and instincts which are higher, deeper and broader than mere mental culture . . . She is a generic being, nearer to the race and should not allow herself to lapse to a cheap idolatry of intellect.'[54]

179

Among the evolutionary explanations for sex differences, those of Geddes and Thompson particularly influenced Hall's thoughts on the matter. Their views, which extended Spencer's interpretation of the Law of Conservation,[55] were widely circulated in England, France and the USA through the publication of *The Evolution of Sex*.[56] While Spencer had claimed that 'for every individual there is an inevitable issue between the demands of parenthood and the demands of self', Geddes and Thompson asserted that this was particularly so in the female, 'being that in it a higher proportion of the vital energy is expended upon or conserved for the future and, therefore, necessarily, a smaller proportion for the purposes of the individual'.[57] Males, they deduced from their animal studies, demonstrated a highly active metabolism (katabolic) which had, since the beginning of evolution, led to larger brains and the development of greater intelligence and a stronger ability to grasp generalities. In contrast, they explained, 'females incline to sluggishness and passivity (anabolic) and possess a more quiescent metabolism with less variation and a tendency toward emotional and irrational behaviour'. Metabolically less active than men, women must consequently be psychologically less active as well.[58] In sum, this meant that 'man thinks more, woman feels more'.[59] Thus they concluded that the social order with its separate sexual spheres and characteristics was based firmly upon anabolic-katabolic biology which could not be reversed.[60] Hall readily concurred. No mortal interference in evolutionary development could obviate the biological trend towards ever greater sexual differentiation through heredity, sexual selection and acquired characteristics.[61]

The importance of adolescence: the chrysalis years

Although the links Hall perceived between ancestral evolution and individual development illustrated the historical and widening divergences in the physical and intellectual growth of men and women, they in no way contradicted the essential soundness of his five basic principles of human development or their application to the promotion of healthy growth and correct education of girls. His views concerning the critical importance of adolescence, a required deference to nature, the need for catharsis at each developmental stage, the pre-eminence of physical over cognitive growth, and the occurrence of physical growth as saltatory rather than gradual and continuous all provided important guidelines for understanding, 'first to know and then to control', female development for the betterment of mankind.[62]

To Hall, female development during childhood was largely con-temporaneous with that of boys and sexual divergence did not begin till early adolescence.[63] Thus he focused all his aspirations for the thrust to a higher plane of evolution upon adolescence – that 'golden period of life', the time of 'second birth' – and placed particular emphasis upon assisting the natural progress of female adolescence. 'Woman at her best,' he noted, 'never outgrows adolescence as man does, but lingers in it, magnifies and glorifies this culminating stage of life.' At this time, he continued, 'the floodgates of heredity seem opened and we hear from our remote forebears and receive our life dower of energy. . .Passions and desires spring into vigorous life.'[64]

The sexual development of adolescent girls rendered their physical health the focus of his chief concern, specifically the establishment of regularity in the menstrual cycle that he called the sexual rhythm. Since early adolescence was the nascent period of maximum female growth, all energies had to be conserved for the critical development of reproduc-tive maturity.[65] The first few menstruations had a particularly large influence upon the brain and the soul, and only having passed safely through the turbulent early stages of menstrual irregularity could the young woman be 'born anew'. With the healthy birth of the 'function' at adolescence, she would become 'vigorous, energetic, joyful, well . . . at the very top of her condition, most brilliant, beautiful [and] attractive to men'.[66] Miss Findlay, a firm Hall supporter, aptly termed these years the 'chrysalis years of womanhood'.[67]

The signs of adolescence occurred earlier in girls than in boys, and the changes appeared to be more marked. 'Between the ages of twelve and fifteen the girl undergoes a more or less rapid evolution from the common to the feminine type,' explained Dr Mary Scharlieb, 'while the boy remains more or less a child up to the age of fifteen and even then alters both more slowly and less completely.'[68] Hall offered two explana-tions as to why girls had a rapid growth spurt earlier than boys and ceased development earlier. Part of the sudden and early increment in girls was a trace of ancient but now deferred maternity due originally to premature male aggression. Alternatively, the larger size of girls at early adolescence might represent natural selection of those who had had the strength to resist fertilization and had acquired an instinct for coyness.[69] Whichever the explanation, however, nature (through the Law of Con-servation) decreed that girls, starting with less strength than boys and using it up more rapidly in early adolescence, would be left with less energy than boys for intellectual growth at this time. Whatever energy remained at the disposal of the female adolescent must be, according to Saleeby, 'in no small degree pledged for special purposes of the highest importance from which we cannot possibly divert them if we desire that she shall indeed become a woman'.[70]

The rapidity with which female development proceeded at this nascent stage and the uneven growth of different body parts constituted a special danger from overstimulation and excessive physical and/or mental effort. Immature tissues and organs were believed to be peculiarly unstable and more liable to be injured and distorted by overuse or wrong use than those of adults.[71] Overfatigue of any part of the body could lead to the overfatigue of the whole. Should bones grow ahead of muscles, overstrain could occur. Were the growth of the heart to lag behind, girls might fatigue easily or experience frequent fainting spells. Hall, for example, quoted studies in *Adolescence* suggesting that numerous physical disorders, including the development of eye defects and tubercular infection, took root through over-exertion at this time. Mental and nervous troubles were also common, especially hysteria and neurasthenia, which Hall saw as resulting from problems in establishing a correct balance between stored and used energy.[72] Lack of harmony in mental and moral as well as physical development also tended to cause difficulties. 'We have learnt,' reminded Scharlieb, 'that it is worse than useless to expect that girls whose mental powers are overtaxed can yet retain vigour and health of body.'[73]

Although overemphasis on mental development was held to be harmful for both sexes, it seemed to be peculiarly vicious in the case of the girl. 'Excessive intellectualism,' said Partridge, writing about the ideas of his mentor Hall, who had himself recaptured with renewed fervour the arguments of Clarke some three decades earlier, 'inculcates wrong ideals about life, and leads the girl away from the simple, plain life of home and the ideals of motherhood and wifehood without which she is certain to be neither morally nor physically a complete woman.'[74] 'The more scholastic the education of women,' Hall argued, 'the fewer children and the harder, more dangerous and more dreaded is parturition.'[75] Hall's student, Cattell, underlined Hall's anxiety. 'It is probably not an exaggeration to say that to the average cost of each girl's education must be added one unborn child.'[76]

It was at adolescence, then, in their transition to healthy womanhood, that girls were seen by Hall to be in the direst need of educational support and regimen from society. 'To understand a woman's body and soul,' he remarked, 'is a larger problem than to understand a man's, because reproduction plays a larger role in her life . . . The quality of motherhood has nowhere a more critical test than in meeting the needs of this epoch.'[77] At no time, therefore, was the correct maintenance of the relation of female body to mind, of reproduction to production, feelings to intellect, intuition to reason, evolution to devolution and nature to civilization more critical.

. . . and then to control: toward a science of education

At the presidential address of the British Child Study Association in 1905, Professor Muirhead praised the remarkable scientific findings of President Stanley Hall of Clark University and claimed that the study of the human being in his growth from early infancy up to manhood and womanhood had laid solid foundations for a science of education.[78] 'None save utter strangers to the vital ideas of Hall,' continued Geddes the same year in his review of Hall's monumental treatise, *Adolescence*, 'can fail to comprehend . . . that the Paper Age of mere book learning has virtually ended and that a new world of balanced education, of life and health, of growth and action has fully begun.'[79]

The new world of education that G. Stanley Hall conceived was an enterprise designed to give education what it had long lacked – a truly scientific basis.[80] Although attacking the deductive system builders in the name of modern science, Hall was committed to building a unified science of education through a comprehensive scheme to advance evolution by respecting nature and facilitating the human development process that he had so painstakingly outlined. By the turn of the century his criticism of traditional schooling had matured into a detailed programme of reforms for educational practice from the kindergarten to the high school.[81] Inept institutions, Hall explained, must be improved or melded into new ones in accord with the primal racial character of mankind.[82] Thus in 1901, in an address to the National Educational Association, he presented his conception of 'The ideal school as based on child study', and followed this with his views on secondary education in 'The high school as a people's college', and in his two volumes on *Adolescence*, published in 1904.

His message to educators underscored the need to follow nature, to 'see to it that education does not obstruct but rather facilitates "natural" evolution'.[83] 'The guardians of the young should strive first of all to keep out of nature's way,' he insisted, 'for a pound of health, growth and heredity is worth a ton of instruction.'[84]

One of nature's decrees was that children were endowed with very different capacities. Not all were fit to be educated or capable of intellectual effort and the sexes clearly had different capacities and functions in life.[85] 'I would bring discrimination down to the very basis of our educational pyramid', Hall stated, thus supporting sorting (though not separation of the sexes) at the earlier levels and justifying separate education for girls and boys at the high school (as well as streaming into vocational training or academic specialization). Boys, said Hall, 'are eager for specialized knowledge, while girls are not suited to it'.[86]

Early in life, kindergarten was to provide for both sexes a healthy environment for free play, exercise and idleness with special attention to nature study, music, dancing, storytelling, and training of the large muscles.[87]

> Here the body needs most attention and the soul least. . . . The child needs more mother and less teacher, freedom rather than restriction and outdoor activity more than small muscle work. Writing and even reading should be neglected before eight.[88]

Although he claimed that supreme attention to health and vigour was to be continued in the elementary school, Hall saw the years between eight and twelve as uniquely suited to 'drill, habituation and mechanism'. Muscle training of every kind was to be accomplished through manual training and games as children rehearsed the range of physical activities of their ancestors. Show and tell was to be the method of choice, not explanation. Girls and boys thus 'were to be encouraged to express cathartically their boorish impulses, drill and exercise their minds, but avoid explanations and thinking'.[89] Plentiful activity was to be the keynote of educational life rather than 'mere knowing'. The big muscles deserved the larger share of attention at this time. These years were also the time when skilful movements were most easily learned and small muscles trained. Small muscle work was best accomplished through industrial handwork for the boys and home-making activities for girls. 'This is, in fact, the one time of life when muscular power may be acquired and habits formed and made stable.'[90] 'In fine,' said Hall, 'this is the age for training, with plenty of space and time for spontaneity and voluntary action' for a 'child's animal spirits are the most reliable cues to begin his or her educability.'[91] It was also the time to begin to fit each sex for its next stage of development and to place girls under care of teachers of their own sex as their childhood drew to a close.

Hall viewed the high school not as a preparation for college but as a people's college, designed to serve both the natural interests of youth and the future needs of society.[92] Fitting for college, he claimed, was not the same as fitting for life.[93] At adolescence, natural development should be re-emphasized, particularly for girls:

> In the ideal school system, the sexes will now . . . pretty much part company. They are beginning to differ in every cell and tissue, and girls for a time need some exemption from competition. They have more power than boys to draw upon their capital of physical energy and to take out of their system more than it can afford to lose, for the individuals of one generation can consume more than their share of vigor at the expense of posterity. In soul and body, girls are more conservative; males vary, differentiate and are more radical. Reproduction requires a far larger proportion of body and function in females . . . Every girl should be educated primarily to become a wife and mother.[94]

In some respects the education for wifehood and motherhood which he espoused so strongly at the high-school level was more a series of biological or medical injunctions than a pedagogical plan.[95] In moulding the girl into the fittest possible individual for racial improvement, the emphasis became one of bodily service rather than intellectual development. 'The one word now written across the very zenith of the educational skies,' wrote Hall, 'is the word service . . . the supreme goal of all pedagogic endeavour, the standard by which all other values are measured.'[96]

Since service could not be supported without health and muscle, and the production of health depended upon sexual maturation, physical education and hygienic instruction rested at the apex of Hall's high school curricula for girls.[97] 'When her health for her whole life depends upon normalizing the lunar month', the school must provide a fitting environment 'to let Lord Nature do its beautiful, magnificent work of efflorescence'.[98] Such an environment was to be characterized by an appropriate balance of rest and physical activity, with intellectual study held to a minimum.

The all-important balance to be struck between rest and muscular activity was a critical lesson to be taught to adolescent girls through physical training and health instruction. In early adolescence particular harm could be done by overpressure in exercises and games. Supporters of Hall's views such as Mary Scharlieb commented that girls at this age 'who had hitherto enjoyed and profited from strenuous exercise ceased to profit and did their exercises languidly and badly during the time when the most momentous developments were occurring'.[99] Arabella Kenealy, too, publicly agreed with Hall that a girl at adolescence became

185

a complex of disabilities. Should she be strained by vigorous activity, sterility, dwarfed structure, blighted emotions and warped instincts might result. There was clearly a direct relation between athletic pursuits and extinction of womanly qualities.[100] One example was the contention that hockey playing could deprive girls of the future ability to breastfeed.[101] It seemed clear that although muscular activity of any kind was not to be condemned, caution was indicated:

> [for] all muscular exercise is expenditure of energy in those outward directions which are not characteristic of womanhood and which must always be subordinated . . . Exercise is excessive and should be immediately curtailed if it leads to the diminution of [the] reproductive function. This is particularly important in relation to the 'muscles of motherhood'.[102]

Excessive development of the musculatory system appeared to hurt the reproductive process. Some, as we have seen, considered bicycling a culprit.[103] On the other hand, inadequate development or atrophy of the abdominal muscles also appeared to be unfavourable to maternity and here the corset was held partly to blame.[104]

Hall drew frequent attention to establishment physicians' warnings concerning the importance of outdoor, though not excessive, physical culture. He noted with approval Clouston's popular warnings about the peculiar power of women to take more out of themselves than they could bear with too systematic exercise.[105] *Festina lente* must be the watchword for teachers of adolescent girls, he explained, agreeing with Taylor's rejection of systematic physical culture in favour of individual games, 'self-bathing in cold water [and] deep-breathing exercises once or twice a day'.[106] Swedish gymnastics were, therefore, to be abandoned along with other indoor, uniform-type exercises, and replaced by outdoor walks, free play and games in the fresh air. Boating and basketball were allowable, but without the competitive element. A girl performs her best service in her true role of sympathetic spectator rather than as fellow player, reminded Hall. All purposeful, though preferably unorganized games rather than exercises, he noted, were to be recommended, for exercises were sometimes only 'ridiculous and empty parodies invented by men rather than nature's own way of acquiring skill'.[107] Explained Saleeby in support, 'games and play of all sorts are incomparably superior to the use of dumb bells and developers. Systems of physical training are good in proportion as they approximate to play.'[108] Thus, games were to be light and exhilarating rather than strenuous and competitive.[109] Dancing (creative and folk rather than ballroom) was especially recommended, for 'no girl is educated who cannot dance'.[110]

Indeed, properly taught, dancing seemed, to Hall, far more suited to girls than many of the exercises and games borrowed from boys and deployed inappropriately in the schools. Dance, echoed his student Partridge, 'makes the best of all systems of physical culture for girls'.[111]

This glorification of motherhood and childrearing through physical education and instruction in health and sex hygiene required a sustained attack upon the notion that female secondary education was a preparation for college. True education for women, said Hall, began and ended in adolescence; the teachers of the people's college should assist nature by reaffirming the priority of the body over the mind and of procreation over intellectual development. 'Health, stamina, the capacity for play, service and procreativity were the criteria for educability.'[112] At the high school girls, now segregated from boys, 'were given the great commission to . . . take to themselves healthy mates, and obey posterity's supreme command to procreate'.[113]

If some saw Hall's conception of education as a science, others viewed it as a series of fads and crazes, coloured by his fascination for evolutionary ideas and his interest in physiology, and strung together by numerous compromises to accommodate or cope with his perceptions of the 'acids of modernity'.[114] In the final words of his autobiography, *Life and Confessions of a Psychologist*, Hall wrote, 'I have laid aside more of the illusions and transcended more of the limitations with which I started than most.'[115] Certainly, comment Burgess and Borrowman, his opportunistic tendencies outweighed his ability to remain loyal to one faith.[116] Although he may have believed himself to be a realist dedicated to scientific truths, said Josiah Royce in 1919, he had in fact constructed an explicitly idealistic theory understandable only to himself.[117]

Hall's illusions were in large measure a product of the progressive era's anxious conviction that American society had degenerated, through rapid urbanization and uncontrolled industrialization, to the point where it was facing a physical and moral emergency necessitating an urgent salvage plan of bodily renovation.[118] Hall was only one of numerous proponents of physical education at the end of the nineteenth-century and in the first decades of the twentieth who envisioned physical improvement as the necessary basis of moral and mental elevation and attempted to make explicit a form of scientific, 'muscular Christianity'.[119] Seeing soul and mind as inseparable from body, Hall elevated physical culture to the heights of religious duty. The sentiment of reverence, dependence and acquiescence, nourished in a healthy, hence dependable body, was (to him) of foremost pedagogical importance.[120] Effective education for women, therefore, was essentially a question of a healthy body, and Hall dreamed of programmes of physical training which might improve the race and lay the foundation for a policy of selective breeding. In our day, he said, 'there are many new reasons to believe that the best nations of the future will be those which give the most intelligent care to the body'.[121]

The role of women in Hall's superstate – the ultimate goal of education

America, Hall perceived in the twilight of his professional career, had allowed its delusions about the sanctity of individualism to give the nation a weak body for an otherwise healthy mind. In his utopia, Atlantis, female 'heart-formers' would correct this state of affairs by encouraging adolescent girls to develop health and stamina for their chief end in life – 'the responsibility to transmit the holy torch of life undimmed to the innumerable unborn'.[122] In sweeping Fichtian terms, Hall thus saw the ultimate goal of education as the sublimation of self for the larger good, requiring the primacy of physical culture for the service of the state over intellectual training for personal development.[123] Knowledge, in sum, was dangerous for any but rare moral geniuses, those supermen who would oversee the perfect educational state and guide the social destiny of the masses according to nature's noble purposes.[124] This, of course, meant the control and guidance by a male elite of all women who, in a historical paradise, would concentrate their energies upon becoming Nietzsche's race of superwomen.[125]

Unlike Nietzsche, however, who believed that it was only through perpetual struggle that growth occurred, and that a natural antagonism between the sexes or among opposing groups was always necessary, Hall ultimately came to view the role of his supermen as somewhat less ruthless, more compassionate and more co-operative.[126] In the 'Fall of Atlantis', reflecting his anxiety over the excesses of German militarism, Hall saw his own ideal society eventually disintegrating because of creeping individualism which destroyed the collective self.[127] Indeed, he explicitly stated that:

> I never expect to see this German system adopted as a whole in this country. Its centralization makes it forever impossible here; but the momentous lesson for us is that the one source of vitality in every educational system is at the top and not at the bottom.[128]

The power of the university, urged Hall, gave it a unique role in society and evolution, for it would train, according to nature's principles, the modern specialist, the expert who was coming to govern the modern world.[129]

Nature had demonstrated that women were not among those who should be found at the top of the educational system. Admitting that many women could possess the ability to succeed in research and in the professions, Hall none the less promoted an educational orientation for women which consistently emphasized the physical at the expense of the intellect, academic specialization and the pursuit of a professional career.[130]

Hall's legacy

In attempting to shift the focus of late nineteenth and early-twentieth-century educational endeavour from mind to body, and in the extraordinary emphasis which he placed upon health, growth and heredity and the uniqueness of the sexes, Hall provided critical support for the forces of anti-intellectualism as well as anti-feminism. 'Not a crackpot,' Stephen Gould reminds us, but 'America's premier psychologist', G. Stanley Hall extended arguments from social Darwinism, especially recapitulation, to justify a broad spectrum of elitist and sexist educational practices.[131] Long before the theory of recapitulation finally collapsed in 1920, Hall, invoking the traditional prestige and objectivity of science, had nailed notions from biological determinism to the conservative mast of educational thought and practice for females. Such notions have proved difficult to dislodge.

Lawrence Cremin has said of G. Stanley Hall that 'he injected into the mainstream of American educational thought some of the most radical and I happen to think, virulent doctrines of the twentieth-century, and there is no understanding the present apart from his contribution'.[132] Strickland and Burgess note that his educational ideas were ominously parallel to twentieth-century totalitarianism. Neither conservative nor liberal, 'he saw no more hope in holding fast to the status quo than in a forward movement along traditional lines of democratic faith'.[133]

In the choice between a school for happy, healthy people and one designed to turn out free and democratic citizens, he chose the former. 'Most people are not fit for freedom,' he argued.

> For most of us the best education is that which makes us the best and most obedient servants. This is the way of peace and the way of nature, for even if

we seriously try to keep up a private conscience at all . . . the difficulties are so great that most hasten . . . to put themselves under authority again.[134]

Hall's words, says Karier, were echoed by another charismatic leader little more than a decade after his death. Hall, like Hitler, saw the bulk of humanity as eager and willing to escape from freedom.[135] 'I am freeing man,' said Hitler, 'from the demands of a freedom and personal independence that only a few can sustain.'[136] Thus, with almost uncanny prophetic vision, Hall blue-printed National Socialism at least a decade before it was realized in Germany.[137] The role of women in what became a ruthless anti-feminist regime mirrored Hall's basic beliefs in motherhood, the family and women's special sphere. In the brave new *Volksgemeinschaft* the extreme consequences of Hall's developmental and educational theories for women could be seen in action, as anti-intellectualism, the glorification of the body and frenetic pro-natalism overwhelmed the moral sensibilities of an entire generation.[138]

Reflections of Hall's ideas in twentieth-century education stand pale by comparison, but Cremin is one of a number of historians to remind us that they have made a significant impact upon educational thought. Hall has been called a 'Darwin of the mind', a peculiar genius, madman, manic depressive, self-absorbed and sex-obsessed, a king-maker, a priestly prophet and an incurable romantic.[139] Clearly, says Karier, he was a complex person who viewed humanity, not from afar, but from a sensual biological inside.[140] This was the earthy essence (William James called it a sort of palpitating influence) with which Hall left his mark upon educational thought, lending force, with his mixed bag of science and spirit and his profound distrust of reason, individualism and democratic egalitarianism, to those conservative aspects of the American educational system which, at their extreme, have nurtured the social, racial, sexist and economic bigot.[141] His developmental theories, naturalistic views and deterministic beliefs about female uniqueness, compounded with the special cult of adolescence that he fixed so firmly in the public mind, contributed to rigid gender images about appropriate physical activities and sporting competition and to the promotion of sexist physical education practices in the high school which have demonstrated remarkable staying power, in spite of massive legislative efforts to dislodge them.

Haley's truism that 'no topic more occupied the Victorian mind than health', was particularly apt in the case of Hall.[142] The extraordinary emphasis which he placed upon adolescent female health and vigour as

190

the focus of educational endeavour is now reflected in a renewed enthusiasm for health prescriptions, aerobic fitness and life-style guidance activities in the school curriculum. Hall's 'heart-formers' can be found in high schools as health and guidance counsellors, assisting girls to cope with new 'acids of modernity' and their special physical and emotional needs in today's 'stressful' society (again, stressing female differences and unique needs compared to the male, who is always the standard).[143] His recommendation for individual life and health books to be kept as a standing witness to youth's progress and fitness for advancement also rings a modern bell.[144] Health passports, fitness profiles, calorie counters and body-weight norms are popularly furnished to adolescents in physical education classes to foster intense and, at times, narcissistic interest in their physical development, vital signs and body statistics.[145]

Although his own brand of primitivism and romantic idealism and his determination to impose a 'curious bio-logos on nature' were scorned by many of his peers, his desire to stimulate a general popular interest in body culture is echoed in the popular health and fitness trends of the last two decades.[146] The concepts of health and holiness, will and muscle culture which informed his turn-of-the-century theories, and the glorification of physical vigour and juvenile idealism over intellect and mature judgement serve admirably to support many of the tenets of the current fitness boom and to heighten interest in the health and conditioning aspects of female physical education and guidance in the schools. Sooner or later, Hall said:

> everything pertaining to education must be . . . judged from the standpoint of health, for health is what gives womanhood to woman. Physical conditioning is the best preparation for any and every new achievement. Live up to the top of your condition. In this state alone can we face, and not flee from reality.[147]

Notes

1 T.H. Huxley, 'On the natural inequality of men', *Nineteenth Century*, XXVII, Jan. 1890, p. 1.
2 Mark H. Haller, *Eugenics. Hereditarian Attitudes in American Thought*, Rutgers University Press, New Jersey, 1963, p. 3.
3 Theodore Roosevelt, 'Birth reform, from the positive, not the negative side', *Complete Works of Theodore Roosevelt*, Scribner, New York, Vol 19, 1926, p. 161; Filene, *Him/Her/Self*, pp. 41–42; Eugenic anxieties were equally strong in England. For an excellent discussion of the relationship of the Eugenics movement to the promotion of scientific motherhood through education; see Davin, 'Imperialism and motherhood'; Dyhouse, 'Social Darwinistic

ideas', and 'Good wives and little mothers'.

4 Hall, *Adolescence*, II, p. 609; for an account of Hall's ideas on the education of women, see 'Address on Founder's Day at Mt. Holyoke College', *The Mount Holyoke News*, VI, November 1896, pp. 64–72; for a complete bibliography of Hall's prolific writings see 'Bibliography of the published writings of G. Stanley Hall', Edward L. Thorndike, *Bibliographical Memoir of Granville Stanley Hall, 1846–1924*, National Academy of Sciences, Washington, DC, XII, 1928, pp. 155–180; for a useful selection of Hall's published works see Dorothy Ross, *G. Stanley Hall, the Psychologist as Prophet*, University of Chicago Press, Chicago, 1972, pp. 441–450; also, Hall's autobiography, *Life and Confessions of a Psychologist*, D. Appleton & Co., New York, 1923, which contains a list of his works, pp. 597–616.

5 Bleier, *Science and Gender*, p. 12. Bleier explains that this is so both because such theories are seriously flawed and basically scientifically meaningless and because essentialist thinking has always functioned as a central feature of ideologies of oppression. Gerda Lerner, *The Creation of Patriarchy*, Oxford University Press, Oxford 1986, pp. 12–13, demonstrates the process of oppression. What Hall said in 'Co-education in the High School' was that 'neither sex should copy nor set patterns to the other but all parts should be played harmoniously and clearly in the great sex symphony'. Lerner notes that men and women indeed live on a stage in which they act out their assigned roles, equal in importance, but the stage set is conceived, painted, defined by men. Men have written the play, directed the show, interpreted the meanings of the action. They have assigned themselves the most interesting, the most heroic parts, giving women the supporting roles. History is the story of such repeated performances.

6 Arguments based upon biological-deterministic reasoning have proven remarkably resilient. Freud, whom G. Stanley Hall introduced to America, gave renewed strength to the female anatomy-is-destiny argument, and E.O. Wilson's *Sociobiology* has reaffirmed Hall's traditionalist views on genetic heritage. Patricia Vertinsky has shown how recurring enthusiams for biological determinism have affected physical education opportunities for girls and responses to demands for equity in the world of sport. 'Biological determinism: Medicine's accomplice in defining the exercise needs of women', paper presented at Aapherd, Las Vegas, April 1987. See also pertinent chapters in Mangan and Park, eds, *Fair Sex*.

7 Swindells, *Victorian Writing and Working Women*, p. 23.

8 G. Stanley Hall, 'Coeducation in the high school', National Educational Association, *Addresses and Proceedings*, 1903, pp. 446–451.

9 G. Stanley Hall, 'The fall of Atlantis', in *Recreations of a Psychologist*, D. Appleton & Co., New York, 1920, p. v; G. Stanley Hall, 'Can the masses rule the world', *Scientific Monthly*, XVIII, 1924, pp. 456–463; see also, G. Stanley Hall, *Morale: The Supreme Standard of Life and Conduct*, D. Appleton, New York, 1920; Hall's complex feelings about his mother and his reverence for her piety, self-sacrificing and saintly nature clearly contributed to his life-long image of women as pure, madonna-like and maternal.

10 G. Stanley Hall, untitled and undated MSS., Clark University Archives, Hall Collection, Articles 1, Addresses, 1902–1917, Box 29, Folder 1, p. 24.

11 Merle Curti, *The Social Ideas of American Educators*, Pageant Books, New Jersey, 1959, p. 410.

12 G. Stanley Hall, *Educational Problems*, I, D. Appleton, New York 1911, Vol 1, p. 200; Hall, *Adolescence*, Vol II, p. 610; 'To educate girls to be self-supporting is wrong and vicious, for nature demands that every girl should be educated primarily to become a wife and mother.' G. Stanley Hall, 'The ideal school as based on child study', *The Forum*, XXXII, September 1901, p. 35.

13 Foucault, *The History of Sexuality*, pp. 146–7. See also, John O'Neill, *Five Bodies. The Human Shape of Modern Society*, Cornell University Press, London, 1985, p. 132.

14 G. Stanley Hall, 'Education of the will', *Princeton Review*, X, November 1882, p. 321; Clarence J. Karier, 'G. Stanley Hall: A priestly prophet of a new dispensation', *The Journal of Libertarian Studies*, VII, no. 1, Spring 1983, p. 54.

15 G. Stanley Hall, 'Child study and its relation to education', *The Forum*, XXIX, August 1900, p. 702. G. Stanley Hall, 'New departures in education', *North American Review*, CXL, February 1885, p. 147.

16 Robert E. Grinder, 'The concept of adolescence in the genetic psychology of G. Stanley Hall', *Child Development*, XL, June 1969, pp. 355–369.

17 Ross, *G. Stanley Hall*, pp. 290–291; for a thorough discussion of the development of Hall's image of adolescence, see John Demos and Virginia Demos, 'Adolescence in historical perspective', *Journal of Marriage and the Family*, XXXI, November 1969, pp. 632–638; Robert E. Grinder and Charles E. Strickland, 'G. Stanley Hall and the social significance of adolescence', *Teachers College Record*, LXIV, February 1963, pp. 390–399; Grinder, 'The concept of adolescence'. Joseph Kett places Hall's work within a broader view of the development of the concept of adolescence in America. 'Weird and pseudo-scientific in retrospect, Hall's concept had a profound impact in his day. A parade of books on the teen years, the awkward age, the high school and the juvenile delinquent followed while a virtual profession of advisers on the tribulations of youth emerged.' 'Adolescence and youth in nineteenth-century America', *Journal of Interdisciplinary History*, II, Autumn 1971, p. 283.

18 Curti, *The Social Ideas*, p. 427.

19 Karier, 'Priestly prophet', p. 56.

20 Charles Darwin, *The Origin of the Species*, John Murray, London 1959: Facsimile edition, E. Mayr (ed.), Harvard University Press, 1964; *The Descent of Man*, 2 vols. John Murray, London 1871; Stephen Jay Gould, *Ever Since Darwin, Reflections in Natural History*, W.W. Norton, New York, 1977, p. 12.

21 Peter J. Bowler, 'Varieties of evolution, essay review', *History and Philosophy of the Life Sciences*, VIII, Spring, 1986, pp. 113–119.

22 J.B. Lamarck, *Zoological Philosophy: An Exposition with Regard to the Natural History of Animals*, Macmillan, London, 1809.

23 Loren Eiseley, *Darwin's Century. Evolution and the Men Who Discovered it*, Anchor Books, New York, 1958, pp. 146–147 and 252.

24 George W. Stocking, Jr. 'Lamarckianism in American social science: 1890–1915', *Journal of the History of Ideas*, XXIII, 1962, p. 243.

25 Ernest Haeckel, *Evolution of Man*, Vol. II, Kegan Paul, London 1879, Vol 2, Ch. 26; Herbert Spencer, *The Principles of Sociology*, D. Appleton & Co., New

York, 1876–97, 3 vols; Spencer's contribution to neo-Lamarckianism is discussed in Alpheus Packard, *Lamarck, the Founder of Evolution: His Life and Work*, New York, 1901, pp. 384–385, and in Richard Hofstadter, *Social Darwinism in American Thought, 1860–1915*, University of Pennsylvania Press, Philadelphia, 1944, pp. 18–36.

26 See G.S. Hall's, 'A synthetic genetic study of fear', *American Journal of Psychology*, XXV, April–July 1914, pp. 149–200, 321–92; 'A glance at the phyletic background of genetic psychology', *American Journal of Psychology*, XXI, April 1908, pp. 149–212; and 'A study of fears', *American Journal of Psychology*, VIII, January 1897, pp. 147–249; One should bear in mind, notes Stocking, 'Lamarckianism', that the spread of ideas about Lamarckianism and recapitulation were not the result of any one man, such as Hall, but were widely held and indeed reflected a widespread popular scientific attitude whose roots lay deep in the Western European cultural tradition.

27 Charles Ellwood, 'The theory of imitation in social psychology', *American Journal of Sociology*, VI, 1901 pp. 731–736.

28 Hall, *Life and Confessions of a Psychologist*, pp. 361–362.

29 Mendel's 1865 data on the hybridization of the sweet pea, revealing that hereditary changes occurred in large rather than minute variations, cast doubt on the Lamarckian view that gradually accumulated experiences in one generation could be passed on to the next. For a rudimentary understanding of Mendelian genetics, see L.C. Dunn and T. Dobzhansky, *Heredity, Race and Society*, rev. ed., Mentor Books, New York, 1946.

30 Hofstadter, *Social Darwinism in American Thought*.

31 Ross, *G. Stanley Hall*, p. 374.

32 Using excerpts from Hall's *Adolescence* on physical, cognitive and social development, Grinder, 'The concept of adolescence', has illustrated how he fashioned five major principles into a science of human development.

33 Hall, *Adolescence*, II, pp. 94 and viii.

34 C. Resek, *Lewis Henry Morgan: American Scholar*, University of Chicago Press, Chicago 1960.

35 This idea of course was Rousseau's who talked about the concept of adolescence as second birth in *Emile*, Book IV, in 1762. Strickland and Burgess note that, although Hall never admitted the close parallel between his thought and that of Rousseau, their descriptions of natural education were very close in spirit and practice. Charles E. Strickland and Charles Burgess, *Health, Growth and Heredity. G. Stanley Hall on Natural Education*, Teachers College Press, New York, 1965.

36 Hall, *Adolescence*, II, p. 303; Indeed, Hall further explained, 'for those prophetic souls interested in the future of our race the field of adolescence is the quarry in which they must seek to find both goals and means'. *Adolescence*, I, p. 50.

37 Strickland and Burgess, *Health, Growth and Heredity*, p. 20.

38 Each stage, explained one of Hall's students, 'is different from that which precedes and follows it , as though it were intended to be a final stage'. G.E. Partridge, *Genetic Philosophy of Education. An Epitome of the Published Educational Writings of G. Stanley Hall of Clark University*, Sturgis & Walton, New York 1912, p. 72.

39 Grinder, 'The concept of adolescence', p. 359.
40 Children were to be encouraged to relive primitive experiences to their full-est through healthy, vigorous and egotistical behaviour which might take the form of 'barbaric associations ... and other savage, reversionary combina-tions', though Hall did waver on insisting upon the necessity of direct cathartic action such as childish cruelty. *Adolescence*, I, pp. 226 and 408.
41 Hall, note Burgess and Strickland, *Health, Growth and Heredity*, could never bring himself to believe that the common man could really think. He viewed the mass of humanity as a 'great army of incapables ... for whose mental development heredity decrees a slow pace and early arrest'. *Adolescence*, II, p. 510; His conception of intellect was that of a superstructure built upon the more complex life of the unconscious. Partridge, *Genetic Philosophy*, p. 60.
42 Hall, *Adolescence*, I, p. 131. Hall considered Schopenhauer's *The World as Will and Idea* as 'the most brilliant and in many respects, the most insightful piece of modern philosophical literature'. G. Stanley Hall to Mr. Arnett, Clark University Papers, 31 October 1902.
43 'Knowledge,' Hall insisted, 'can never save individuals or nations. There is only one language and that is willed action ... the only organs of which are muscles.' 'Christianity and physical culture', *Pedagogical Seminary*, IX, September 1902, p. 378. Indeed, cognitive growth was to be discouraged in children for 'the only duty of young children is implicit obedience.' 'Dressur,' said Hall, 'should be the all-pervading aim and method. School should be made work and not all play. There should be a drudgery, effort, hardness in it, and not too much pleasure or recreation.' 'The Ideal School as Based on Child Study', 1901, p. 482. 'At adolescence, however, the mind at times grows in leaps and bounds ... and a kind of reasoning mania is easily possible.' *Adolescence*, II, pp. 451, 533. Thus Hall assigned to adolescent intellect a critical role in his scheme to promote a superstate but in no way did he feel that intellectual development and the fostering of creativity should ever approach the importance of healthy physical growth.
44 Hall, 'Co-education in the high school', p. 447.
45 Hall, *Adolescence*, I, p. 131.
46 'A knowledge of the nascent stages and the aggregate interests of different stages of life,' Hall observed, 'is the best safeguard against very many of the prevalent errors of education and life'. *Adolescence*, I, p. viii.
47 Hall, *Adolescence*, I, p. 128; Dismissing the first stage of growth at early child-hood as relatively insignificant, Hall considered the prepubescent period of childhood between about eight and twelve or thirteen years of age to be a relatively stable phase marked by a decreased rate of growth. During these years children could use their sum of energy to move vigorously through, and exploit with play, all the physical survival activities of primitive man; climbing trees, throwing objects, fishing, hunting, chasing and swimming. Partridge, *Genetic Philosophy*, p. 29; See also, Charles E. Strickland, 'The child, the community and Clio: The uses of cultural history in elementary school experiments of the eighteen nineties', *History of Education Quarterly*, VII, Winter 1967, p. 492; and G. Stanley Hall, 'The new psychology as a basis of education', *The Forum*, XVII, August 1894, pp. 710–20; G. Stanley Hall, *Youth, Its Education, Regimen and Hygiene*, D. Appleton, New York 1906.

48 Hall, *Adolescence*, I, p. 48; 'Christianity and physical culture', pp. 374–378.

49 Hall, 'Coeducation in the high school', p. 446.

50 The basis of sex-typing was established early in the history of race. 'We have abundant evidence,' said Hall, 'that the race has had a sexual consciousness', *Adolescence*, II, p. 99.

51 Spencer, *Education: Intellectual, Moral and Physical*.

52 Miss M.E. Findlay, 'The education of girls', *Paidologist*, VII, January, 1905, p. 93; Webster (ed.), *Biology, Medicine and Society, 1840–1940*, writes of the persistent convenience with which Darwinism has come to the aid of social and educational causes, opposition to feminism and support for the traditional order.

53 Herbert Spencer, 'Psychology of the sexes', *Popular Science Monthly*, IV, 1873, p. 31. For further discussion of Spencer's views on women and biological determinism, see Newman, ed., *Men's Ideas, Women's Realities*, pp. 1–11; Delamont and Duffin (eds.), *The Nineteenth-Century Woman*, and Sayers, *Biological Politics*, pp. 32–38.

54 Hall, 'Coeducation in the high school', p. 451.

55 The law of conservation of matter which was derived from Newtonian principles was held to be a universal law of nature throughout the nineteenth century and was the foundation upon which Herbert Spencer based his philosophy of evaluation in *Principles of Biology*, 1864–67. Although the idea of the body as a closed energy system came under attack in the early 1900s, the belief retained wide currency. Robert Woodworth, 'Psychiatry and experimental psychology', in *Psychological Issues: Selected Papers of Robert S. Woodworth*, Columbia University Press, New York, 1939. It continued to be popularized by Hall, Havelock Ellis and then Sigmund Freud well into the twentieth century. V.B. Ross, 'The Human Body as a Machine', *Popular Science Monthly*, LVII, September 1900, pp. 491–499; Paul Robinson, *The Modernization of Sex: Havelock Ellis, Alfred Kinsey, William Masters and Virginia Johnson*, Harper and Row, New York 1976, pp. 15–16; Harvey Green, *Fit for America: Health, Fitness, Sport and American Society*, Pantheon Books, New York, 1986, pp. 167–180, also discusses sport and anxieties over loss of energy.

56 Patrick Geddes and J. Arthur Thompson, *The Evolution of Sex*, Walter Scott, London 1889. Sayers notes in *Biological Politics*, p. 41, that so serviceable did Geddes and Thompson's arguments seem to the anti-feminist cause that they were still in circulation sixty years later when De Beauvoir criticized them in *The Second Sex*.

57 Saleeby, *Woman and Womanhood*, p. 65, discussing Spencer's *Principles of Biology*, and Geddes and Thompson's *The Evolution of Sex*.

58 For an interesting discussion on the influence of Geddes' work, see Jill Conway, 'Stereotypes of femininity in a theory of sexual evolution', Martha Vicinus, ed., *Suffer and Be Still. Women in the Victorian Age*, Indiana University Press, Bloomington, 1972, pp. 140–154.

59 Mosedale, 'Science corrupted', p. 36; See also Helen Bradford Thompson, *The Mental Traits of Sex: An Experimental Investigation of the Normal Mind in Men and Women*, University of Chicago, Press, Chicago, 1903 for a discussion of popular beliefs about sex differences in 1900. Also, Rosenberg, *Beyond*

Separate Spheres, explains that 'belief in masculine and feminine uniqueness had never been so marked as it was in 1900. There was great strength in society's belief in sexual polarity', p. 69.

60 Geddes and Thompson, *The Evolution of Sex*, pp. 268–271.

61 G. Stanley Hall, 'The feminist in science', *New York Independent*, March 22, 1906, pp. 661–662.

62 Hall, 'Child study', p. 702.

63 Saleeby stated this succinctly: 'Psychology inclines to the view that small children are of neither sex.' C.W. Saleeby, 'The psychology of parenthood', *Eugenics Review*, I, 1909–10, p. 40; Havelock Ellis corroborated the view that fundamental differences of practical importance between the two sexes before twelve are not to be found. *Man and Woman: A Study of Secondary and Tertiary Sexual Characters*, Houghton Mifflin, Boston 1894.

64 Hall, *Adolescence*, II, p. 624; I, p. 308.

65 For an elaboration of these aspects of the menstrual disability theory, see Patricia A. Vertinsky, 'Exercise, physical capability, and the eternally wounded woman in late nineteenth-century North America', *Journal of Sport History*, XIV, Spring 1987, pp. 7–27.

66 Hall, *Adolescence*, I, p. 492.

67 Findlay, 'The education of girls', p. 84.

68 Mary Scharlieb, 'Adolescent girlhood under modern conditions with special reference to motherhood', *The Eugenics Review*, I, April 1909 – January 1910, p. 174.

69 Hall, *Adolescence*, I, pp. 42–43.

70 Saleeby, *Woman and Womanhood*, p. 101.

71 Scharlieb, 'Adolescent girls', p. 176.

72 Hall, *Adolescence*, I, pp. 250–253, 257 and 267.

73 Scharlieb, 'Adolescent Girls', p. 179.

74 Partridge, *Genetic Philosophy*, p. 361. Dr Edward Clarke's highly influential book, *Sex in Education*, had fully outlined the Spencerian argument that women's unique physiology limited their educational capacity. Endowed with smaller and simpler brains and greater emotionality, women could not tolerate intellectual exertion as men could. Higher education imposed an undue strain on women's minds and caused irreparable damage to their bodies. Thus Clarke explicitly linked the physiological demands of an academic education to the reproductive impairment of the nation's future mothers.

75 Hall, *Youth: Its Education*, p. 280.

76 J. McKeen Cattell, 'The School and the family', *Popular Science Monthly*, LXXI, January 1909, p. 91.

77 Hall, *Adolescence*, I, pp. 505 and 504.

78 Professor Muirhead, 'The scope and object of child-study', *Paidologist*, VII, January, 1905, pp. 66–73.

79 Patrick Geddes, 'Adolescence', *Paidologist*, VII, January, 1905, p. 40.

80 For a discussion on the quest for a science of education in the nineteenth century, see James R. Robarts, 'The quest for a science of education in the nineteenth century', *History of Education Quarterly*, VIII, Winter 1968, pp. 431–446.

81 Strickland and Burgess, *Health, Growth and Heredity*, p. 114.
82 Hall, *Adolescence*, II, p. 571; 'Educational Problems', I, p. 200. Hall 'perceived that education was in a sad way and he did not hesitate to say so', noted his biographer, Lorine Pruette, *G. Stanley Hall. A Biography of a Mind*, D. Appleton & Co., New York 1926, p. 111.
83 Hall, *Adolescence*, I, p. xi.
84 Hall, 'The ideal school', p. 24.
85 Hall advocated a policy of weeding out the unfit and the slow at every grade level and sending them to 'dullard' schools. 'Only the few have the genius and talent to improve through mental training.' Hall, 'Child study', p. 717. G. Stanley Hall, 'Editorial', *Pedagogical Seminary*, II, 1892, p. 4.
86 G. Stanley Hall, 'The New Movement in Education', Address delivered to the school of pedagogy, University of the City of New York, December 1891; G. Stanley Hall, 'Feminization in school and home', *World's Work*, XVI, May 1908, pp. 1037–44; What counted most of all, however, in deciding who was worth educating and how specialised such education should be, was health. 'I almost believe that the boy or girl who has not enough vigor to play a good deal is hardly worth educating at all.' G. Stanley Hall, *New York Tribune*, V, February 5, 1905, p. 1.
87 G. Stanley Hall, 'Some defects of the kindergarten in America', *The Forum*, XXVIII, January 1900b, pp. 579–91.
88 Hall, 'Ideal school', pp. 488–9.
89 Grinder, 'The concept of adolescence', p. 364; The emphasis on discipline was not the contradiction it seemed, note Strickland and Burgess, *Health, Growth and Heredity*, for Hall equated natural with formal education for children of this age, arguing that formal methods suited the nature of the pre-adolescent. Thus his interpretation, with the exception of the emphasis on healthy play, corresponded with later images of the child-centred school.
90 Partridge, *Genetic Philosophy*, pp. 125–6.
91 Hall, 'The ideal school as based on child study', p. 481.
92 Hall, 'The high school as the people's college', pp. 260–268; 'How far is the present high school and early college training adapted to the nature and needs of adolescents?'
93 Hall, *Adolescence*, I, p. 510.
94 Hall, 'Ideal school', p. 482.
95 Burgess and Borrowman note that Hall paid little more attention to the academic side of adolescent girls' curriculum than Rousseau paid to Sophie's education. Charles Burgess and Merle L. Borrowman, *What Doctrines to Embrace. Studies in the History of American Education*, Scott, Foresman & Co., Illinois 1969, p. 84. Lynda Lange has developed an interesting argument to demonstrate how Rousseau's work contains a justification for the inequality of men and women and their respective educations. 'Rousseau: Women and the general will', L.M.G. Clark and L. Lange, eds., *The Sexism of Social and Political Theory*, University of Toronto Press, Toronto, 1979, pp. 41–52.
96 Hall, *Educational Problems*, II, p. 668.
97 Hall, *Adolescence*, II, p. 637. Education in sex-hygiene for girls was particularly critical to address the dwindling birthrate and increasing rate of infant mortality. Thus, at adolescence, the chief need of girls was for hygienic

instruction concerning their monthly regimen. G. Stanley Hall, 'Education in sex hygiene', *Eugenics Review*, I, 1909–10, p. 247.

98 Hall, 'Coeducation in the High School', pp. 181–182.

99 Scharlieb, 'Adolescent girlhood', p. 179.

100 Kenealy, *Feminism and Sex-Extinction*, pp. 179, 120 and 139.

101 Murray Leslie, 'Women's progress in relation to eugenics', *Eugenics Review*, II, 1910–11, p. 286.

102 Saleeby, *Woman and Womanhood*, pp. 101, 8 and 119.

103 Sir Halliday Croom, quoted in Saleeby, *Woman and Womanhood*, p. 119, 'used to criticize cycling as tending towards local rigidity unfavourable to child birth'.

104 Hall, *Adolescence*, II, p. 571. Said Saleeby, *Woman and Womanhood*, p. 120, 'Holding the abdomen together by means of a corset may serve its own purpose, but does less than nothing in the crisis of motherhood. The corset indeed conduces to the atrophy of the most important of all the voluntary muscles for the most important crisis of a woman's life.' Mel Davis, 'Corsets and conception: Fashion and demographic trends in the nineteenth century', *Comparative Studies in Society and History*, XXIV, October 1982, pp. 611–641, recently presented sociological evidence suggesting that the tightlaced corset did indeed contribute to a decline in nineteenth-century middle-class fertility as Hall and others feared.

105 Clouston, 'Female education from a medical point of view', January 1884, p. 321.

106 J. Madison Taylor, 'Puberty in girls and certain of its disturbances', *Pediatrics*, July 15, 1896.

107 The ultimate educational environment for girls' health, of course, was Hall's Rousseauian romantic view of the country 'in the midst of the hills, the climbing of which is the best stimulus for heart and lungs; there should be water for boating, bathing and skating, aquaria and aquatic life; gardens both for kitchen vegetables and horticulture; good roads, walks and paths that tempt to walking and wheeling; playgrounds and space for golf and tennis; all that can be called environment is even more important for girls than boys', *Adolescence*, II, pp. 636–7; Hall claimed that because girls specialized less than boys they preferred unorganized games, *Adolescence*, I, pp. 224 and 230.

108 Saleeby, *Woman and Womanhood*, p 110.

109 Kenealy, *Feminism and Sex-Extinction*, p. 139.

110 Hall, *Adolescence*, II, p. 630.

111 Partridge, *Genetic Philosophy*, p. 370.

112 Hall, 'The fall of Atlantis', p. 45.

113 Burgess and Borrowman, *What Doctrines to Embrace*, p. 91.

114 Hall himself wrote, in a personal letter, 'I sometimes think my life has been a series of fads or crazes. At any rate I have had various vocational ideas.' In her biography of Hall, Pruette further notes that 'the word evolution charmed him and the evolutionary concept fascinated him to the end, colouring all his interpretations of life'. *G. Stanley Hall*, p. 109.

115 Hall, *Life and Confessions of a Psychologist*, p. 595.

116 Burgess and Borrowman, *What Doctrines to Embrace*, p. 76. For the historian,

says Hall's biographer Ross, 'Hall's double-dealing is a marvelous revelation of the complexities of his age [for he] belonged to the late-Victorian, post-Darwinian era whose very name expressed its transitional nature', *G. Stanley Hall*, p. xiv. In many ways Hall picked up and exposed the intellectual and cultural conflict of his era.

117 Josiah Royce, *Lectures on Modern Idealism*, Yale University Press, New Haven, 1919, p. 236.

118 Whorton, *Crusaders for Fitness*, p. 286.

119 Whorton, *Crusaders for Fitness*, pp. 289–90, notes that in as concise a statement of muscular christianity as can be found, Hall spoke for Progressive physical educators as a group. 'We are soldiers of Christ, strengthening our muscles not against a foreign foe but against sin within and without us.' Hall, 'Christianity and physical culture', p. 377. Biological engineers such as Sargent, Hartwell, Anderson, Gulick and Tait McKenzie all devised their physical education systems as antidotes to the evils and alienation of city life and provided much support to Hall's own broad claims for physical education. See also, Joel H. Spring, 'Mass culture and school sports', *History of Educational Quarterly*, XIV, Winter 1974, pp. 483–499. Gulick especially subscribed to Hall's psychological theories, arguing that maintenance of order in modern society depended on the proper channelling of adolescent sexuality, and that juvenile delinquency could often be attributed to a lack of athletics. To this end, he developed physical training programmes for the Y.M.C.A. and promoted groups of boy scouts and the camp-fire girls in which athletics could play the role set out by genetic psychology of providing release for primitive instinctual drives and sublimating sexuality. Luther Gulick, 'Play and democracy', *Proceedings of the First Annual Playground Congress*, New York, 1907, pp. 11–16.

120 Burgess and Borrowman, *What Doctrines to Embrace*, p. 72; Hall, 'Editorial', *Pedagogical Seminary*, I, 1891, p. 120.

121 Hall, *Adolescence*, I, p. 202.

122 Hall, 'The fall of Atlantis', p. 82.

123 Hall was initially filled with admiration for the ideas of Johann Fichte who had called for an educational state in Germany, governed by an elite and dedicated to the cultural perfection of mankind. Hall believed that the German social order had 'actualized the Platonic Republic'. G. Stanley Hall, 'The moral and religious training of children', *Princeton Review*, X, January 1882, p. 27; For further discussion, see Grinder and Strickland, 'G. Stanley Hall and the social significance of adolescence', p. 391, and Burgess and Borrowman, *What Doctrines to Embrace*, pp. 93–94.

124 Hall, 'The education of the will', p. 321.

125 Nietzsche's ambivalence about women led him to make a strong claim for the value of the forced repression of woman to make her 'unconditionally submit'. Clark & Lange (eds.), *The Sexism of Social and Political Theory*, p. 120. This repression was necessary, he believed, since if women were not dominated and did not have to struggle, they would lose the energy necessary for the main function as biological mothers. In attacking feminism, he claimed that education destroyed their Dionysian instinct and caused sterility. 'Aut liberi, aut libri' (either children or books,) he demanded.

'Everything about woman has one solution. It is called pregnancy.' In *Thus Spoke Zarathustra* (tr. Hollingdale.), Harmondsworth, 1969, pp. 92–3, women are told 'Let your hope be: May I bear the superman'; Nancy Huston, 'The matrix of war: Mothers and heroes', Suleiman (ed.) *The Female Body in Western Culture*, pp. 119–138, explicates the analogy between warmaking and childbearing, motherhood and the military, which has long saturated Western culture and which G. Stanley Hall intuitively felt. He pointed with insistence, for example, to the initiation rites of primitive peoples to explain the evolutionary progression to separate spheres through pain incurred on behalf of the group. Ritual rites of passage assisted girls to learn that only the pain of motherhood could make women of them; boys were taught that only the blood of war could make men of them. Said Hall, just as man must be ready to lay down his life for his country, so woman needs a heroism of her own to face the pain, danger and work of bearing and rearing children, *Adolescence*, II, p. 609.

126 Hall, 'Educational problems', II, p. 207.
127 Hall, 'The fall of Atlantis', pp. 1–127.
128 G. Stanley Hall, 'The educational state; or the methods of education in Europe', *Christian Register*, LXIX, November 1890, p. 719.
129 Address delivered at the opening of Clark University, in *Clark University, Worcester, Massachusetts: Opening Exercises*, October 2, 1889, pp. 19, 24; For a discussion of Hall's conception of the university, see Ross, *G. Stanley Hall*, p. 200.
130 At Clark, Hall allowed women to become graduate students but they worked in the shadow of his hostility to any criticism of traditional views of sex differences. Rosenberg, *Separate Spheres*, p. 68. See also Ross, *G. Stanley Hall*, p. 416.
131 Gould, *The Mismeasure of Man*, p. 118.
132 Lawrence A. Cremin, Preface to Strickland and Burgess, *Health, Growth and Heredity*, p. viii.
133 Strickland and Burgess, *Health, Growth and Heredity*, p. 25; Karier also suggests that Hall's scale for measuring progress towards a new order was clearly a totalitarian one and that the conditions which gave rise to such convictions bear further intensive examination. 'Priestly prophet', p. 55.
134 Hall, 'The education of the will', pp. 321–322.
135 Karier, 'Priestly prophet', p. 52.
136 Quoted in Herbert J. Muller, *Issues of Freedom*, Harper and Row, New York, 1960, p. 36.
137 Clarence J. Karier, *Man, Society and Education. A History of American Educational Ideas*, Scott, Foresman and Co., University of Rochester, 1967, pp. 156–57; It was no accident that Hall's sensitive unconventional mind should anticipate many of the functional constructs of National Socialism, notes Karier, for he had integrated into his personal life numerous primitive beliefs of the 'Volkische Kultur', many of which were antecedents to the later rise of National Socialism in Germany. For an understanding of 'Volk' see George L. Mosse, *The Crisis of German Ideology*, Grosset and Dunlap, New York, 1964.
138 Claudia Koonz, *Mothers in the Fatherland: Women, the Family and Nazi Politics*,

Cape, London 1987.

139 Lawrence Cremin, in Strickland and Burgess, *Health, Growth and Heredity*, p. viii. For a fairly benign view of Hall's long-term influence, see, for example, Merle Curti's chapter, 'G. Stanley Hall, evolutionist, 1846–1924', *The Social Ideas of American Educators*, Pageant Books, New Jersey, 1959, pp. 396–428; In a recent book honouring the research traditions established by Hall at Johns Hopkins University, Hulse and Green note that 'Hall scattered in America the seeds of an experimental approach to the study of mind and its courier, human and animal action – which revolutionized behavioural science in the Western world.' Stewart H. Hulse, and Bert F. Green, Jr., (eds.), *One Hundred Years of Psychological Research in America. G. Stanley Hall and the Johns Hopkins Tradition*, The Johns Hopkins University Press, Baltimore, 1986, p. xi; On the other hand, claim Boring and Boring, Hall left no 'hallians' behind nor did he leave a systematic body of ideas to future psychologists. Mollie D. Boring and E.G. Boring, 'Masters and pupils among the American psychologists', *American Journal of Psychology*, LXI, 1948, pp. 527–34; Mortimer Herbert Appley, summing up Hall's influence, notes that his legacies were more significant in terms of structures and emphases and attention to the developmental process. 'G. Stanley Hall: Vow on Mount Owen', Hulse and Green, *One Hundred Years of Psychological Research*, pp. 3–20; In his autobiography Hall mentioned the hope that his life work, although now only a trail, would sometime become a royal highway, *Life and Confessions*, p. 3. In fact, it was ideas of Hall's contemporaries such as William James's radical empiricism and his *Principles of Psychology* as applied to education and John Dewey's instrumental philosophy which gave to education a role of first importance in achieving a more democratic society, that took pride of place on the highway Hall coveted. Yet it was Hall, rather than James, 'who created adolescence as a distinct discipline of psychology' and in some respects it has been the conservative traditions expounded by Hall rather than Dewey's liberal ideas that have had the greater influence upon American educational practice. Although Dewey was the great synthesizer of American experience, he failed basically, claims Karier, to translate his philosophy into concrete educational practices, *Man, Society, and Education*, p. 148.
140 Karier, 'Priestly Prophet', p. 50.
141 C.J. Karier, 'Elite views on American Education', W. Laqueur and G.L. Mosse (eds.), *Education and Social Structure in the Twentieth Century*, Harper and Row, New York, 1967, p. 151; Is, for example, Hall's thought typical of an impulse of progressivism which we may too often ignore, asks E.V. Johanningmeier, and 'does Hall typify a position as restrictive and oppressive as Presbyterianism?' 'Presbyterians, democracy and demography, essay review', *History of Education Quarterly*, XI, Summer 1971, p. 208.
142 Haley, *The Healthy Body and Victorian Culture*, p. 3.
143 Heart-formers, the psychologists in Atlantis, concentrated especially upon the sex education of adolescents. Female heart-formers led the girls through the sacred mysteries of sex and later arranged matings for marriage and procreation. Hall, 'The fall of Atlantis', pp. 1–127.

144 Hall, 'Child study', p. 709.
145 But see John C. Burnham's 'Change in the popularization of health in the United States', *Bulletin of the History of Medicine*, LVIII, no. 2, 1984, pp. 183–197, who illustrates dramatic changes in the 'context and cultural functions of the popularization of health, the separation of health from science, and a loss of coherent rationale as to the best manner of life. Whorton, *Crusaders for Fitness*, p. 348, on the other hand, discusses the resurgence of the core philosophy of health wholism and the promotion of a hygienic ideology of self-actualization – again, different from Hall's dream of health for service.
146 Wilson R. Jackson, 'Essay review I – Dewey's Hegelianism', in William H. Goetzmann, ed., *The American Hegelians; An Intellectual Episode in the History of Western America*, Dickson Pratt, New York 1973, quoted in *History of Education Quarterly*, XIV, Spring 1975, p. 90.
147 G. Stanley Hall, 'Editorial', *Pedagogical Seminary*, II, 1892, p. 7; 'The first aim which should dominate every item, pedagogic method and matter,' said Hall, 'should be health.' *Adolescence*, II, p. 637. The health of women is more important for the welfare of the race than that of man and the influence of her body upon her mind is greater and, therefore, should be supreme and primary. *Life and Confessions*, p. 283; As a fitting testimony to Hall's emphasis on the health aspects of physical education, 'in 1924 the guardians of school health joined with the gym teachers to form the Department of Health and Physical Education of the National Educational Association'. Ross, *G. Stanley Hall*, p. 365.

7

The new woman and nervous illness:
Charlotte Perkins Gilman

Everyone who possesses a strong mind in a sane body is heir presumptive to the kingdom of this world.[1]

Hard as G. Stanley Hall and the male medical establishment might try to restrain the growing demands of the 'new woman', and insist that she adhere to traditional injunctions about femininity, a swelling group of feminists pressed rebelliously against the boundaries of their allotted sphere. Indeed, a growing number of women struggled to further their intellectual capacity and extend the parameters of their physical capabilities within a patriarchal tradition of female confinement and subordination.[2] Although they encountered controlling ideologies and rigid role prescriptions which had the effect of subduing their initiatives, a number of feminists expressed a growing desire to control their own bodies and reproductive lives by pursuing health and wholeness. They demanded release from the rigid behavioural expectations which large numbers of males and doctors determined to be their birthright and sought to escape from the social script that women had both internalized and performed in response to social expectations. Demanding new roles and opportunities, these feminists aspired to become not simply equal to men but 'new women'.

A prominent (though by no means typical) example of the 'new woman' was Charlotte Perkins Gilman. An exceptional woman of considerable talent, Gilman became a major intellectual force in turn-of-the-century America. As a result of her prolific writing and lecturing on the theory of the evolution of gender relations and women's need to become socially useful in the larger world of production, she became known worldwide as a feminist theorist and iconoclastic social critic.[3]

Until recently Charlotte Gilman's literary contributions to critical aspects. of the 'woman question' of the late nineteenth and early twentieth centuries have remained relatively unexamined. Currently, however, feminist historians and literary critics have begun interpreting her actions and writings as paradigmatic of critical tensions between the sexes at the turn of the century, especially of female struggles for creative fulfilment and physical autonomy. The context and substance of her writings, suggests Cottom, are 'sites of historical struggles well worthy of investigation and analysis'.[4] Gilman's writings have been interpreted as a parable of female literary confinement, and as a dramatic illustration of the potential sexual violence of both the Victorian familial bedroom and the male doctor's relationship with his female clients. They also reflect her substantial life-long preoccupation with physical fitness and the importance she placed upon good health practices and unrestricted physical mobility as critical components of an emancipated womanhood.

Gilman's life experiences and her prolific writings were inextricably linked. One has only to examine the texts of Charlotte Perkins Gilman in light of her personal history to appreciate the extent to which this is so. Analyses of her feminist writings, fiction, poetry, diaries and auto-biography all provide rich historical insight into her strivings for both physical autonomy and intellectual freedom. Although the way Gilman tried to live her life was in some ways deviant (and at least one historian has claimed she was truly neurotic), her notions of mind–body rela-tionships illustrate dominant modes of thought about female health and autonomy in the late nineteenth century.[5]

To understand Charlotte Gilman it is necessary to examine more closely the prevailing attitudes of her era towards female health and the mind–body relationship. The attempted emergence of Gilman as a 'new woman' can best be understood as her break away from the accepted medical paradigm based upon the competition of mind and body for a limited endowment of energy, and her forging of a radically new mind–body concept as synergistic. The tragedy of Gilman's life lay in the fact that personally she was never completely able to liberate herself from the grasp of the traditional medical paradigm with its somatic emphasis.

The role of physical culture in Gilman's life-style

Born in 1860, Gilman declared early in life that physical fitness could function as an important strategy for emancipation, since embracing physical culture seemed one clear way to remove the badge of female dependence. 'It is apparent,' she reflected in her autobiography, 'that a careful early training in physical culture lasts a life time [and] in this line of improvement I was highly ambitious . . . and absolutely vain of my physical strength and agility.'[6]

Gilman's dedication to physical fitness derived partly from her ongoing feeling, intensified at adolescence, that she needed strength to cope with what she was beginning to perceive as the female burden of economic dependence and a confining domestic role. The seeds of her desire to transcend these restrictions were rooted, one of her biographers suggests, in Gilman's earliest struggles for independence and self-assertion against the repressive discipline of her mother, Mary Perkins, who had been deserted by her father, Frederick Beecher Perkins, and who 'unwittingly taught her daughter about the false security and spurious deceit of wife-mother myths'.[7] They were also nourished by her Beecher heritage. Charlotte Gilman was the grandniece of Catharine Beecher, Harriet Beecher Stowe and Henry Ward Beecher, all of whom promoted exalted and energetic images of themselves as self-assertive reformers during her many visits to them as a child. Henry Ward Beecher had an extremely fine physique and was enormously energetic. Catharine Beecher, in particular, had already demonstrated the importance of promoting health and fitness as a means for middle-class women to combat myths about female frailty, improve their functional efficiency and expand their influence in the home and society at large.[8] She provided a stimulating model of vigorous self-dependence during Gilman's formative years, and Gilman later named her only daughter Katharine after her great-aunt.

The early separation of her own parents had, for Gilman, resulted in an oppressive environment. 'Because my childhood had no father', she complained, the family was frequently in debt, and constantly on the move, thwarting any continuity in her education.[9] Her formal schooling was unusually brief and not particularly memorable. During her time at the Young Ladies School in Providence, only the physical fitness classes sparked her interest, especially the exercise programmes run by Dr John Brooks, gymnastics teacher, physician and director of the Providence gymnasium. Encouraged by her great-aunt Catharine Beecher's health treatises, John Brook's practical coaching and a memorable physical culture lecture attended during her adolescent years, she channelled much of her energy towards improving her health through rational dress, fresh air, cold baths and 'every kind of attainable physical exercise'.[10]

Gilman later described her adolescence as a time of constant conflict between her feminine and masculine elements.[11] She resented being hemmed in by her mother's stern restrictions, drab routine, coldness and unbending discipline, and she felt victimized by the demands and difficulties of living in a single-parent household. Seeing conventional femininity as symbolized by her mother's dependence and vulnerability, she viewed her father's traits of creativity, strength, independence and worldliness as infinitely more desirable, even though he largely ignored his family.

Gilman described how she dealt with the disappointments caused by her mother's intransigence and her father's indifference by practising rigid forms of self-discipline, especially rigorous physical exercise and spartan habits. She was constantly preoccupied with physical fitness and followed 'Blaikie every night with greatest assiduity'. The 1879 edition of William Blaikie's highly popular layperson's guide to health and fitness, *How to Get Strong and How to Stay So*, preached judicious, daily physical exercise for both sexes and all ages but gave special attention to women's needs. Physical fitness for women, wrote Blaikie, was:

> the key to sanity and mental power; to self-respect and high purpose; to sound health and vigorous enduring health . . . Let every intelligent girl and woman in this land bear in mind that, from every point of view, a vigorous and healthy body, kept toned by rational systematic daily exercise, is one of the greatest blessings which can be had in this world.[12]

Claiming Blaikie's book as 'her bedside Bible, her Atalanta guidebook for the coming race', Gilman practised his recommendations daily. She lifted weights, practised gymnastics and ran the seven-minute mile. 'Girls should all learn to run', said Blaikie, so each day Gilman 'ran a mile, not for speed but wind'. 'I could vault and jump,' she wrote, 'go up a knotted rope, walk on my hands under a ladder, kick as high as my head, and revel in the flying rings. But best of all were the travelling rings, those wide spaced, single ones, stirrup-handled, that dangled in a line the length of the hall.'[13]

In 1881, when Gilman was twenty-one, she sought more systematic training in a gymnasium and persuaded Dr John Brooks, the local gymnastic teacher, to start a women's gymnasium for herself and a group of friends. The same year she boasted in her diary that 'my health was splendid, I never tired . . . [I was] . . . as strong as a horse.' 'I could easily have been an acrobat,' she wrote later, 'having good nervous coordination, strength, courage and excellent balancing power.'[14] So pleased was she with her experiences at the Providence Ladies'

Gymnasium that she advertised its merits in the *Provincial Daily Journal*:

> For Ladies' Gymnasiums it may be said that the laws of health cover both sexes and that there can be little beauty without harmonious physical development. . . . Our gymnasium is located in a hall that leaves little to be desired, a large, light airy hall 65 x 45 and 25 feet high . . . It is thoroughly stocked with apparatus selected by Dr Sargent of Harvard University . . . Each [lady] is weighed, measured and gauged before beginning, and again at the end of the season; and the increase in strength and beauty has been most encouraging. Special work is given to counteract special deficiencies and it is glorious, to see the backs straighten, shoulders fall into place, narrow chests expand and weak muscles grow firm and round. Women who are weak and ailing can regain strength and for young girls . . . there is room for hearty enjoyment and acquisition of health and strength that lasts far into the future.[15]

From health to illness: the price of nonconformity

Gilman's growing desire for personal autonomy pressed her to consider rejecting a conventional future of domesticity. 'I have decided I'm not domestic and I don't want to be. I can work now to some purpose, wait with some patience, guard my health and strength with an end in view.' The objective, as far as she could articulate it, was to strengthen herself to repress any inclinations to develop 'merely as a woman or that useful animal, a wife and mother'.[16] 'I insist upon a life of comparative freedom and great activity', she wrote in her diary, and in her letters she gloated about her determination and physical strength; 'I, the strong and impregnable; I, the budding athlete, and Chief Performer at the Providence Ladies' Sanitary Gymnasium; I, the surefooted and steady eyed. . .'[17]

Her determination to resist a conventional future of marriage was soon put to the test, however, by Charles Walter Stetson's marriage proposal.[18] After much vacillation she accepted his proposal but soon revealed her misgivings in her diary. Realizing she was choosing the duty to submit and endure rather than a duty to rebel, she anticipated, at times, a future of failure and suffering.[19] 'Children sickly and unhappy. Husband miserable because of my distress; and I . . .!' Believing that she might counter such forebodings about her forthcoming confinement in marriage by distracting herself through exercise, which would also maintain her strength to resist total entrapment, she redoubled her physical fitness efforts, improved her diet and resumed her gymnasium classes. Greater vigour might dispel, she hoped, the mental gloom descending upon her. She was delighted to find that, despite her anxieties, she could still go up the rope and on the rings, 'run forty laps, vault six and lift three rings on the ladder'! In her diary she recorded her pleasure at exercising hilariously, cavorting wildly, enjoying the gymnasium intensely and doing more than usual. Yet, despite her pleasure at her increased physical fitness, she felt that she was losing control over other aspects of her life, especially her ability to make the right decisions about the future. In her diary she constantly displayed her indecision:

> Can I, who suffer from the wild unrest
> Of two strong natures claiming each its due,
> And cannot tell the greater of the two; [20]

Ultimately she did, however, agree to marry Charles Stetson. Soon she became pregnant, and depression followed quickly. Pregnancy and mothering proved bitter experiences. The physical incapacity and loss of the body tone acquired through hours in the women's gymnasium disturbed her and, Berkin suggests, 'no doubt contributed to her sense of unnatural lethargy and of a passivity she held in contempt'.[21] 'Nothing was more utterly bitter than this,' she wrote as her depression intensified, 'that even motherhood brought no joy.'

> I could not read nor write nor paint nor sew nor talk nor listen to talking nor anything. I lay on the lounge and wept all day. The tears ran down into my ears on either side. I went to bed crying, woke in the night crying, sat on the edge of the bed in the morning and cried from sheer continuous pain.[22]

Guilt and shame exacerbated her condition. 'That a heretofore markedly vigorous young woman should collapse in this lamentable manner was inexplicable,' she wrote:

> You did it yourself. You had health and strength and hope and glorious work before you and you threw it all away. No good as a wife, no good as a mother, no good at anything . . . I, the ceaselessly industrious, could do no work of any kind.[23]

She blamed herself for her weakness and her husband for pressing her into marriage without understanding her needs. 'Men are attracted by women's femininity and charm,' she wrote, 'but care not a whit for their real personalities and concerns.'[24] As their relationship deteriorated, she visited California in an attempt to recoup her health and strength. Indeed, away from her family she soon found herself feeling vigorous and youthful again.[25]

The reappearance of her depression upon her return to her family confirmed her underlying resentment of her husband, who obviously cherished traditional notions of wife, home and motherhood, and her own feelings about the confining role of housewife and mother. The resentment also coloured her early writing. In her poem, *The Answer*, later published in the *Woman's Journal* in 1886, she articulated her feelings about the repressive aspects of marriage:

> A maid was asked in marriage. Wise as fair,
> She gave her answer with deep thought and prayer,
>
> Expecting in the holy name of wife,
> Great work, great pain and greater joy in life.
>
> Such work she found as brainless slaves might do,
> By day and night, long labour, never through;
>
> Such pain no language can such pain reveal; It had no limit
> but her power to feel;
>
> Such joy life left in her sad soul's employ,
> Neither the hope nor memory of joy.
>
> Helpless she died, with one despairing cry, 'I thought it good;
> How could I tell the lie?'
>
> And answered Nature, merciful and stern,
> I teach by killing; let the others learn.[26]

As her marital relationship deteriorated, Gilman tried to overcome her difficulties by reinstating her therapeutic gymnastics programme and demonstrating anew her belief that exercise could counterbalance mental depression. 'Still feel poorly,' she wrote in her diary, but 'depart at six for the gymnasium, speedily make friends, and . . . find myself happy to the verge of idiocy at being there again.'[27] She also rowed. Charles Stetson wrote admiringly in his diary about one expedition up the Seekonk River where his wife rowed over four miles in less than fifty minutes without tiring.[28]

Gymnastics and other physical activities, however, did not prevent her continued despondency and she soon found herself 'back to the edge of insanity again'.[29] Her husband wrote despairingly of her 'spasms of horror'. 'After making herself and me miserable for four or more years [Charlotte] has found her real strength, which is weakness. My patience is about exhausted.' In particular, Stetson was tired of his wife's absorption in the woman question, her feminist meetings and activities. 'It is very noble and to an extent proper, but it seems a wee bit unhealthy, feverish.'[30] In desperation, and with Gilman a willing participant, he enlisted in 1887 the help of Dr Weir Mitchell whose rest cure it was hoped would return his wife to the normalcy he expected in the marriage relationship.[31]

Despite her initial enthusiasm, Gilman later decided that this eminent physician 'was well versed in two kinds of nervous prostration; that of the business man exhausted from too much work, and the society woman exhausted from too much play. The kind I had was evidently beyond him.'[32] Dr Mitchell, however, was confident in his diagnosis of neurasthenia and of his cure for Charlotte Gilman. By now highly specialized in the treatment of female neurasthenics, 'those sensitive creatures whose destiny if not handled properly was the shawl and the sofa', he treated Gilman as an aggressive, dominating and manipulative woman. Such women, he believed were like 'vampire[s] sucking the blood of the healthy people of a household', and, therefore, deserving of little sympathy.[33] In mapping out the cure for Gilman's nervous depression Dr Mitchell reflected well the attitudes of a number of leading establishment male physicians of his era towards the 'new woman'.

Medicine as an instrument of social control: the doctor and the 'new woman'

Late nineteenth-century medicine, as we have seen, relied heavily upon systems of gender differentiation and was important in constructing sexual ideology and in illuminating social perceptions of 'woman as body'. Fear of female independence and competition and the movement of nineteenth-century medicine towards somaticism inclined doctors (who were mostly male) to concentrate even more closely upon the supervision of female patients' bodies (and hence minds) and the regulation of all aspects of women's lives. Limited female energy, the doctors proclaimed, was meant for the altruism of home and posterity, not unsanctioned activity of mind, body and other augmentations of individuality which could only lead to ill health.

The tension between the medical paradigm, which restricted physical mobility and creative endeavour, and the new momentum in women's search for self-development and a creative outlet was evident in claims of a disturbing increase in female nervous disorders.[34] Confronted with what they perceived to be an epidemic of nervous afflictions, male doctors, especially an articulate group of neurological specialists, pronounced anorexia nervosa, hysteria and neurasthenia the result of the 'new woman's' indifference to marriage and motherhood and attempted incursion into the male intellectual and public world. 'Woman's efforts,

211

acted out rashly and foolishly,' wrote a leading establishment physician in 1890, 'made her ultimately unfit for active life because of the perilous injury brought on by the deleterious irritation of the outside world'.[35] Neurasthenic women, said another doctor, were those who led faulty lives and required for correction a radical change in life-style.[36] For many female intellectuals in the late nineteenth century, the attempted transition from a domestic to a professional life was characterized by nervous disorders and periodic depression. 'New women' and nervous illness seemed to go together, and neurologists readily fashioned treatments which were designed to ease the anxieties of female patients by defusing their ambitions and resocializing them to their traditional sphere and its familiar obligations.[37]

The eminent neurologist Dr Weir Mitchell used his own studies on the physiology of the cerebellum to provide himself with a neurological explanation for the apparent breakdown of mind and body that led to female hysteria and neurasthenia. He ascribed female neurasthenia to 'reflex irritation' wherein irritations of the reproductive organs were transmitted electrically via nerve impulses to the brain, causing lesions in the brain cortex.[38]

Convinced that neurotic phenomena had a somatic base, Mitchell sought to heal the mind by first restoring the body to health.[39] The view that one's general wellbeing depended first and foremost upon the wellbeing of the body, and that a systematic training of the body assured a robust mind (the popular Victorian interpretation of 'mens sana in corpore sano') was based more upon Herbert Spencer's interpretation of evolutionary theory than upon Juvenal's ancient phrase.[40] Had neurologists been impressed by Plato's insistence that a healthy body could not in itself produce a healthy mind, they might have placed less store upon the somatic basis of mental problems.[41] As it was, they focused upon the physical causes of mental depression and concentrated upon restoring mental health through physical interventions.[42] Disease was inconceivable without some underlying physical basis and functional disorders such as neurasthenia, in which there was apparently tissue dysfunction without structural abnormality, were seen to be rooted in 'real if unrecognized physical processes'.[43] 'You cure the body,' Mitchell said 'and somehow the mind is also cured.'[44]

The rest cure

The key to cure, and the basis of Mitchell's famous rest cure, logically lay in regulating individual habits and restoring balance to the patient's daily life. Mitchell's observations caused him to believe in conserving energy through enforced rest followed by the provision of a complete and carefully specified moral and physical re-education.[45] For a typical female neurasthenic patient such as Gilman, complete rest, seclusion and excessive feeding began once she relinquished total control to her physician.[46] Dr Mitchell made use of 'every grade of rest . . . from repose on a lounge for some hours up to entire rest in bed for up to eight weeks'.[47] During this time the patient was only gradually allowed to sit up, use her hands or read. Various passive exercises such as massage and electricity were prescribed to offset the deleterious effects of prolonged confinement in bed.[48] Gentle, carefully controlled but never excessive exercise was allowed only in brief excursions from the bed. 'You must get the effect of exercise without its ills', said Mitchell.[49] The massage treatment, which covered the whole body, could last up to an hour each day.[50] Tonics such as pints of milk and fattening foods were presented as strengtheners which generated surplus fat to 'fight moral or mental strain and fevers'.[51]

The enforced rest and feeding took place well away from the patient's home and relatives and friends were excluded while moral and physical re-education took place. After building up her health, re-education focused primarily upon teaching the patient how to regain and preserve domination over her emotions. This was carried out by a well-trained female nurse who was the unquestioning agent 'firmly implementing the orders of the more distant and totally authoritative male, the doctor in charge'.[52] In this way the patient was gradually taught not to yield to hysterical behaviour but to display order, control and self-restraint. She was expected to become 'less hysterical and more obsessional', and perform her female role in a structured manner with dutiful attention to rules and detail.[53] In short, the rest cure was a behaviour modification treatment designed to make nervous, overactive and dissatisfied women more passive, feminine and healthy, and to help them learn that domesticity was the cure, not the cause, of their problems. The female neurasthenic was thus 'returned to her menfolk's management, recycled and taught to make the will of the male her own'.[54]

For some women the remedy was an agent of regeneration, and they reported feeling better for the enforced rest and the opportunity to withdraw temporarily from life's demands and sorrows. At least they had gained weight and colour, and some felt more relaxed. Yet, by depriving some women patients of those activities which were most important to them, and by suspending their active and intellectual life, the rest cure could also become a potent form of punishment in the process of social control. Deprived of reading or writing, freedom of vigorous activity in the open air, and ready access to understanding friends, the mental and physical incarceration imposed by the rest cure became a devastating medical experience from which some women never recovered.[55]

Gilman and the rest cure

When Charlotte Perkins Gilman came, in 1887, to Dr Weir Mitchell's practice on 1524 Walnut Street in Philadelphia she was confident that the rest cure would alleviate the severe nervous depression which had ensued in the aftermath of her marriage.[56] Unable to cope with life's circumstances, Gilman saw the rest cure as a last resort in her belief that medical therapy was necessary to cure the brain fever which was 'her form of neurasthenia'.[57] Viewing the doctor as a necessary link to the outside world of health and activity, Gilman was acknowledging that her own attempts to maintain a mind–body balance through years of attention to physical culture and systems of self-development had failed.[58]

Absorbing the popular medical belief that physical health would engender mental stability, Gilman believed that the depressions which plagued her would be eased should she strive for a high level of physical fitness. She saw her own life as one where the physical must overcompensate for the mental during her frequent bouts of anxiety. What she learned from her disastrous experience with Mitchell's rest cure was that a strong and healthy body was a necessary but not a sufficient condition for mental health. Mental and physical health, she conjectured, were so intimately connected that true growth could only occur when both aspects were allowed to develop. Whereas many medical specialists advocated fixed amounts of energy being apportioned to tasks and activities stipulated by social prescription, Gilman eventually realized (as did many other feminists in the 1890s and early years of the twentieth century) that mind and body could continue to grow in strength and harmony were they both put to use in a productive enterprise.[59] Seen in this light, health became 'more an experiment than a blueprint', a search in which unrestricted physical energy was an important key to personal autonomy and a useful support in escaping from the private to the public sphere.[60] Feminists thus saw that the use of physical exertion to strive against and overcome obstacles could bring with it a sense of conquest out of which the identity of the 'new woman' could emerge. This, however, was just a starting point because the new identity could become concrete only if the mind was also ready to jettison traditional encumbrances to welcome new challenges and creative growth.

When Dr Mitchell, in his cure for neurasthenia, restricted physical and mental avenues of growth through enforced rest, Gilman almost lost her sanity. In the rest cure the complete suspension of physical activity, intellectual work and social contacts deprived her of all that she held most important. The therapy brought neither health nor serenity and seemed to dampen all hopes for a meaningful future. While rest and solicitous attention may have proved useful to the overworked and exhausted late-nineteenth-century neurasthenic man or woman, it became a form of punishment and an imprisonment to 'new women' like Gilman struggling to overcome the difficulties of breaking away from a meaningless existence.

Mitchell's final prescription for Gilman was to concentrate upon living as domestic a life as possible. 'Have your child with you all the time. . . .Lie down an hour after each meal. Have but two hours of intellectual life a day. And never touch pen, brush or pencil for as long as you live.'[61] Nothing could have had a more disastrous effect. She went home, followed those directions rigidly for months, and believed she came perilously near to losing her mind.[62] As her depressions worsened she decided that it was better for her to leave a husband sane than to stay with him insane.[63] The final breakdown helped Gilman both escape her marriage and find in her work an excuse for possible failure.[64] It also inspired 'The Yellow Wallpaper', a Poe-esque short story in which Gilman recalled her bitter experience with Dr Weir Mitchell's rest cure.[65] Initially the story was rejected by the editor of the *Atlantic* who wrote that he could not forgive himself if he made others as miserable as he had made himself by reading it.[66] In 1892, however, it was published in the *New England Magazine*.[67]

Although 'The Yellow Wallpaper' is now considered the best of Gilman's fiction, it was originally read as a chilling horror story rather than as an examination of the social roots of mental illness and an exploration of male–female relationships in the late nineteenth century.[68] In the story, the narrator, a writer, finds herself increasingly depressed and nervously ill. Her loving and well-meaning husband, who is also a 'censorious and paternalistic physician', believes that she needs complete rest and a cessation of her work if she is to recover. He takes her to a house in the country and lovingly consigns her to enforced idleness in an upstairs room, a former nursery with faded yellow-patterned wallpaper, bars on the windows and a large bed nailed to the floor. The setting thus becomes both a forced retreat into childhood and a prison, cutting her off from the regular processes needed to shape women's lives.[69] She is constantly told to rest and sleep, use her willpower to overcome her depression and avoid 'silly fancies'. With nothing left to occupy her mind, the yellow wallpaper eventually becomes the only aspect of interest in the narrator's life which she wants to control.[70] Behind the pattern of the wallpaper she begins to visualize a trapped woman stooping down and creeping about:

> Sometimes I think there are a great many women behind, and sometimes only one, and she crawls around fast, and her crawling shakes it all over.
> Then in the very bright spots she keeps still, and in the very shady spots she just takes hold of the bars and shakes them hard.
> And she is all the time trying to climb through. But nobody would climb through that pattern – it strangles so; I think that is why it has so many heads. They get through, and then the pattern strangles them off and turns them upside down, and makes their eyes white![71]

Her obsession becomes the rescue of that shadow woman from the paper pattern that bars her own self-realization. One night she finally sets about freeing the trapped woman and hence herself. 'I pulled and she shook, I shook and she pulled, and before morning we had peeled off yards of that paper.' In her final descent into madness the narrator begins to creep and crawl about the room. With the climax of the story her husband breaks down the door and faints as she triumphantly crawls over his body exclaiming, 'I've got out at last . . . in spite of you and Jane. And I've pulled off most of the paper, so you can't put me back.'[72] Thus the heroine's triumph over the rest cure, husband and doctor comes at the expense of her mind.

Gilman later wrote that her protest against Mitchell's rest cure through 'The Yellow Wallpaper' was designed to convince the Doctor of the errors of his ways.[73] It was also an effort to portray 'a nightmare vision of sick women dependent on male doctors who used their professional superiority . . . to prolong their patients' sickness, and consequently the supremacy of their own sex.'[74] In 'The Yellow Wallpaper', Gilman presented insanity as an ultimate form of rebellion, where madness was the only creative act available to one doomed to submit to society's standards.[75]

Freedom or not: the flowering of Gilman's literary career

> Perhaps one way to define madness is to say that it is the affliction of those who take the basic premises of the society they live in too literally and pursue the logical consequences of that society's underlying assumptions with too single-minded a determination.[76]

Feminist interpretations of Gilman's writings and life until her breakdown view her near descent into madness (as described in 'The Yellow Wallpaper') as a subtle form of growth – a way to health and a rejection of and escape from an insane society.[77] By interpreting madness as a higher form of sanity one could read Gilman's story as a quest for her own identity. In her mad sane way, they suggest, she saw her own situation and that of all women for what it really was, and madness became her only freedom and her ultimate road to health.[78] By identifying with the woman behind the wallpaper and helping her to escape, Gilman is seen to effect her own liberation from disease and find that she, too, has entered 'the open space of her own authority'.[79]

Gilman's breakdown and the failure of Dr Weir Mitchell's rest cure helped facilitate her escape from the traditional domestic role so objectionable to her. Although emotionally painful, her refusal to be returned 'cured' to her confined sphere by a loving family and a leading physician encouraged a measure of personal growth and a new ability to identify and deal with rather than avoid conflict.[80] Gilman finally realized that she could never be truly 'healthy' in the traditional female role. Abandoning the role that had caused her such pain and disclaiming a prevalent male medical model that had tried to refit her for that role, she began a new search for self-definition and wholeness as a female writer. Confident that self-assertion and personal growth through reading, writing, exercising and meeting and talking with other women provided a better chance than medical intervention of improving her health, she left her husband and moved to California in 1888.[81] Forced to become self-dependent, she developed a base for her 'professional living', a writing and public-speaking career.

As Gilman became increasingly popular among feminist reformers in California, she and Stetson initiated divorce proceedings. Intimating her lack of womanliness, newspapers covering the divorce emphasized that among the husband's complaints was her overzealous pursuit of physical fitness, to the point that 'she became very muscular'![82] Stetson clearly associated her frequent visits to the gymnasium with those suffrage meetings that had, in his opinion, exacerbated her resentment of the domestic sphere. Following the divorce, Gilman's former husband decided to marry her life-long friend Grace Channing and Gilman allowed her daughter Katharine to live with them.

No longer tied to husband and daughter, Gilman grasped the freedom she believed she needed for health and self-fulfilment. Yet the family break-up left her with a life-long guilt and sadness often exposed in her stories.[83] As Filene notes, when such women tried to bring theory to life, practising it in their daily lives, they inevitably experienced frustration, confusion and existential pain.[84] 'These were years,' Gilman wrote, 'that I could never see a mother and child together without crying.'[85] The social disapproval which accompanied her freedom depressed her, and during the period of adjustment she believed her lot must for ever be emancipation without joy. Later she wrote that she must be unfit to live with since she was so busy and so engrossed in 'being me'.

Her divorce and separation from her child left her, she noted, with a 'lasting loss of power . . . the necessity for a laboriously acquired laziness foreign to both temperament and conviction, a crippled life'.[86] Yet, despite her debilitating exhaustion, she increasingly found the strength to rededicate herself to self-development and write about suffrage issues. She aligned herself to two movements in particular, non-Marxian socialism as espoused by Edward Bellamy and the social purity concerns of the women's movement. Socialism, she believed, was the most practical form of human development, while the equality of the sexes was the most essential condition of that development. It was an evil, she lectured, to conceal the facts of sex and allow the rigid conventions of society to restrict one's daily life.[87]

The influence of Bellamy's *Looking Backward* (1888), especially his consideration of women's place in a future egalitarian order, was particularly apparent in Gilman's first major study and her most important work, *Women and Economics*.[88] Bellamy's utopian novel had drawn a world in the year 2000 where co-operation was the norm, women had political and economic equality, and childbearing and domestic matters were supported by the state. Public kitchens, dining rooms and nurseries released women for other activities. In the educational system particular prominence was accorded physical culture, and proficiency in athletic feats and games was given equal importance with scholarship. In the novel a leading character, Dr Leete explained to Julian West, Bellamy's visitor from the nineteenth-century, that:

> [the] magnificent health which distinguishes our women from those of your day who seem to have been so generally sickly, is owing largely to the fact that

all alike are furnished with healthful and inspiring occupation. . .It is in giving full play to the differences of sex rather than in seeking to obliterate them, as was apparently the effort of some reformers in your day, that the enjoyment of each by itself are alike enhanced. . .We have given [women] a world of their own with its emulations, ambitions and careers, and I assure you they are very happy in it. It seems to us that women were, more than any other class, the victims of your civilization [with] their ennuied, undeveloped lives, stunted at marriage, their narrow horizon, bounded so often physically by the four walls of home and morally by a petty circle of personal interests. Such an existence would have softened men's brains or driven them mad.[89]

This delineation of the economic basis of women's freedom was precisely the message that Gilman framed so forcefully in *Women and Economics*.[90] Contrasting women's current oppression with Bellamy's utopian notions, she demanded economic reorganization to allow women full participation in society's affairs. Her thesis was in many ways an elaboration of her great-aunt Catharine Beecher's argument thirty years earlier that women should unite to establish their economic independence to demand dignity and respect for their domestic labour.[91] Society confused women's sexual and economic roles, Gilman posited, by denying women access to wage-earning jobs and forcing them to use sex to earn their keep.[92] The family perpetuated female enslavement and degradation, wasted women's energies in the mundane tasks of cooking, cleaning and personal service, and made women psychologically and physically dependent upon men's demands. Forced to emphasize sexuality at the expense of humanity, woman had to prove her capacity for submission to the dominant male.[93]

Gilman's radical 1898 assault on the inequalities of marriage and the patriarchal restrictions on women's intellectual and physical development attracted immediate and wide attention on both sides of the Atlantic and made her the leading intellectual in the women's movement.[94] *Women and Economics* was widely acclaimed as a brilliant theoretical attack upon conservative interpretations of political economy.[95] It was, said *The Nation*, 'the most significant utterance on the subject of women since Mill's *The Subjection of Women*'.[96]

Gilman's social vision

Though Gilman rebelled against the constraints of an oppressive patriarchal system, she was no revolutionary. Like many of her contemporary feminists, her life was confused and contradictory. She remained, in many ways, loyal to the old order, suffering from an inability to reconcile her conformist tendencies towards the traditional, domestic role of the Victorian middle-class woman with her desire to transcend the limitations of female experience. Indeed, the characterization of Charlotte Gilman as a 'militant madonna' by an auditor at one of her lectures was astute. While promoting radical changes to the female condition in her writings and experimenting with alternative domestic arrangements in her own life, she never denied the differences between the sexes or denigrated the importance of wifehood and motherhood.[97] Rather, she tried 'to reverse traditionally-negative connotations of femininity by emphasizing the virtues of womanhood. . . Woman's uniqueness was her strength and glory, her mother-love a countervailing force within the baneful androcentric culture.'[98]

Sociologist Lester Frank Ward provided appropriate ammunition for these beliefs though his gynaecocentric theory.[99] Gilman claimed that Ward's gynaecocentric theory was 'the greatest single contribution to the world's thought since evolution'.[100] In 'Our better halves', published in 1888, Ward argued that from an evolutionary perspective the female sex was always primary and the male secondary.[101] Evolutionary study showed that the first male function was simply to enable the female to produce and that the female, the primary source of life, was of superior importance. Although environmental and hereditary forces had combined to enfeeble temporarily the naturally productive inclinations of women, this did not mean that they could not or should not resume their natural role in progress to the future. On the contrary, since women were, by instinct, altruistic, nurturant and co-operative, they were clearly better fitted than males for certain types of leadership in society, because males were inherently aggressive, competitive and destructive. Thus, 'fundamental to the evolutionary process was woman's inherent responsibility (and unique talent) for the preservation of the race, the selection of a mate, and the nurturance of children'.[102] Indeed, said Ward, 'true science teaches that the elevation of woman is the only sure road to the evolution of man'.[103]

In a cornucopia of poetry, fiction and reform tracts,[104] Gilman developed her general social vision upon Ward's gynaecocentric theory and drafted a social blueprint in which the emerging 'new woman' would play a leading role. The prototype of this 'new woman' was outlined initially in *Women and Economics*. She was 'honester, braver, stronger, more healthful and skilful and able and free, more human in all ways'.[105] No less female than women from earlier days, she was wholesome, healthy and physically emancipated, a companion to men rather than a dependent. She remained dedicated, however, to the highest ideals of duty to family, womanhood and social betterment.

In keeping with these beliefs about womanhood and her own personal passion for physical culture, female health, strength and independence were constantly revisited themes in Gilman's writings. She believed that central to the promotion of meaningful work for women was their right to pursue health and maintain physical fitness for both their own benefit and the common good. 'As human beings they will want human bodies . . . and human bodies need human exercise to develop them.' 'Improving the physical condition,' she wrote repeatedly, and 'building up a clean and noble body', were vital factors in social advancement.[106] In 'The Primal Power', for example, she urged women to become 'full-grown mothers, brave and free', with 'splendid bodies, trained and strong'.[107] Then, she noted, they would be able to 'gradually rear a new race of men, with minds large enough to see in human beings something besides males and females'.[108]

Gilman was particularly successful in dramatizing these ideas in her feminist utopian novel, *Herland*, first serialized in *The Forerunner* in 1915.[109] The history of Herland revealed an evolutionary process where all males were gradually killed off and a female community began to flourish through parthenogenesis (a virgin birth process which produced only female children). Dedicated to growth through life-giving and nurture, the women of Herland concentrated on preserving and improving the quality of life through eugenics and family limitation (one child per mother). 'Thus, defects of mind and body are bred out and the family becomes stronger and increasingly more intelligent, innovative, imaginative and physically beautiful.'[110]

Challenging the assumption that women were weak and in need of male protection, Gilman focused upon the way female agility could defeat the temptations and advances of masculine exploitation.[111] In Herland, 'each [woman] was in the full bloom of rosy health, erect, serene, standing sure-footed and light as any pugilist . . . athletic, light and powerful'. 'Fishwives and market women might show similar strength,' wrote Gilman, 'but it was coarse and heavy.'[112] By contrast, Gilman's utopian women maintained their strength and agility through lifelong acrobatics and athletic dancing, living that life of freedom and activity for which the author herself had always yearned. In their gymnasia, 'there were no spectacular acrobatics, such as only the young can perform, but for all-around development they had a most excellent system'. Furthermore, such exercises were only a small part of their physical culture. They ran like marathon winners and leaped like deer, raced and played games, climbed trees, swung on ropes. Children were taught to use and control their own bodies. They could swim before they walked and were sure-footed, steady-handed and clear-headed. This stalwart race of tall, strong and healthy women personified human motherhood in full working use, mother love raised to its highest power. Life to the mothers of Herland was growth. Everything was beauty, order, perfect cleanness and the pleasantest sense of home over it all.[113]

Here, then, was Gilman's view of the fruition of Lester Frank Ward's gynaecocentric theory of evolutionary progress, a world of women experiencing the meaningful work, economic independence and equal human love that Gilman believed was so necessary to full health. 'We had expected hysteria,' said the three male visitors to Herland, 'and instead found a standard of health and vigor [and] a calmness of temper . . . .'[114]

Since literary utopias depict the state of mind or ideals desired by their authors, reading them helps obtain a sense of history-as-experienced that statistics or political documents cannot provide.[115] Gilman's feminist utopian novel *Herland* was less a social blueprint than the demonstration of a set of values and experiences which she considered superior to those allowed in a patriarchal society. The female citizens of Herland were not restricted physically or mentally. They transcended the traditional female limitations and were in full control of their lives. They were 'free from the rape of their minds as well as their bodies', and their female-only society was engaged in a continual growth.[116] Herlanders were healthy women in a healthy society.

For Gilman, the calm healthfulness of the feminist utopia Herland, with 'the best kind of people . . . [kept] . . . at their best and growing better', stood in sharp contrast to her earlier description of enforced passivity and female mental disintegration in 'The Yellow Wallpaper'.[117] Her feminist utopia offered turn-of-the-century women an alternative model of female puberty and growth which directed the girl into a full and free adulthood, not the constraining world of 'The Yellow Wallpaper' which maintained the woman in a childlike state.[118]

During the decades which separated her writing of these vastly different portrayals of female real and potential experience, Gilman, by frequently confronting her life through resolutions achieved in her work, attempted to experience her own sense of personal transformation and growth.[119] The emphasis upon physical mobility in all Gilman's fiction was a direct comment on the barriers blocking women from physical mobility in the real world. 'Whosoever lives always in a small dark place,' she warned, and 'is always guarded, directed and restrained, will become inevitably narrowed and weakened by it.'[120] Thus the desire to transcend these limitations of female experience was as evident in her life-style as in her writings, and her interest in physical fitness as a means to gain personal autonomy remained with her throughout her life.

Gilman's inspiration came largely from her efforts to transform personal contradictions and difficulties into legitimate insights into social problems (and the institutions and ideologies that caused them). Bridging the gap from personal experience to social understanding, her experiences of health, illness, physical fitness and perceived confinement found lucid expression in her writings.[121] An analysis of these writings helps the social historian assess the impact of behavioural expectations on nineteenth-century women more successfully than examining role prescriptions in isolation.[122]

Gilman never regained the vigorous health of her early adult years, however, and despite her persistence in trying to maintain a well-trained physique through sport and exercise, she experienced 'grey fogs' – bouts of uncontrollable mental depression – for the rest of her life.[123] 'You must understand,' she told an acquaintance who once commented upon her healthy appearance, that 'what ails me is a weak mind in a strong body.' But, said Gilman, her acquaintance did not understand. 'They never do', she added.[124] One is left to speculate whether Gilman's perceived inability to achieve complete health was indicative of her difficulties in accepting the views she propounded publicly on women's emancipation. Gilman's ambivalence about her own abilities as a mother, for example, pressed her to imagine a utopian world of socialist mothers where one could learn to be a mother as she had never been taught, and where one could experience giving and receiving the mother-love that she had never experienced or felt competent to give. If, as she so often wrote, female fulfilment came from 'human motherhood in full working use', then she had failed to achieve it. Despite maintaining the physical fitness she believed necessary for an emancipated life, she therefore believed that she had not achieved the holistic state of health she considered necessary for true growth.[125] In her quest for self-possession she had not become the 'new woman' sound in mind and body, but remained in a transitional zone split within herself and torn between the old and the new world.[126] Physical culture had helped her to survive, to feel happier, more vigorous and in greater control of her body.[127] It had not, however, been the key to sanity and mental power that William Blaikie had promised his many nineteenth-century female readers. Convinced that she did not possess a strong mind in her healthy body, she believed that she could never personally inherit Margaret Fuller's kingdom. Through her literary contributions to feminism, however, she suggested to future generations of women that an integrated self was attainable.

Notes

1 Margaret Fuller, *Life Without and Life Within, or Reviews, Narratives, Essays and Poems* (Boston:Roberts Brothers, 1874), 116.

2 Feminists, of course, had expressed such anxieties consistently throughout the nineteenth century. Margaret Fuller, for example, criticized a society in which men were too selfish and vain to allow women to become independent. 'Women must realize,' she said, that 'a house is no home unless it contains food and fire for the mind as well as for the body.' Without confidence in themselves, she believed that middle-class women could never find out what they were fit for, and instead of seeking strength and learning to stand alone, they tended to repress their impulses, doubt their instincts and become paralyzed in their actions. *Woman in the Nineteenth Century and Kindred Papers Relating to the Sphere, Condition and Duties of Women*, 1845: rept., W.W. Norton, New York, 1971, p. 35; See also Roberta J. Park, 'The attitudes of leading New England Transcendentalists toward healthful exercise, active recreations and proper care of the body: 1830–1860', *Journal of Sport History*, IV, no. 1, Spring 1977, pp. 46–47.

Fuller's theme was revisited with increasing frequency during the last three decades of the century. Feminist Jane Croly complained that 'within the household, there is neither reward nor promotion. The more strictly and conscientiously a woman fulfills her duty ... the more narrow and contracted her life becomes. Marriage is a refuge of some, but it has been the grave of many clever women.' Jane Croly, *For Better or Worse: A Book for Some Men and All Women*, Boston, 1874, p. 61; Elizabeth Cady Stanton also decried the restrictions on physical activity and intellectual stimulation and pointed out the high demands and low rewards of married life. Such constraints upon self development, she believed, led inevitably to mental and bodily strain. Elizabeth Cady Stanton, 'The health of American women', *North American Review*, CXXXV, Dec. 1882, p. 513.

Condemned by marriage to dependence, seclusion and intellectual sterility, in addition to the arduous burdens of child-bearing and child-rearing, many bright and ambitious women did become nervous and depressed. Some were driven to madness. Florence Nightingale's Cassandra, for example, showed vividly how isolation, physical restriction and lack of intellectual stimulation within the Victorian middle-class family could be totally maddening to an intelligent woman. 'One would think we had no heads or hearts by the total indifference of the public towards them. Our bodies are the only things of consequence.' Nightingale, 'Cassandra', p. 405.

Virginia Woolf later commented on the same frustrating phenomenon: 'It needs little skill in psychology to be sure that a highly gifted girl who had tried to use her gift for poetry would have been so thwarted and hindered by other people, so tortured and pulled apart by her own contrary instincts that she must have lost her own health and sanity to a certainty.' Virginia Woolf, *A Room of One's Own*, 1929, Harbinger Books, New York, rpt., 1957, p. 127.

3 B. Berch, 'Charlotte Perkins Gilman', in John Eatwell, Murray Milgate and Peter Newman, eds., *The New Palgrave. A Dictionary of Economics*, Vol. II, The MacMillan Press, London, 1987, p. 528.

4 Daniel Cottom, *Social Figures; George Eliot, Social History and Literary Representation*, University of Minnesota Press, Minneapolis, 1987, p. 211.

5 Bell and Offen, *Women, the Family and Freedom*, II, p. 9; Morantz, *Clio's Consciousness*, p. 43.

6 Mary A. Hill, *Charlotte Perkins Gilman: The Making of a Radical Feminist, 1860–1896*, Temple University Press, Philadelphia, 1980, p. 117; Charlotte Perkins Gilman, *The Living of Charlotte Perkins Gilman: An Autobiography*, D. Appleton Century Co., New York, 1935, pp. 67 and 64.

7 Hill, *Radical Feminist*, pp. 13 and 22. The break-up of the Perkins marriage, thought Gilman, had much to do with the reproductive difficulties of her mother who after numerous difficult pregnancies and losing two children, was advised to have no more.

8 Kathryn Kish Sklar, *Catharine Beecher: A Study in American Domesticity*, Yale University Press, New Haven, 1973; Patricia Vertinsky, 'Sexual equality and the legacy of Catharine Beecher', *Journal of Sport History*, VI, Spring 1979, pp. 35–49. Gilman, suggests Nancy Woloch, was the Beecher's last and greatest contribution to American feminism. *Women and the American Experience*, Alfred A. Knopf, New York, 1984, p. 399.

9 Gilman, *Autobiography*, p. 8.

10 Hill, *Radical Feminist*, pp. 42–43; Gilman, *Autobiography*, p. 28; Fellman and Fellman, *Making Sense of Self*, p. 58.

11 Gilman, *Autobiography*, p. 29; Hill, *Radical Feminist*, p. 45, notes that Gilman's autobiography is misleading to the extent that she remembered herself as a passive victim more than a lively rebel sport, and that her diaries present more accurate information about her youthful activities.

12 Charlotte Perkins Gilman, Diary, 27 October 1879, Arthur and Elizabeth Schlesinger Library, Charlotte Perkins Gilman Collection, Radcliffe College, Cambridge, Massachusetts (hereafter called the AESL collection); William Blaikie, *How to Get Strong and How to Stay So*, Harper and Bros., New York, 1883, pp. 272, 48, 72 and 73. Although Blaikie quoted Dr S. Weir Mitchell's suggestion that vigorous muscular exercise was the very thing to quiet the excited nerves and brain, Mitchell, in fact, increasingly restricted exercise in his rest cure and substituted passive methods and bed rest.

13 Hill, *Radical Feminist*, p. 65; Blaikie, *How to Get Strong*, p. 272; Gilman, *Autobiography*, pp. 66–67.

14 Gilman, *Autobiography*, p. 71.

15 Charlotte Perkins Gilman, 'The Providence Ladies Gymnasium', *Providence Journal*, VIII, 23 May, 1883, p. 2.

16 Hill, *Radical Feminist*, pp. 73–74; See also Charles C. Eldredge, *Charles Walter Stetson: Color and Fantasy*, University of Kansas Press, Kansas, 1982, pp. 25–26.
17 Hill, *Radical Feminist*, p. 101; Eldredge, *Charles Walter Stetson*, p. 32.
18 Karen Horney provides one perspective on avoiding adulthood, in 'The flight from womanhood: The masculinity complex in women as viewed by men and women', *Psychoanalysis and Women*, Jean Baker Miller, ed. Penguin Books, Middlesex, 1973, pp. 5–20.
19 On the notion of woman's duty, George Bernard Shaw was particularly eloquent. 'Unless woman repudiates her womanliness, her duty to her husband, to her children, to society, to the law, and to everyone but herself, she cannot emancipate herself... Therefore, woman has to repudiate duty altogether. In that repudiation lies her freedom.' George Bernard Shaw, *The Womanly Woman From the Quintessence of Ibsenism*, London, 1891, rpt 1913, p. 52.
20 Diary entry for Jan. 1, 1884. AESL Collection; Diary entries for Jan. 30, 11, Feb. 20, March 24, 1884. AESL Collection; Diary entry for April 1, 1883.
21 Carol Ruth Berkin, 'Private woman, public woman: The contradictions of Charlotte Perkins Gilman', in *Women of America: A History*, C.R. Berkin and M.B. Norton, eds. Houghton Mifflin, Co., Boston, 1979, p. 161.
22 Gilman, *Autobiography*, pp. 89–92 and 101.
23 Gilman, *Autobiography*, p. 91.
24 Charlotte Perkins Stetson, 'On advertising for marriage', *Alpha*, II, no. 1, Sept 1, 1885, p. 7.
25 Hill, *Radical Feminist*, pp. 132–3.
26 Charlotte Perkins Gilman, 'The answer', *Woman's Journal*, XVII, October 2, 1886, p. 313. Carroll Smith-Rosenberg, Elaine Showalter and other leading feminist historians suggest that Gilman, and others like her, were attempting to escape from their traditional role of housewife and mother and cope with the stress of real or perceived situational anxieties by adopting depressed or hysterical behaviour. Ehrenreich and English support such an explanation by pointing out that Jane Addams, Margaret Sanger, Eleanor Marx, Olive Shreiner, Ellen Swallow and Charlotte Gilman's miseries and their crippling indecisiveness upon entering womanhood was common among tens of thousands of women. It was as if they had come to the brink of adult life and then refused to go on. Some women, like Gilman, they explain, transformed their numbness into anger and became activists in reform movements but many remained permanently depressed, bewildered or sick. Barbara Ehrenreich and Deidre English, *For Her Own Good*, pp. 2–3. Smith-Rosenberg, 'The hysterical woman', in *Disorderly Conduct*, p. 207; Showalter, *The Female Malady*; Morantz-Sanchez, *Sympathy and Science*; John S. Haller Jr., 'Neurasthenia. The medical profession and the 'new woman' of late nineteenth century', *New York State Journal of Medicine*, Feb. 15, 1971, pp. 473–482.
27 Hill, *Radical Feminist*, p. 143.
28 Mary Armfield Hill, *Endure: The Diaries of Charles Walter Stetson*, Temple University Press, Philadelphia, 1985, p. 313; Hill notes that in Gilman's later fiction there were a number of heroines who not only enjoyed rowing but

did so faster and more effectively than men.
29 Diary entry for 20 March 1887. AESL collection.
30 Hill, *Endure*, p. 333.
31 By the 1880s, Dr Mitchell had become the most prominent neurologist in America and was widely known on both sides of the Atlantic. Richard D. Walter, *S. Weir Mitchell M.D. Neurologist, A Medical Biography*, Charles C. Thomas, Springfield, Ill, 1970, p. 141. He reputedly made $70,000 in a good year, much of it in consulting fees. Barbara Sicherman, 'The uses of a diagnosis: Doctor's patients and neurasthenia', *Journal of the History of Medicine and Allied Sciences*, XXXII, 1977, pp. 33–54.
32 Gilman, *Autobiography*, p. 95.
33 S. Weir Mitchell, *Wear and Tear: Or Hints for the Overworked*, Lippincott, Philadelphia, 1871, p. 28; S. Weir Mitchell, *Doctor and Patient*, Lippincott, Philadelphia, 1888, p. 45.
34 Verbrugge, *Able-Bodied Womanhood*, p. 106; See also Showalter, *The Female Malady*, p. 131.
35 C. Bennett, *The Modern Malady, or Sufferers from Nerves*, E. Arnold, London, 1890, p. 168; G.M. Hammond, 'Nerves and the American woman', *Harper's Bazaar*, XL, 1906, p. 591.
36 H.J. Hall, 'The systematic use of work as a remedy in neurasthenia and allied conditions', *Boston Medical and Surgical Journal*, CLII, 1905, p. 29.
37 Men, of course, were also at risk from nervous exhaustion brought on by overwork and the overzealous pursuit of success (though it was thought they had superior nervous stores to women) and many became candidates for a variety of therapies for neurasthenia. George Beard was especially eager to legitimize neurasthenia as a disease for men who had a deficient energy system from worry and overworking. Therapies usually allowed men the opportunity to carry out business activities between resting periods, and the moral aspect of the treatment was lacking. Increasingly, however, male specialists built their practices around the plentiful supply of female neurasthenics whose difficulties from the 'revolutions' of menstruation, child-bearing and menopause made them prone to serious nervous irritability. Gosling notes that the view that nervous symptoms in women were directly linked to female biology became a tenet of gynaecological practice during this period and influenced gynaecological thought well into the twentieth-century. Francis G. Gosling, 'Neurasthenia in Pennsylvania: A perspective on the origins of American psychotherapy, 1870–1910', *Journal of the History of Medicine and Allied Sciences*, XL, Spring, 1985, p. 193. See also T. Diller, 'Some observations on neurasthenia', *Pennsylvania Medical Journal*, V, 1902, pp. 646–650; Weir Mitchell, *Lectures on Diseases of the Nervous System*; Douglas Wood, 'The fashionable diseases', p. 225. To many neurological specialists it seemed that much neurasthenia was simply a result of women becoming sick because they gave too much energy and attention to selfishly bettering their own sex. 'Co-education and the Higher Education of Women A Symposium', by Professors William Goodell, M.D., T. Gaillard Thomas, M.D., James R. Chadwick, M.D., S. Weir Mitchell, M.D., M. Allen Starr, M.D., and J.J. Putnam, M.D., *Medical News*, LV, 1889, pp. 667–673.

38 Silas Weir Mitchell, 'Researches on the physiology of the cerebellum', *American Journal of Medical Science*, LVII, 1869, pp. 320–338. Among the studies that have been made of Dr S. Weir Mitchell's physiological research are W. Bruce Fye, 'S. Weir Mitchell. Philadelphia's frustrated physiologist and triumphant reformer', *The Development of American Physiology. Scientific Medicine in the Nineteenth Century*, The Johns Hopkins University Press, Baltimore, 1987; Richard D. Walter, *S. Weir Mitchell, M.D. Neurologist, A Medical Biography*, Charles C. Thomas, Springfield, Ill., 1970; Ernest Earnest, *S. Weir Mitchell, Novelist and Physician*, University of Pennsylvania Press, Philadelphia, 1950. See also discussion in Fellman and Fellman, 'Brain and Mind in Sickness and Health', *Making Sense of Self*, pp. 55–72.

39 Mitchell clearly relied upon the explanations of George Beard, who first applied the term 'Neurasthenia' to nervous disorders in the 1860s. Beard, in *American Nervousness. Its Causes and Consequences*, G.P. Putnam, New York, 1881, pp. 7–9, explained that since nervousness was a physical, not a mental state it could be treated with physical methods. Insanity was a physical ailment as much as a broken leg, he said, and this held true for all nervous disorders. To secure his cause, notes Rosenberg, 'he called with impartiality upon physics, neurophysiology and technology, upon Herbert Spencer, Thomas Edison and Herman V. Helmholz for the building blocks with which to construct a mechanistic model exploring the pathology of nervous exhaustion'. Charles E. Rosenberg, 'The place of George M. Beard in nineteenth-century psychiatry', *Bulletin of the History of Medicine*, XXXVI, No. 3, May–June 1962, p. 249.

Although neurasthenia was originally seen as an American disorder by George Beard in the 1860s, English psychiatrists were quick to adopt the neurasthenia diagnosis as pertinent to English nervous disorders. British neurologist Dr Playfair was the first to transport Dr Beard's ideas and Dr Weir Mitchell's treatment for neurasthenia to England. See Suzanne Poirier, 'The Weir Mitchell rest cure: doctors and patients', *Women's Studies*, X, 1983, p. 33, and W.S. Playfair, *The systematic treatment of nerve prostration and hysteria*. Henry C. Lea, Philadelphia, 1883.

40 Haley, *The Healthy Body and Victorian Culture*, p. 254

41 Plato, *The Republic of Plato*, trans. and ed. F.M. Cornford, Oxford University Press, New York, 1945, pp. 312 and 97.

42 Earnest, *S. Weir Mitchell*, p. 229.

43 David Armstrong, *Political Anatomy of the Body*, Cambridge University Press, Cambridge, 1983, p. 20.

44 Silas Weir Mitchell, 'The treatment of rest, seclusion etc, in relation to psychotherapy', *Journal of the American Medical Association*, L, June, 1908, p. 2037. In retrospect, says Sicherman, it is clear that what was called Neurasthenia actually comprehended a range of conditions that included depressive, obsessive and phobic states later classified as psychoneuroses; mildly psychotic and borderline states; palpable physical ills that could not then be adequately diagnosed; and a host of symptoms that are today considered psychophysiological. 'The uses of a diagnosis', p. 34.

45 Silas Weir Mitchell, *Fat and Blood. An Essay on the Treatment of Certain Forms of Neurasthenia and Hysteria*, 10th ed., J.B. Lippincott Co., Philadelphia, 1877.

46 H.J. Byford, *Manual of Gynecology*, 2nd ed. P. Blakiston, Philadelphia, 1897, pp. 180–185.
47 Ellen L. Bassuk, 'The rest cure', p. 247; Mitchell, *Fat and Blood*, p. 71.
48 Mitchell, *Lectures on Diseases of the Nervous System*, pp. 217–233;
49 S. Weir Mitchell, 'Rest in nervous disease: It's use and abuse', *A Series of American Clinical Lectures*, E.C. Seguin, ed., I, 1875, p. 86.
50 Ann Douglas Wood, 'The Fashionable Diseases', p. 225.
51 Silas Weir Mitchell, *Fat and Blood and How to Make Them*, 8th ed., Lippincott, Philadelphia, 1900, p. 288; Showalter suggests that the weight gain accompanying the forced feeding was a kind of pseudo-pregnancy. Elaine Showalter, *A Literature of Their Own*, Princeton University Press, Princeton, 1977, p. 274.
52 Ben Barker-Benfield, 'Sexual surgery in late-nineteenth century America', *International Journal of Health Services*, V, No. 2, 1975, p. 294.
53 Bassuk, *The Rest Cure*, p. 250; 'You get her to promise to fight every desire to cry or twitch, or grow excited', said Mitchell. S. Weir Mitchell, 'True and false palsies of hysterics', *Medical News and Abstract*, XXXVIII, Feb. 1880, p. 71.
54 Barker-Benfield, 'Sexual Surgery', p. 294.
55 Charlotte Gilman and Jane Addams were among Mitchell's most conspicuous failures. G.J. Barker-Benfield, ' "Mother Emancipator:" The meaning of Jane Addams' sickness and cure', *Journal of Family History*, IV, Winter 1979, pp. 395–420.
56 Gilman, *Autobiography*, pp. 93–95.
57 Gilman, *Autobiography*, p. 95.
58 Elizabeth Stuart Phelps was yet another example, who, as her health broke down, and she began to lose her faith in her ability for vigorous independence, began to define sickness as needing the male/doctor. Christine Stansell, 'Elizabeth Stuart Phelps: A study in female rebellion', Lee Edwards, Mary Heath and Lisa Baskin, eds., *Woman: An Issue*, Little, Brown and Company, Boston, 1972, pp. 239–259.
59 Jane Addams, for example, said that to be put to bed and fed milk was not what a frustrated woman required. 'What she needs is simple health-giving activity, which, involving the use of all her faculties, shall be a response to all the claims which she so keenly feels.' Jane Addams, *Democracy and Social Ethics*, Macmillan, New York, 1902, p. 87.
60 Verbrugge, *Able-Bodied Womanhood*, p. 195.
61 Gilman, *Autobiography*, p. 96.
62 Eldredge, *Charles Walter Stetson*, p. 45.
63 Hill, *Radical Feminist*, p. 152; Marriage, Gilman decided was incompatible with freedom. In one of her stories, she poignantly declared that 'a woman could have love and lose life, or she could have life and lose love, but never could she have them both. That was the woman's problem.' Charlotte Perkins Gilman, 'Three women', *Success*, Vol II, Aug. 1908, pp. 490–491, 522–526.
64 Beate Schopp-Schilling, 'The Yellow Wallpaper: A rediscovered realistic story', *American Literary Realism*, VIII, Summer 1975, p. 286.
65 Elaine Hedges discusses this point in her afterword to Charlotte Perkins Gilman, *The Yellow Wallpaper*, The Feminist Press, the City University of New

York, 1973, p. 39. (Rept. of 1899 ed. Small, Maynard, Boston).

66 Horace Scudder, editor of the *Atlantic* quoted in Vivian Gornick, 'Twice told tales', *The Nation*, CCXXVII, September 23, 1978, p. 278.

67 Charlotte Perkins Stetson, 'The Yellow Wallpaper', *New England Magazine*, V, Jan. 1892, pp. 647–659.

68 Lane, *The Charlotte Perkins Gilman Reader*, p. xvi.

69 Gilman vividly saw the connection between independent space and women's creative work, as did Virginia Woolf in *A Room of One's Own*, 1929; for an extended discussion see also, Gilbert and Gubar, *The Madwoman in the Attic*.

70 Loralee MacPike, 'Environment as psychological symbolism in "The yellow wallpaper" ', *American Literary Realism*, VIII, Summer 1975, p. 288.

71 Gilman, 'The yellow wallpaper', p. 30, Hedges, p. 108.

72 Stetson, 'The yellow wallpaper', *New England Magazine*, pp. 647, 656.

73 Gilman, *Autobiography*, p. 121.

74 Wood, 'The fashionable diseases', p. 230; Regina Morantz rightly insists upon caution in viewing the existence of Victorian women solely from the perspective of male domination, especially medical men. 'It is true that Mitchell was very much the Victorian patrician ... but can Wood honestly overlook the fact of Gilman's neurosis and its role in structuring her response to Mitchell ... must our heroines be utterly free from blemishes ...? Should one not pay more attention to the dysfunctional aspects of female socialization in this period?' Morantz, 'The lady and her physician', pp. 42–44.

75 In this sense, says MacPike, Gilman anticipated R.D. Laing's notion that in an insane world, only the mad are sane. MacPike, 'Environment', p. 288.

76 Dijkstra, *Idols of Perversity*, p. 221.

77 Jean E. Kennard, 'Convention coverage or how to read your own life', *New Literary History*, XIII, Autumn 1981, p. 77.

78 Elaine Hedges, 'Afterword', in Charlotte Perkins Gilman, *The Yellow Wallpaper*, ed. Elaine Hedges, Feminist Press, Old Westbury, New York, 1973, p. 39.

79 Janice Haney-Peritz, 'Monumental feminism and literature's ancestral house: Another look at "The Yellow Wallpaper" ', *Women's Studies*, XII, 1986, p. 121.

80 Bassuk, 'The rest cure', p. 256.

81 Hill, 'Charlotte Perkins Gilman' p. 514.

82 A newspaper report said that Stetson had complained that 'she had picked up her dress reform duds, her Bellamy writings, and her muscular development and put off for California'. *San Francisco Examiner*, 19 December 1892.

83 See, for example, Charlotte Perkins Gilman, 'The unnatural mother', *The Forerunner*, November 1916, pp. 281–285. 'No mother that was a mother', said Mis' Briggs, 'would desert her own child for anything on earth.'

84 Filene, *Him/Her/Self*, p. 64.

85 Hill, *Radical Feminist*, p. 231.

86 Gilman, *Autobiography*, p. 100.

87 Carl N. Degler, Introduction, *Women and Economics*, ed. Charlotte Perkins Gilman, Harper & Row, New York, 1966, p. xii; Hill, *Radical Feminist*, pp. 4–5.

88 Charlotte Perkins Gilman, *Women and Economics: A Study of the Economic Relation Between Men and Women as a Factor in Social Evolution*, Harper and Row, New York, 1966, 1st pub., 1898; Charlotte Anna Perkins Gilman wrote under successive names as she married, divorced and married again. Born Charlotte Perkins, she married Charles Walter Stetson in 1884 and later divorced him. In 1900, she married George Houghton Gilman and used his name for the rest of her literary career.
89 Edward Bellamy, *Looking Backward, 2000–1887*, Ticknor, Boston, 1888, pp. 248–250.
90 Buhle, *Women and American Socialism*, pp. 76–77.
91 Sklar, *Catharine Beecher*, p. 267; For a discussion of her plans to socialize domestic work, see Dolores Hayden, 'Two Utopian feminists and their campaigns for kitchenless houses', *Signs*, IV, no. 2, 1978, pp. 274–290.
92 Gilman, *Women and Economics*, pp. 110–126.
93 Clinton, *The Other Civil War*, p. 192.
94 Alice Rossi, ed., *The Feminist Papers: From Adams to De Beauvoir*, Bantam, New York, 1971, pp. 566–572; Jean E. Friedman & William S.G. Shade, eds., *Our American Sisters: Women in American Life and Thought*, D.C. Heath & Co., Lexington, 1982, p. 322.
95 Clinton, *The Other Civil War*, p. 191.
96 *The Nation*, 8 June 1899, p. 443.
97 Degler, Introduction, *Women and Economics*, pp. xvii and xxiv; In *The Man-Made World of Our Androcentric Culture*, Charlton Co., New York, 1911, Gilman attempted to draw a line between the real distinctions of sex and those artificially imposed by society. Games of skill, for example, were inherently masculine 'from the snapped marble of infancy to the flying missile of the bat ... the basic masculine impulse to scatter, to disseminate, to destroy, is shown. Certain sports,' she continued, 'that involve the throwing of a ball will never appeal to women because they are only masculine not human.' p. 114.
98 Hill, 'Charlotte Perkins Gilman', p. 523; Maternàlist theory, notes Gerda Lerner, *The Creation of Patriarchy*, pp. 26–28, is built upon the acceptance of biological sex differences as a given and stems from J.J. Bachofen's highly influential work, *Das Mutterecht*, Stuttgart, 1861. Bachofen's work on evolutionism and Darwinian thought strongly influenced Gilman although she assigned a higher significance to the maternal function.
99 William Doyle claims that Gilman's approach to the woman question was derived essentially from Lester Ward. Charlotte Perkins Gilman and the Cycle of Feminist Reform, Ph.D. Diss., University of California, Berkeley 1960, pp. 175, 161. Hill believes that the intellectual as well as the experiential bases of Gilman's views were so rich and varied that Ward should be viewed as only one important influence among them. Hill, *Radical Feminist*, p. 270.
100 Gilman, *Autobiography*, p. 187.
101 Lester Frank Ward, 'Our better halves', *Forum*, VI, November, 1888, pp. 266–275.
102 Hill, 'Charlotte Perkins Gilman', p. 524; See also, Gilman, *The Man-Made World* for a discussion of women's place in the evolutionary process.
103 Ward, 'Our Better Halves', p. 275.

104 Carl Degler calculates that Gilman published six non-fiction books, a full-length utopian novel, a volume of poetry, two volumes of fiction, seven volumes of a monthly magazine, *The Forerunner*, the contents of which she wrote entirely by herself – scores of articles, poems and short stories in the popular and scholarly periodicals, and an autobiography published post-humously in 1935. C.N. Degler, 'Charlotte Perkins Gilman on the theory and practice of feminism', *American Quarterly*, VIII, no. 1, Spring 1956, p. 22, fn. 6; A.J. Lane's introduction to Gilman's *Herland*, 1979, p. x. Gary Scharnhorst has developed a comprehensive bibliography of all of Gilman's works. *Charlotte Perkins Gilman. A Bibliography*. Scarecrow Press, New Jersey, 1985.

105 In *Women and Economics*, pp. 148–9, Gilman pointed to the popular Gibson girl of the 1890s as her prototype of the new woman; yet as Lois Banner points out, the Gibson girl was only partly a reform figure. She was rarely portrayed in any feminist or reform activity and in many ways her independence did not go much beyond playing sports, wearing natural clothing and looking self-reliant. Possessing a wholesome athletic air that did not smack too much of athletics; she was more a happy combination of the old and new than the personification of the 'new woman'. Lois Banner, *American Beauty*, Alfred A. Knopf, New York, 1983, pp. 156–7; For a further discussion of this 'type', see Banta, *Imaging American Women*, pp. 85–91.

106 Charlotte Perkins Gilman, 'Homework and athletics', *Woman's Journal*, XXXVI, March 5, 1906, p. 75; Charlotte Perkins Gilman, 'Mending morals by making muscles', *Saturday Evening Post*, May 19, 1900, p. 1078; Gilman, *The Man-Made World of Our Androcentric Culture*, Charlton Co., New York, 1911.

107 Charlotte Perkins Gilman, 'The Primal Power', *His Religion and Hers*, The Century Co., New York, 1923, pp. 96–97.

108 Gilman, quoted in Glenda Riley, *Inventing the American Woman. A Perspective on Women's History 1865 to the Present*, Vol. II, Harlan Davidson, Inc., Arlington Heights, Ill, 1986, p. 154.

109 The first truly feminist work in the American utopian tradition *Herland* was serialized in *The Forerunner* in 1915 and did not appear in book form until 1979; See Lucy M. Freibert, 'World views in utopian novels by women', *Journal of Popular Culture*, XVII, Summer 1983, pp. 49–60; Charlotte Perkins Gilman, *Herland: A Lost Feminist Utopian Novel*, Pantheon Books, New York, 1979 [1915].

110 Friebert, 'World Views in utopian Novels', p. 51.

111 Christopher P. Wilson, 'Charlotte Perkins Gilman's steady burghers: the terrain of Herland', *Women's Studies*, XII, 1986, p. 271.

112 Theoretically, notes Hill, Gilman was an egalitarian, though in fact she was typically middle-class, condescending, elitist and often racist, viewing immigrants as coarse and culturally and racially inferior. Hill, *Radical Feminist*, pp. 172–3.

113 Gilman, *Herland*, pp. 128, 22, 30, 32, 107, 66 and 19;

114 Gilman, *Herland*, p. 114.

115 Frank E. Manuel and Fritzie P. Manuel, *Utopian Thought in the Western World*, Belknap/Harvard, Cambridge, 1982, pp. 23–24; See also Carol Farley Kessler, ed., *Daring to Dream: Utopian Stories by United States Women, 1836–1919*, Pandora Press, Boston, 1984.

116 Carol Pearson, 'Coming home: Four feminist utopians and patriarchal experience', *Future Females: A Critical Anthology*, Marlene S. Barr, ed., Bowling Green State University Popular Press, Ohio, 1981, p. 64.

117 Charlotte Perkins Gilman, 'With her in Ourland', Serialized in *The Forerunner*, VII, 1916, p. 297.

118 Joanna Russ, 'Recent feminist utopias', *Future Females*, p. 80.

119 After her marriage to her cousin George Houghton Gilman, Charlotte pursued what Ann J. Lane calls 'that ideal of desirable quality that personified her life and work'. Lane, Introduction to *Herland*, p. xxii.

120 Charlotte Perkins Gilman, *The Home, Its Work and Influences*, Charlton Co., New York, 1910, p. 3.

121 Berkin, 'Private woman, public woman', pp. 152, 165; Banner, *American Beauty*, p. 206.

122 Norton, 'The Paradox of women's sphere', *Women of America; A History*, p. 147; Mary Ellis Gibson, 'Book Review: Charlotte Perkins Gilman: The making of a radical feminist, 1860–1896'. Mary A. Hill, ed., *Signs*, VII, Summer 1981, pp. 753–757.

123 Degler, Introduction, *Women and Economics*.

124 Gilman, *Autobiography*, p. 104.

125 Gilman, *Herland*, 66; 'Growth,' she re-iterated in *The Man-Made World*, 'is the eternal law,' p. 258.

126 Sarah Slavin Schramm, *Plow Women Rather than Reapers: An Intellectual History of Feminism in the United States*, The Scarecrow Press, Metuchen, N.J., 1979, p. 42. For a discussion of how women represent themselves as fragmented and lacking a sense of true autonomy see Emily Martin, *The Woman in the Body. A Cultural Analysis of Reproduction*, Beacon Press, Boston, 1987, p. 194.

127 The heroines in Gilman's fiction all believed their first line of survival lay in maintaining their health and strength, exercising, studying nutrition and getting fresh air; Lane, *Charlotte Perkins Gilman Reader*, p. xxxii.

Epilogue

The worst fear of G. Stanley Hall was that human advancement might cease with women's independence. Such fears did not exist for Charlotte Gilman, who foresaw in women's economic advancement the path to a regenerated world. The twentieth century, she optimistically believed, would be the century of women, a hope which was expressed repeatedly in the feminist literature of the time. Gilman's prolific writing and lecturing on the theory of evolution in gender relations pointed up the need for women to become physically and socially useful in the larger world of production. The task of feminist thinkers, therefore, became one of pressing society to view women not as serviceable functionaries, but as developed persons capable of controlling their own destiny.

The twentieth century has not been the century of women, nor does their world yet contain some of the male privileges early feminists fought for. Few cultures, noted Margaret Mead, have devised the means to encourage women to quest as well as to bear children, while most cultures have devised ways to satisfy men in their constructive activities without distorting their sense of masculinity.[1] Society's encouragement of women to become productive mothers, while recognizing them as active participants in ensuring future progress, has traditionally interfered with female emancipation by confining women to a singular purpose, submerging their importance as individuals in their generative function.[2] In the sense that socio-cultural expectations of women have forced them in one direction rather than another, feminists have argued that women are not really free to choose among life goals with quite the same ease as men. Despite glaring evidence to the contrary, many kinds of discriminatory practices against women continue to be justified by the claim that they follow from the biological limits placed upon women's capacity to work and play. In other words, women's capacity to become pregnant invariably leaves her physically disabled in comparison to men.[3]

In sport and physical activity practices Mead's observation becomes particularly acute. Much of the professional discourse on female health, exercise and sport during the twentieth century is still contaminated by deterministic views which focus on the biological mission of the female. Feminists consider that the medical system, in becoming the guardian of reproduction technology and medicalizing crucial female biological life events – pre-menstrual syndrome, menarche, pregnancy, childbirth and menopause – has been instrumental in furthering female oppression, especially in the arena of physical activity.[4] Claiming to know best how to steer women through their crucial reproductive life events, the medical profession has too often interpreted natural events as medical problems requiring life-style restrictions which limit personal options. Critics suggest that doctors have thus assisted not only in rendering women dependent upon the health care system, but also in poisoning their concept of physical self by causing them to perceive their natural processes as deviant and as a continuing burden.[5] Conservative members of the medical profession continue to play a central role in the realm of physical activity, discouraging women in the quest for higher and broader levels of human performance by highlighting potential risks to the female reproductive system. It is true that the health hazards of high performance or risky sports for men are also noticed and discussed by medical experts, but it is the risk to their performance or sporting career, rather than to their ability to father children and to parent that tends to be underlined. Where women athletes are concerned, the risks of reproductive impairment rarely go unmentioned. Says Hubbard, it is as though fertile women are at all times potential parents, and men never.[6]

Indeed, over a hundred years after the heyday of the menstrual disability theory, medical research studies continue to add new grist to traditional anxieties that vigorous exercise might be harmful to the female's reproductive function. Medical scientists remain fascinated about the effect of exercise on a pregnant woman, reported a recent article in the *New York Times*. New evidence associating endurance-type exercise with changes in the menstrual cycle and ovulation disruption is being used to refocus attention on the natural (biological) limits of female activity.[7] Studies explain that the teenager who begins an intensive physical exercise programme prior to normal menarche may experience a delay in the onset of her first period of several years. It is noted that amenorrhoea and infertility are common among female ballet dancers, gymnasts, cross-country skiers, swimmers and distance runners. Physicians and exercise physiologists complain that, to achieve optimum performance, many female athletes are going to extraordinary lengths to reduce their body-fat stores, with severe consequences to their general health and possible problems for their reproductive health.[8] Indeed, the relationships between exercise, body-fat and the onset and persistence of menstruation are being explored from a variety of disciplinary viewpoints due, in part, to a perceived increase in the incidence of pathogenic weight-control behaviours considered alarming among girls and women.[9]

There is a growing and well-articulated fear among medical authorities that females, especially athletes, in pushing back the frontiers of corporeal existence in a quest for self-identity and distinctiveness through physical activity, may close off options available to normally functioning females and damage their reproductive health for the sake of fitness.[10] Within this anxiety do we hear perhaps the echo of Dr Clouston's warning to adolescent girls rebounding? 'Women,' he wrote in 1884, 'have a peculiar power of taking out of themselves more than they can bear. All should carry a reserve to meet emergencies and not use up all their power and thus rob future generations.'[11]

In an ironic twist to medical preoccupation with potential reproductive risks to elite athletes, some sporting authorities are now claiming that motherhood may have a positive effect on sports performance. 'A look at the record books shows a surprising number of top athletes have given stellar performances after bearing children', claims *Sports Illustrated*.[12] Psychologists suggest that the demonstration of femininity and/or the development of new mental strengths from the experience of pregnancy may relieve the pressure upon female athletes and allow them to perform better. Physiologists conjecture that pregnancy may improve cardiovascular and metabolic functioning of female athletes and there have been dark reports of Eastern bloc athletes becoming pregnant before major competitions only to abort later.

The medical tendency to reduce women to their biological category continues to have an effect on older women also. Due to the fact that so many more women are surviving well beyond their reproductive years, life after reproduction has necessarily taken on a much greater meaning for an increasing segment of female society. Now that the average age of menopause is around fifty years, nearly a third of a woman's life expectancy is left to be lived after she has reached the end of her ability to reproduce. Yet a number of medical doctors, by continuing to place emphasis upon the reproductive system as a woman's raison d'être, have contributed to the on-going association of female old age with loss and a set of disease symptoms. Viewing older women as set on the path to inevitable biological and emotional decline, widely read physicians such as Wilson and Wilson suggested not too long ago that after menopause 'we no longer have the whole woman – only the part woman'.[13]

The medicalization of menopause and the continued connection of ageing to the biomedical model of inevitable and irreversible decline associate getting old with negative connotations such as ill health, disability and conspicuous frailty. The ageing women is socialized to take on the role that society expects, despite the possibility that factors of diet, exercise and the like may have been underestimated or ignored as potential moderators of the ageing process.[14] Convinced that ageing is all too often accompanied by inevitable frailty and physical deterioration, the older woman becomes inclined to withhold attempts to be fit and strong and accedes to sedentary dependency. Having learned to view herself as inherently diseased, she is hardly likely to quest for health and wholeness through physical activity and adventurous leisure pursuits. Despite increasing evidence that suggests that the elderly who exercise have a reduced susceptibility to illness, are more productive in their work, more active and relaxed, with better self-concepts and lower levels of psychological stress, older women often worry that vigorous activity will render them fragile and in need of medical care.[15] They tend to spend very little time engaged in physical activity, and the physical activity they do select can be too low in intensity to improve their functional capacity.[16] Many older women tend vastly to exaggerate the health risks involved in vigorous exercise after middle age, overestimate the benefits of light and occasional exercise which they may take and underrate their own physical abilities and capabilities.[17] As activity levels decrease with age, the use of health care services rise, and the physician becomes an even more important source of influence on female attitudes toward physical activity.[18] Encouraged to view themselves as sick, older women adopt 'disability behaviour', visiting doctors and hospitals more frequently than men and using more prescription drugs and more psychiatric services.[19]

Elderly women thus learn that they are likely to become sick because they are old and female, and that, doomed to inevitable ill health, they need therapy and body repair from their physicians rather than life-style enhancing prescriptions for sport, exercise and other physical activities, as well as encouragement to regenerate their health and vigour. They learn to want medicine rather than health and eventually their capacity for independent living is jeopardized.[20]

Boutilier and San Giovanni claim that by enhancing women's physical and psychosocial wellbeing, exercise and sport may function to challenge conventional medical definitions of what constitutes the healthy female person at all ages.[21] They suggest that the emergence of the physically active woman presents an opportunity for medical doctors and related health professionals to rethink conventionally accepted definitions of and responses to women's reproductive functioning and the ageing process. Such professionals could then generate informed policy designed to expand women's access to health-enhancing sport and exercise.

Public policy, however, no matter how well motivated, cannot obliterate tensions related to inherently unequal relations between the sexes in the family, the professions or in the sporting arena. Laws that purport to help women often end up doing them more harm than good.[22] Women have many times been the victims of policies designed to protect them, since the very nature of protection has denied them the opportunity to make their own decisions and take responsibility for their own actions. Sex-specific laws, medical therapeutic practices and other policies thus risk perpetuating old prejudices about women's incapacity to control their own bodies and lives.

For women, control over the means of reproduction and control over definitions of body self are crucial. In the long run it is women's perceptions of themselves and their physical capabilities that are ultimately important in affecting their sporting and exercise behaviour. Public policy cannot legislate to encourage competitive inclinations among women or demand their assertion of mastery in the domain of physical skill, strength and endurance activities and other physical pursuits. Women will have to demonstrate their own capacity to make life choices by continuing to cast off persistently held gender images about appropriate sports and physical activities and by working to remove barriers, reverse stereotypes and dispel myths. Thus the physically competent 'new woman' of the late twentieth century will no longer be vulnerable to suggestions that her activities should be delimited because she is 'eternally wounded'.

Notes

1 Sarah Slavin Schramm, *Plow Women Rather than Reapers: An Intellectual History of*

Feminism in the United States. The Scarecrow Press, Metuchen, New Jersey, 1979, p. 115.

2 Delamont and Duffin, *The Nineteenth-Century Woman*, p. 58.

3 Ruth Hubbard, 'Science, facts and feminism', *Hypatia*, III, no. 1, Spring 1988, p. 7.

4 Ehrenreich and English, *Complaints and Disorders*, p. 5. Jacqueline N. Zita, 'The Premenstrual Syndrome: "Dis-easing" the Female Cycle', *Hypatia*, III, no. 1, Spring 1988, pp. 77–99.

5 Sheryl Burt Ruzek, *The Women's Health Movement. Feminist Alternatives to Medical Control*, Praeger Pubs, New York, 1978, p. 14.

6 Hubbard, 'Science, facts, and feminism', p. 8.

7 American College of Sports Medicine, 'Opinion statement on the participation of the female athlete in long-distance running', *Medicine and Science in Sports and Exercise*, IV, no. 11, 1979, pp. ix–xi; Jerilyn Prior and Yvette Vigna, 'Reproductive responses to endurance exercises in women: From corsets to shin splints', *Canadian Women's Studies*, IV, no. 3, Spring 1983, pp. 35–39; R. Bloomberg, 'Coach says running affects menstruation', *The Physician and Sports Medicine*, V, no. 9, 1977, p. 15; E. Dale, D.H. Gerlach, & A.L. Wilhite, 'Menstrual dysfunction in distance runners', *Obstetrics and Gynecology*, LIV, 1979, pp. 47–53; B. Schwartz, D.C. Cumming, E. Riordan, H. Selye, S.S.C. Yen, & R.W. Rebar, 'Exercise-associated amenorrhea: A distant entity?', *American Journal of Obstetrics and Gynecology*, CXLI, 1981, pp. 662–670.

8 Recent studies show that menarche occurs at a significantly later age in the American female athlete than in her non-athletic counterpart. Frisch, R.E. cited by Sullivan in 'New Studies link exercise to delays in menstruation and less cancer'. *New York Times*, Feb. 16, 1988; R.M. Malina, W.W. Spirduso, C. Tate and A.M. Baylor, 'Age at menarche and selected menstrual characteristics in athletes at different competitive levels and in different sports', *Medicine and Science in Sports*, X, 1978, pp. 218–222; Robert M. Malina, Albert B. Harper, Henrietta H. Avent & Donald E. Campbell, 'Age at menarche in athletes and non-athletes', *Medicine and Science in Sports*, V, 1973, pp. 11–13; M. P. Warren, 'The effects of exercise on pubertal progression and reproductive function in girls', *Journal of Clinical Endocrinology and Metabolism*, LI, 1980, pp. 1150–1157; J.H. Wilmore, C.H. Brown & J.A. Davis, 'Body physique and composition of the female distance runner', *Annals of the New York Academy of Sciences*, XXXII, 1977, pp. 764–776; J.L. Cohen, P.B. May, C.S. Kim & N.J. Ertel, 'Exercise and amenorrhea in professional ballet dancers', *Clinical Research*, XXVIII, no. 1 1980, p. 23.

9 Lionel W. Rosen, Douglas B. McKeag, David O. Hough, and Victoria Curley, 'Pathogenic weight-control behaviour in female athletes', *The Physician and Sports Medicine*, XIV, no. 1, January 1986, pp. 79–86; N.J. Smith, 'Excessive weight loss and food aversion in athletes simulating anorexia nervosa', *Pediatrics*, LXVI, July 1980, pp. 139–142. The suppression of menstruation is a distinguishing feature of anorexia nervosa, which is a phobic fear of fat. It is known that the initiation of menses depends upon the attainment of a critical body-weight and composition, and it is suspected that a lack of food and/or a large energy drain of habitual physical activity delays menarche. Rose E. Frisch and Janet W. McArthur, 'Menstrual cycles: Fatness as a determinant of

minimum weight for height necessary for their maintenance or onset', *Science*, CLXXXV, September 1974, pp. 942–949. Thus fat and the female reproductive system cannot be separated physiologically, for the art of starvation not only promises control of the shape that distinguishes the female body, but leads to a cessation of menstruation as well. See, for example, Noelle Caskey, 'Interpreting anorexia nervosa', *Poetics Today*, I–II, 1985, pp. 259–273; and Kim Chernin, *The Obsession: Reflections on the Tyranny of Slenderness*, Harper and Row, New York, 1981; Susan Bordo suggests that the 'rising incidence of eating disorders, increasing dissatisfaction and anxiety among girls and women concerning how they look, and [their] compulsive regimens of bodily "improvement" can be viewed as the waging of a political battle over the energies and resources of the female body'. Bordo, 'The body and reproduction of femininity', p. 28.

10 Frans de Wachter, 'The symbolism of the healthy body: A philosophical analysis of the sportive imagery of health', *Journal of the Philosophy of Sport*, XI, 1985, pp. 56–62.

11 Clouston, 'Female education', 1884, pp. 319–334.

12 Shannon Brownlee, 'Moms in the fast lane', *Sports Illustrated*, May 30, 1988; p. 57.

13 Robert A. Wilson and Thelma H. Wilson, 'The fate of the non treated post-menopausal woman: A plea for the maintenance of adequate estrogen from puberty to the grave', *Journal of the American Geriatric Society*, 11, 1965, pp. 351–356.

14 William J. Evans and Carol N. Meredith, 'Exercise and nutrition in the elderly', H.M. Munro and D.E. Danford, eds., *Nutrition, Aging and the Elderly*, Plenum Publishing Co., New York, 1989, pp. 89–126.

15 Patricia Vertinsky and J. Auman, 'Elderly women's barriers to exercise, Part I: Perceived risks', *Health Values*, XII, No. 4, July/August 1988, pp. 13–20; E.J. Bassey, 'Age, inactivity and some physiological responses to exercise', *Gerontology*, XXIV, 1976, pp. 66–67; Bonnie G. Berger, 'The role of physical activity in the life quality of older adults', W.W. Spirduso and H.M. Eckert, eds., *Physical Activity and Aging*, American Academy of Physical Education Papers No. 22, Human Kinetics Inc., 1989, pp. 42–58.

16 R.J. Shephard, 'Factors influencing the exercise behaviour of patients', *Sports Medicine*, II, no. 5, 1985, pp. 348–366; A.C. Ostrow and D.A. Dzewaltoswki, 'Older adults perceptions of physical activity participation based on age-role and sex-role appropriateness', *Research Quarterly for Exercise and Sport*, LII, no. 2, 1981, pp. 216–227.

17 Sidney, K.J. and R.J. Shephard, 'Perception of exercise in the elderly, effects of aging, modes of exercise and physical training', *Perceptual and Motor Skills*, XLIV, 1977, pp. 999–1010.

18 Patricia Vertinsky and J. Auman, 'Elderly women's barriers to exercise Part II: The physicians role', *Health Values*, XII, No. 4, July/Aug. 1988, pp. 20–25.

19 T.N. Chirikos and J.T. Nickel, 'Socioeconomic determinants of continuing functional disablement from chronic disease episodes', *Social Science and Medicine*, XXII, 1986, pp. 1329–1335; L.M. Verbrugge, 'Sex differences in complaints and diagnoses', *Journal of Behavioural Medicine*, III, 1980, pp. 327–55; L.M. Verbrugge, 'Female illness rates and illness behaviour: testing

hypotheses about sex differences in health', *Women and Health*, IV, Spring 1979, pp. 61–79.

20 T. Calasanti and A. Bonnano, 'The social creation of dependence, dependency ratios and the elderly in the United States: A critical analysis', *Social Science and Medicine*, XXIII, no. 12, 1986, pp. 1229–1236.

21 Boutilier and San Giovanni, 'Women and Sports: Reflections on health and policy', p. 230.

22 David L. Kirp, M.G. Yudolf, M.S. Franks, *Gender Justice*, The University of Chicago Press, Chicago, 1986, p. 208.

References

Abram, Ruth J. (ed.) 1985. *Send Us a Lady Physician: women doctors in America, 1835–1920.* New York: W. W. Norton.

Adams, W. H. Davenport. 1880. *Woman's Work and Worth in Girlhood, Maidenhood and Wifehood.* London: John Hogg.

Addams, Jane, 1902. *Democracy and Social Ethics.* New York: Macmillan.

Ainsworth, Dorothy. 1930. *History of Physical Education in Colleges for Women.* New York: A. S. Barnes.

Alcoff, Linda. 1987. 'Justifying feminist social science', *Hypatia*, vol. 2 (3), pp. 107–27.

Allan, J. McGrigor 1896. 'On the real differences in the minds of men and women', *Transactions of the Anthropological Society of London*, vol. 7, pp. 195–215.

Allbutt, T. Clifford. 1905. 'Chlorosis', in T. C. Allbutt (ed.), *A System of Medicine*, vol. 3, pp. 474–85. New York: Macmillan.

Allen, Grant. 1889. 'Plain words on the woman question', *Popular Science Monthly*, vol. 36 (December), pp. 170–81.

Allen, M. B., and McGrigor, A. C. 1896. *The Glory of Woman.* Philadelphia, Pa: Elliott Publishing.

Allen, Mary Wood. 1913. *What Every Woman Ought to Know.* Philadelphia, Pa: Vir Publishing.

Allen, Nathan. 1876. 'The normal standard of women for propagation', *American Journal of Obstetrics*, vol 9 (April), pp. 1–39.

— 1889. 'Physical degeneracy', *Journal of Psychological Medicine*, vol. 4, pp. 725–64.

American College of Sports Medicine. 1979. 'Opinion statement on the participation of the female athlete in long-distance running', *Medicine and Science in Sports and Exercise*, vol. 4 (11), pp. ix–xi.

Anderson, Michael. 1984. 'The social position of spinsters in mid-Victorian Britain', *Journal of Family History*, vol. 9 (4), pp. 377–93.

Anderson, W. E. 1887. 'The Physical Side of Education'. Wisconsin State Board of Health Report, quoted in Popular Miscellany, *The Popular Science Monthly*, April 1888, vol. 32, p. 856.

Anderson, William G. 1897. *Anderson's Physical Education.* New York: A. D. Dana.

Appley, Mortimer Herbert. 1986. 'G. Stanley Hall: vow on Mount Owen', in Stewart J. Hulse and Bert F. Green Jr (eds.), *One Hundred Years of Psychological Research in America: G. Stanley Hall and the Johns Hopkins tradition*, pp. 3–20.

References

Baltimore, Md: Johns Hopkins University Press.

Ardener, Shirley (ed.) 1975. *Perceiving Women*. London: Malaby Press.

Arehart-Treichel, Joan. 1982. 'Life expectancy: the great 20th century leap', *Science News*, vol. 121, pp. 186–8.

Aristotle [1943]. *On the Generation of Animals* (trans. A. L. Peck). London: Heinemann.

Armstrong, David. 1983. *Political Anatomy of the Body*. Cambridge: Cambridge University Press.

Atkinson, Paul. 1978. 'Fitness, feminism and schooling', in Sara Delamont and Lorna Duffin (eds.), *The Nineteenth-Century Woman: her cultural and physical world*, pp. 92–133. London: Croom Helm.

— 1985. 'Strong minds and weak bodies: sports, gymnastics and the medicalization of women's education', *British Journal of Sports History*, vol. 2 (1), pp. 62–71.

— 1987. 'The feminist physique: physical education and the medicalization of women's education', in J. A. Mangan and Roberta J. Park (eds.), *From 'Fair Sex' to Feminism: Sport and socialization of women in the industrial and post-industrial eras*, pp. 38–57. London: Cass Publications.

Austin, George L. 1883. *Perils of American Womanhood, or a doctor's talk with maiden, wife and mother*. Boston, Mass: Lee & Shephard.

Bachofen, J. J. 1861. *Das Mutterecht*. Stuttgart: Krais & Hoffman.

Baillie, Gertrude. 1894. 'Should professional women marry?', *Women's Medical Journal*, vol. 2 (February), pp. 33–5.

Bain, Mary Jo. 1976. *Here to Stay: American families in the twentieth century*. New York: Basic Books.

Baker, Elizabeth Renwick. 1984. 'Historical perspectives of research on physical activity and the menstrual cycle', in Jacqueline L. Puhl and C. Harmon Brown (eds.), *The Menstrual Cycle and Physical Activity*, pp. 1–8. Champaign, Ill.: Human Kinetics.

Baker, Rachel. 1946. *The First Woman Doctor: the story of Elizabeth Blackwell, MD*. London: George Harrap.

Baldy, John. 1894. *An American Textbook of Gynaecology*. Philadelphia, Pa: W. B. Saunders.

Bancroft, Jessie Hubbell. 1925. 'Eliza M. Mosher, MD', *Medical Women's Journal*, vol. 32, pp. 122–9.

Bannister, Robert C. 1979. *Social Darwinism: science and myth in Anglo-American thought*. Philadelphia, Pa: Temple University Press.

Banks, J. A., and Banks, Olive. 1964, *Feminism and Family Planning in Victorian England*. New York: Schocken Press.

Banner, Lois, 1983. *American Beauty*. New York: Alfred A. Knopf.

Banta, Martha. 1987. *Imaging American Women: ideas and ideals in cultural history*. New York: Columbia University Press.

Barash, David. 1979. *The Whisperings Within*. New York: Harper & Row.

Barker-Benfield, Ben. 1972. 'The spermatic economy: a nineteenth-century view of sexuality', *Feminist Studies*, vol. 1 (1), pp. 45–74.

— 1975. 'Sexual surgery in late-nineteenth-century America', *International Journal of Health Services*, vol. 5 (2), pp. 279–98.

Barker-Benfield, G. J. 1976. *The Horrors of the Half-Known Life: male attitudes towards women and sexuality in nineteenth-century America*. New York: Harper & Row.

— 1979. 'Mother emancipator': the meaning of Jane Addams' 'sickness and cure', *Journal of Family History*, vol. 4 (4), pp. 395–420.

Barnes, Robert. 1873. 'Lumleian Lectures; report on the convulsive diseases of women', *The Lancet*, vol. 1, p. 622.

Bassey, E. J. 1976. 'Age, inactivity and some physiological responses to exercise', *Gerontology*, vol. 24, pp. 66–71.

Bassuk, Ellen L. 1985. 'The rest cure: repetition or resolution of Victorian women's conflicts?', *Poetics Today*, vol. 6 (1), pp. 245–57.

Beard, George. 1881. *American Nervousness: its causes and consequences*. New York: G. P. Putnam.

de Beauvoir, Simone. 1962 [1949]. *The Second Sex* (trans. H. M. Parshley). New York: Alfred A. Knopf.

Beecher, Catharine E. 1856. *Physiology and Calisthenics for Schools and Families*. New York: Harper & Bros.

— 1972 [1855]. *Letters to the People on Health and Happiness*. New York: Arno Press.

Beedy, Mary E. 1874. 'Girls and women in England and America', in Anna C. Brackett (ed.), *The Education of American Girls Considered in a Series of Essays*, pp. 213–14. New York: G. P. Putnam's Sons.

Bell, J. W. 1899. 'A plea for the aged', *Journal of the American Medical Association*, vol. 33 (9), pp. 1136–8.

Bell, Susan Groag, and Offen, Karen M. 1983. *Women, the Family and Freedom: the debate in documents*, Volume II: *1880–1950*. Stanford, Ca: Stanford University Press.

Bellamy, Edward. 1888. *Looking Backward, 2000–1887*. Boston, Mass: Ticknor.

Benedict, A. L. 1897. 'Dangers and benefits of the bicycle', *Century Magazine* (July), pp. 471–3.

Bennett, A. Hughes. 1870 Correspondence, *The Lancet*, vol. 1, p. 887.

— 1880. 'Hygiene in the higher education of women', *Popular Science Monthly*, vol. 16, pp. 519–30.

Bennett, C. 1890. *The Modern Malady, or sufferers from nerves*. London: E. Arnold.

Berch, B. 1987. 'Charlotte Perkins Gilman', in John Eatwell, Murray Milgate and Peter Newman (eds.), *The New Palgrave: a dictionary of economics*, vol. 2, pp. 528–29. London: Macmillan.

Berger, Bonnie G. 1989. 'The role of physical activity in the life quality of older adults', in W. W. Spirduso and H. M. Eckert (eds.), *Physical Activity and Aging*, pp. 42–58. American Academy of Physical Education Papers no. 22. Champaign, Ill.: Human Kinetics.

Berger, Peter L., and Luckman, Thomas. 1966. *The Social Construction of Reality: a treatise on the sociology of knowledge*. Garden City, NY: Doubleday.

Berger, Peter L., Berger, Brigitte, and Kellner, Hansfried. 1973. *The Homeless Mind: modernization and consciousness*. New York: Random House.

Bergman-Osterberg, M. 1899. 'Physical training as a profession', *Women's International Congress*, 'The making and breaking of a female tradition: women's physical education in England 1880–1980', p. v. quoted by Sheila Fletcher, 1985, *British Journal of Sports History*, vol. 2 (1), pp. 27–39.

Berkin, C. R. 1979. 'Private woman, public woman: the contradictions of

References

Charlotte Perkins Gilman', in Carol Ruth Berkin and Mary B. Norton (eds.), *Women of America: a history*, pp. 150–76. Boston, Mass.: Houghton Mifflin.

Bettelheim, Bruno. 1954. *Symbolic Wounds*. Glencoe, Ill.: Free Press.

Bisland, Margaret. 1889–90. 'Fencing for women', *Outing*, vol. 15, pp. 341–7.

Blackwell, Elizabeth. 1852. *Laws of Life, with special reference to the physical education of girls*. New York: G. P. Putnam.

— 1858. 'Extracts from the *Laws of Life, with special references to the physical education of girls*', *Englishwoman's Journal*, vol. 1, pp. 189–90.

— 1871. *Lectures on the Laws of Life, with special reference to the physical education of girls* (2nd edn). London: Sampson Low, Son & Marston.

— 1871. 'The religion of health', lecture delivered at St George's Hall, London, 9 February, reprinted in Elizabeth Blackwell (ed.), 1972 [1902], *Essays in Medical Sociology*, vol. 2, pp. 213–51. New York: Arno Press.

— 1879. *Counsel to Parents on the Moral Education of Their Children*. Hastings: F. J. Parsons, 1902.

— 1895. *Pioneer Work in Opening the Medical Profession to Women*. London: Longman, Green.

— (ed.) 1972 [1902]. *Essays in Medical Sociology*, 2 vols. New York: Arno Press.

— 1972 [1902]. 'The influence of women in the profession of medicine', reprinted in Elizabeth Blackwell (ed.), *Essays in Medical Sociology*, vol. 2, pp. 1–32. New York: Arno Press.

—1984. 'Elizabeth Blackwell; 1821–1910', in Margaret Forster (ed.), *Significant Sisters: the grassroots of active feminism, 1839–1939*, pp. 55–92. London: Secker & Warburg.

— and Blackwell, Emily. 1860. *Medicine as a Profession for Women*. New York: Tinson.

Blaikie, William. 1883. *How to Get Strong and Stay So*. New York: Harper & Bros.

Bleier, R. 1984. *Science and Gender*. New York: Pergamon Press.

Bledstein, Burton J. 1976. *The Culture of Professionalism: the middle class and the development of higher education in America*. New York: W. W. Norton.

Bliss, W. W. 1869. *Woman and Her Thirty-Year Pilgrimage*. New York: William M. Littell.

Bloomberg, R. 1977. 'Coach says running affects menstruation', *The Physician and Sports Medicine*, vol. 5 (9), p. 15.

Boone, Gladys. 1942. *The Women's Trade Union League in Great Britain and the United States of America*. New York: Columbia University Press.

Bordo, Susan R. 1989. 'The body and the reproduction of femininity: a femininist appropriation of Foucault', in Alison M. Jagger and Susan R. Bordo (eds.), *Gender/Body/Knowledge*, pp. 13–33. New Brunswick: Rutgers University Press.

Boring, Mollie D., and Boring, E. G. 1948. 'Masters and pupils among the American psychologists', *American Journal of Psychology*, vol. 61, pp. 527–34.

Boutilier, Mary, and San Giovanni, Lucinda. 1983. *The Sporting Woman*. Champaign, Ill.: Human Kinetics.

— — 1985. 'Women and sports: reflections on health and policy', in Ellen Lewin and Virginia Olesen (eds.), *Women, Health and Healing: toward a new perspective*, pp. 186–95. New York: Tavistock Publications.

Bowler, Peter J. 1986. 'Varieties of evolution: essay review', *History and Philosophy of the Life Sciences*, vol. 8, pp. 113–19.

References

Brack, Datha Clapper. 1982. 'Displaced – the midwife by the male physician', in Ruth Hubbard, Mary Sue Henifin and Barbara Fried (eds.), *Biological Woman: the convenient myth*, pp. 207–26. Cambridge, Mass.: Schenkman.

Brackett, Anna C. (ed.) 1874. *The Education of American Girls, Considered in a series of Essays*. New York: G. P. Putnam's Sons.

Branca, Patricia. 1975. *Silent Sisterhood: middle-class women in the Victorian home*. London: Croom Helm.

— 1976. 'Image and reality: the myth of the idle Victorian woman', in Mary Hartman and Lois Banner (eds.), *Clio's Consciousness Raised: new perspectives on the history of woman*, pp. 179–91. New York: Octagon Books.

Breslow, L., and Somers, A. R. 1977. 'The lifetime health monitoring program: a practical approach to preventive medicine', *New England Journal of Medicine*, vol. 296, pp. 601–10.

Brieger, G. H. 1972. *Medical America in the Nineteenth Century*. Baltimore, Md: Johns Hopkins University Press.

Brightfield, Myron F. 1961. 'The medical profession in early Victorian England, as depicted in the novels of the period, 1840–1870', *Bulletin of the History of Medicine*, vol. 35 (3), pp. 221–9.

Brownlee, Shannon. 1988. 'Moms in the fast lane', *Sports Illustrated*, 30 May, p. 57.

Brumberg, Joan Jacobs. 1984. 'Chlorotic girls 1870–1920: a historical perspective on female adolescence', in Judith Walzer Leavitt (ed.), *Women and Health in America*, pp. 186–95. Madison, Wisc.: University of Wisconsin Press.

Bryce, James. 1974. 'The American Commonwealth II', in Ernest Earnest (ed.), *The American Eve in Fact and Fiction, 1775 – 1914*, p. 236. Urbana, Ill: University of Illinois Press.

Buhle, Mari Jo. 1981. *Women and American Socialism, 1870–1920*. Urbana, Ill.: University of Illinois Press.

Bullogh, Vern, and Voght, Martha. 1973. 'Women, menstruation and nineteenth-century medicine', *Bulletin of the History of Medicine*, vol. 47 (1), pp. 66–82.

Burdell, John (ed.) 1842. *The Discourses and Letters of Luigi Cornaro on a Sober and Temperate Life*. New York: Fowler & Wells.

Burgess, Charles, and Borrowman, Merle L. 1969. *What Doctrine to Embrace: studies in the history of American education*. Glenview, Ill.; Scott Foresman & Co.

Burnham, John C. 1984. 'Change in the popularization of health in the United States', *Bulletin of the History of Medicine*, vol. 58 (2), pp. 183–97.

Burstall, Sara A. 1894. *The Education of Girls in the United States*. New York: Macmillan.

— 1911. *English High Schools for Girls: their aims, organization and management*. London: Longman.

— 1911. 'Medical inspection', in Sara Burstall and M. A. Douglas (eds.), *Public Schools for Girls*, pp. 220–5. London: Longman.

Burstyn, Joan N. 1973. 'Education and sex: the medical case against higher education for women in England 1870–1900', *Proceedings of the American Philosophical Society*, vol. 117 (2), pp. 79–89.

— 1980. *Victorian Education and the Ideal of Womanhood*. London: Croom Helm.

Butler, Josephine. 1882. *Parliamentary Papers*, ix, Q5379, p. 340. London: HMSO.

References

Byford, H. J. 1897. *Manual of Gynecology* (2nd edn). Philadelphia, Pa: P. Blakiston.

Calasanti, T., and Bonnano, A. 1986. 'The social creation of dependence, dependency ratios and the elderly in the United States: a critical analysis', *Social Science and Medicine*, vol. 23 (12), pp. 1229–36.

Caskey, Noelle. 1985. 'Interpreting anorexia nervosa', *Poetics Today*, vol. 6 (1–2), pp. 259–73.

Cattell, J. McKeen. 1909. 'The school and the family', *Popular Science Monthly*, vol. 71, pp. 91–2.

Census of Great Britain. 1913. *Parliamentary Papers* (Cd 7018) lxxviii, p. 552. London: HMSO.

Chadwick, James Read. 1882. 'The health of American women', *North American Review*, vol. 313, pp. 505–24.

— 1895. 'Bicycle saddles for women', *Boston Medical and Surgical Journal*, vol. 132, pp. 595–6.

Chambers-Schiller, Lee. 1977. 'The single woman: family and vocation among nineteenth-century reformers', in Mary Kelly (ed.), *Woman's Being, Woman's Place: female identity and vocation in American history*. Boston, Mass.: G. K. Hall.

Channing, Walter. 1820. *Remarks on the Employment of Females as Practitioners in Midwifery, by a Physician*. Boston, Mass.: Cummings & Hilliard.

Chavasse, Pye Henry. 1871. *Woman as Wife and Mother*. Philadelphia, Pa.: W. B. Evans & Co.

Checkley, Edwin. 1890. *A Natural Method of Physical Training: a practical description of the Checkley system of physioculture*. New York: W. C. Bryant.

Chernin, Kim. 1981. *The Obsession: reflections on the tyranny of slenderness*. New York: Harper & Row.

Chirikos, T. N., and Nickel, J. T. 1986. 'Socioeconomic determinants of continuing functional disablement from chronic disease episodes', *Social Science and Medicine*, vol. 22 (12), pp. 1329–36.

Chudacoff, Howard P. 1980. 'The life course of women: age and age consciousness, 1865–1915', *Journal of Family History*, vol. 5 (3), pp. 274–92.

— and Hareven, Tamara. 1979. 'From the empty nest to family dissolution: life course transition into old age', *Journal of Family History*, vol. 4 (1), pp. 69–83.

Clark, L. M. G., and Lange, Lynda (eds.) 1979. *The Sexism of Social and Political Thought*. Toronto: University of Toronto Press.

Clarke, Edward H. 1869. 'Remarks to the Graduating Class at Harvard, 1869', *Boston Medical and Surgical Journal*, vol. 81, pp. 345–6.

— 1873. *Sex in Education; or a fair chance for girls*. Boston, Mass: James R. Osgood.

Clay, Charles E. 1888–89. 'Mask and foil for ladies', *Outing*, Vol. 13 (October–March), pp. 313–14.

Cleaves, Margaret A. 1910. *The Autobiography of a Neurasthene as told by one of them and recorded by Richard D. Badger*. Boston, Mass.

Clinton, Catherine. 1984. *The Other Civil War: American women in the nineteenth century*. New York: Hill & Wang.

Clouston, T. S. 1883. 'Female education from a medical point of view I', *Popular Science Monthly*, vol. 24 (December), pp. 214–28.

— 1884. 'Female education from a medical point of view, II', *Popular Science Monthly*, vol. 25 (January), pp. 319–34.

References

— 1884. *Clinical Lectures on Mental Discourse*. Philadelphia, Pa: Henry C. Lee's Sons.

— 1906. *The Hygiene of the Mind*. London: Methuen.

Cohen, J. L., May, P. B., Kim, C. S., and Ertel, N. J. 1980. 'Exercise and amenorrhea in professional ballet dancers', *Clinical Research*, vol. 28 (1), p. 230a.

Cole, Thomas R. 1980. 'Post Meridian: aging and the northern middle class', PhD thesis, University of Rochester.

Comfort, Alex. 1967. *The Anxiety Makers: some curious preoccupations of the medical profession*. Camden, NJ: Thomas Nelson.

Cominos, Peter. 1963. 'Late-Victorian sexual respectability and the social system', *International Review of Social History*, vol. 8, pp. 19–48.

Conway, Jill. 1971–72. 'Women reformers and American culture 1870–1930', *Journal of Social History*, vol. 5 (2), pp. 164–77.

— 1972. 'Stereotypes of femininity in a theory of sexual evolution', in Martha Vicinus (ed.), *Suffer and Be Still: women in the Victorian age*, pp. 140–54. Bloomington, Ind.: Indiana University Press.

Cope, Edward D. 1888. 'The relation of the sexes to government', *Popular Science Monthly*, vol. 33 (October), pp. 721–30.

Cott, Nancy. 1977. *The Bonds of Womanhood*. New Haven, Conn.: Yale University Press.

Cottom, Daniel. 1987. *Social Figures: George Eliot, social history and literary representation*, Minneapolis, Minn.: University of Minnesota Press.

Coulter, Harris Livermore. 1969. 'Political and Social Aspects of Nineteenth-Century Medicine in the United States', PhD thesis, Columbia University.

Cowan, John. 1871. *The Science of a New Life*. New York: Cowan & Co.

Cowan, Ruth Schwartz. 1983. *More Work for Mother*. New York: Basic Books.

Crawford, R. 1915. Editorial. *The Lancet*, vol. 2, pp. 1331–6.

Croly, Jane Cunningham. 1874. *For Better or Worse: a book for some men and all women*. Boston, Mass.: Lee & Shephard.

Currier, Andrew F. 1897. *The Menopause*. New York: D. Appleton.

Curti, Merle. 1959. *The Social Ideas of American Educators*. New Jersey: Pageant Books.

Dale, E., Gerlach, D. H., and Wilhite, A. L. 1979. 'Menstrual dysfunction in distance runners', *Obstetrics and Gynecology*, vol. 54, pp. 47–53.

Darnall, William Edgar. 1901. 'The pubescent schoolgirl', *American Gynecological and Obstetrical Journal*, vol. 18, pp. 490–2.

Darwin, Charles. 1964 [1859]. *On the Origin of Species*. London: John Murray. Fascimile edn. ed. E. Mayr, Cambridge, Mass: Harvard University Press, 1964.

— 1871. *The Descent of Man*, 2 vols. London: John Murray.

— 1874. *The Descent of Man and Selection in Relation to Sex* (2nd edn). Akron, Oh.: Werner.

Datan, Nancy. 1986. 'Corpses, lepers and menstruating women: tradition, transition and the sociology of knowledge', *Sex Roles*, vol. 14 (11/12), pp. 693–703.

Davin, Anna. 1978. 'Imperialism and motherhood', *History Workshop*, vol. 5 (Spring), pp. 9–65.

Davis, Mel. 1982. 'Corsets and conception: fashion and demographic trends in the nineteenth century', *Comparative Studies in Society and History*, vol. 24, pp. 611–41.

Dawkins, R. 1979. *The Selfish Gene*. New York: Oxford University Press.

Degler, Carl N. 1956. 'Charlotte Perkins Gilman on the theory and practice of feminism', *American Quarterly*, vol. 8 (1), pp. 21–39.

— 1966. 'Introduction', in Charlotte Perkins Gilman, *Women and Economics: a study of the economic relation between men and women as a factor in social evolution* (ed. Carl N. Degler), pp. vi–xxv. New York: Harper & Row.

— 1974. 'What ought to be and what was: women's sexuality in the nineteenth century', *American Historical Review*, vol. 79, pp. 1467–90.

Delamont, Sara, and Duffin, Lorna (eds.). 1978. *The Nineteenth-Century Woman: her cultural and physical world*. London: Croom Helm.

Delaney, Janice, Lupton, Mary Jane, and Toth, Emily. 1976. *The Curse: a cultural history of menstruation*. New York: E. P. Dutton.

Delaunay, G. 1881. 'Equality and inequality in sex', *Popular Science Monthly*, vol. 20 (December), pp. 184–92.

Delavan, G. B. 1910. 'The influence of the use of the automobile on the upper air passages', *Medical Record*, 20 August.

Demos, John, and Demos, Virginia. 1969. 'Adolescence in historical perspective', *Journal of Marriage and the Family*, vol. 31 (November), pp. 623–38.

Deutsch, Helene. 1945. *The Psychology of Women*, vol. 2. New York: Grune & Stratton.

Devereux, G. 1950. 'The psychology of feminine genital bleeding', *International Journal of Psychoanalysis*, vol. 31, pp. 237–57.

Dewey, John. 1886. 'Health and sex in higher education', *Popular Science Monthly*, vol. 29, pp. 606–15.

Dickinson, Robert L. 1895. 'Bicycle for women from the standpoint of the gynecologist', *American Journal of Obstetrics*, vol. 31 (January), pp. 24–37.

Dijkstra, Bram. 1986. *Idols of Perversity: fantasies of feminine evil in fin-de-siècle culture*. Oxford: Oxford University Press.

Diller, T. 1902. 'Some observations on neurasthenia', *Pennsylvania Medical Journal*, vol. 5, pp. 646–50.

Donnelly, Mabel C. 1988. *The American Victorian Woman: the myth and the reality*. Westport, Conn.: Greenwood Press.

Douglas, Ann. 1977. *The Feminization of American Culture*. New York: Alfred A. Knopf.

Douglas, Mary. 1966. *Purity and Danger: an analysis of the concepts of pollution and taboo*. Boston, Mass: Routledge & Kegan Paul.

Dove, Jane Frances. 1898. 'Cultivation of the body', in Dorothy Beale, Lucy Soulsby and Jane Frances Dove, *Work and Play in Girls' Schools*, pp. 396–423. London: Longmans, Green & Co.

Doyle, William. 1960. 'Charlotte Perkins Gilman and the Cycle of Feminist Reform', PhD thesis, University of California, Berkeley.

Drachman, Virginia D. 1976. 'Women Doctors and the Women's Medical Movement: feminism and medicine, 1850–1895', PhD thesis, State University of New York at Buffalo.

— 1984. *Hospital with a Heart: women doctors and the paradox of separatism at the New England Hospital, 1962–1969*. Ithaca, NY: Cornell University Press.

References

Dreyfus, Hubert L., and Rabinow, Paul. 1983. *Michel Foucault: beyond structuralism and hermeneutics* (2nd edn). Chicago, Ill.: University of Chicago Press.

Dublin, Louis I., Lotka, Alfred J., and Spiegelman, Mortimer (eds.). 1936. *Length of Life: a study of the life table*. New York: Ronald Press.

Duffey, Eliza Brisbee. 1874. *No Sex in Education, or an Equal Chance for Both Boys and Girls*. Philadelphia, Pa: J. M. Stoddart.

Duffin, Lorna. 1978. 'The conspicuous consumptive: woman as an invalid', in Sara Delamont and Lorna Duffin (eds.), *The Nineteenth-Century Woman: her cultural and physical world*, pp. 26–56. London: Croom Helm.

Dunn, L. C., and Dobzhansky, T. 1946. *Heredity, Race and Society* (rev. edn). New York: Mentor Books.

Dyhouse, Carol. 1976. 'Social Darwinistic ideas and the development of women's education in England, 1888–1920', *History of Education*, vol. 5 (1), pp. 41–58.

— 1977. 'Good wives and little mothers: social anxieties and the schoolgirl's curriculum, 1890–1920', *Oxford Review of Education*, vol. 3 (1), pp. 21–35.

Earnest, Ernest. 1950. *S. Weir Mitchell: novelist and physician*. Philadelphia, Pa: University of Pennsylvania Press.

Edgar, J. C. 1911. 'The influence of the automobile on obstetric and gynecologic conditions', *American Journal of Obstetrics*, vol. 63, p. 1084.

Ehrenreich, Barbara, and English, Deirdre. 1973a. *Complaints and Disorders: the sexual politics of sickness*. Old Westbury, NY: Feminist Press.

— 1973b. *Witches, Midwives and Nurses*. Old Westbury, NY: Feminist Press.

— 1979. *For Her Own Good: 150 years of the experts' advice to women*. Garden City, NY: Anchor Books.

Eiseley, Loren. 1958. *Darwin's Century: evolution and the men who discovered it*. New York: Anchor Books.

Eldredge, Charles C. 1982. *Charles Walter Stetson: color and fantasy*. Lawrence, Kan.: University of Kansas Press.

Elliotson, John. 1840. *Human Physiology* (5th edn). London: Longman, Orme, Brown, Green & Longmans.

Ellis, Havelock. 1894. *Determinants of Puritan Stock and Its Causes*. New York: Charles Scribner's Sons.

— 1894. *Man and Woman: a study of secondary and tertiary sexual characters*. Boston, Mass: Houghton Mifflin.

— 1912. *The Task of Social Hygiene*. London: A & C. Black.

Ellsworth, Edward W. 1979. *Liberators of the Female Mind: the Shirreff sisters, educational reform and the women's movement*. Westport, Conn.: Greenwood Press.

Ellwood, Charles 1901. 'The theory of imitation in social psychology', *American Journal of Sociology*, vol. 6, pp. 731–6.

Emmet, Thomas E. Addis. 1879. *The Principles and Practice of Gynecology*. Philadelphia, Pa: Henry C. Lea.

Engelmann, George. 1900. 'The American girl of today', *American Journal of Obstetrics*, vol. 42 (8), pp. 753–96.

— 1901. 'The American girl of today: the influence of modern education on functional development', *American Gynecological Society*, vol. 25, pp. 8–45.

Engels, Friedrich. 1942. *The Origin of the Family, Private Property and the State in the*

References

Light of Researches of Lewis H. Morgan. New York: International Publishers.

Epstein, Cynthia. 1971. *Woman's Place.* Berkeley, Ca: University of California Press.

Erickson, Eric. 1964. 'Womanhood and the inner space', *Daedalus: Journal of the American Academy of Arts and Sciences,* vol. 2, pp. 582–606.

Evans, Thomas R. 1896. 'Harmful effects of the bicycle upon the girls' pelvis', *American Journal of Obstetrics,* vol. 33, pp. 554–6.

Evans, William J., and Meredith, Carol N. 1989. 'Exercise and nutrition in the elderly', in H. M. Munro and D. E. Danford (eds.), *Nutrition, Aging and the elderly,* pp. 89–126. New York: Plenum Publishing.

Fancourt, Mary St J. 1966. *They Dared to Become Doctors: Elizabeth Blackwell, Elizabeth Garrett Anderson.* London: Longman Green.

Farnham, Eliza. 1864. *Woman and Her Era.* 2 vols. New York: A. J. Davis & Co.

Fausto-Sterling, Anne. 1985. *Myths of Gender.* New York: Basic Books.

Fee, Elizabeth. 1979. 'Nineteenth-century craniology: the study of the female skull', *Bulletin of the History of Medicine,* vol. 53, pp. 415–33.

Feinson, Marjorie C. 1985. 'Where are the women in the history of aging?' *Social Science History,* vol. 9 (4), pp. 429–52.

Fellman, Anita Clair, and Fellman, Michael. 1981. *Making Sense of Self: medical advice literature in late-nineteenth-century America.* Philadelphia, Pa: University of Pennsylvania Press.

Fenton, W. H. 1896. 'A medical view of cycling for ladies', *Nineteenth Century,* vol. 39 (May), pp. 796–801.

Filene, Peter J. 1986. *Him/Her/Self: sex roles in modern America* (2nd edn). Baltimore, Md: Johns Hopkins University Press.

Findlay, M. E. 1905. 'The education of girls', *The Paidologist,* vol. 7, pp. 83–93.

Fisk, George, and Comfort, Anna Manning. 1874. *Woman's Education and Woman's Health: chiefly in reply to 'Sex in Education'.* New York: Syracuse.

Fletcher, Sheila. 1984. *Women First: the female tradition in English physical education, 1880–1980.* London: Athlone Press.

Fluhman, C. Frederic. 1939. *Menstrual Disorders, Pathology, Diagnosis and Treatment.* Philadelphia, Pa: W. B. Saunders.

Foster, Frank I. 1986. *Handbook of Therapeutics.* New York. D. Appleton.

Forster, Margaret. 1984. *Significant Sisters: the grassroots of active feminism, 1839–1939.* London: Secker & Warburg.

Foucault, Michel. 1980. *The History of Sexuality,* Volume I: *An introduction.* New York: Vintage Books.

Freeman, Ruth, and Klaus, Patricia. 1984. 'Blessed or not? The new spinster in England and the United States in the late nineteenth and early twentieth centuries', *Journal of Family History,* vol. 9 (4), pp. 395–414.

Freibert, Lucy M. 1983. 'World views in utopian novels by women', *Journal of Popular Culture,* vol. 17, pp. 49–60.

Freind, John. 1729. *Emmenologia* (translated by Thomas Dale). London: T. Cox.

Freud, Sigmund. 1949. *Outline of Psychoanalysis.* London: Hogarth Press.

Friedman, Jean E., and Shade, Williams S. G. (eds.), 1982. *Our American Sisters: women in American life and thought.* Lexington, Mass: D. C. Heath.

Frisch, Rose E., and McArthur, Janet W. 1974. 'Menstrual cycles: fatness as a determinant of minimum weight for height necessary for their maintenance or onset', *Science*, vol. 185, pp. 942–9.

Fuller, Margaret. 1874. *Life Without and Life Within, or reviews, narratives, essays and poems*. Boston, Mass: Roberts Brothers.

— 1971 [1845]. *Woman in the Nineteenth Century and Kindred Papers Relating to the Sphere, Condition and Duties of Women*. New York: W. W. Norton.

Fye, W. Bruce. 1987. 'S. Weir Mitchell: Philadelphia's frustrated physiologist and triumphant reformer', *The Development of American Physiology: scientific medicine in the nineteenth century*, pp. 54–91. Baltimore, Md: Johns Hopkins University Press.

Galabin, A. L. 1893. *Diseases of Women* (5th edn). Philadelphia, Pa: P. Blakiston, Son & Co.

— 1900. *A Manual of Midwifery*. London: Churchill.

Gannon, Linda R. 1985. *Menstrual Disorders and Menopause: biological, psychological and cultural research*. New York: Praeger Scientific.

Gardner, Augustus Kinsley. 1870. *Conjugal Sins: against the laws of life and health and their effects upon the father, mother and child*. New York: J. S. Redfield.

Garrett, Elizabeth. 1868a. 'Miscellanea, Physical training of girls', *Englishwoman's Journal*, 12 October, pp. 151–20.

— 1870. *The Times*, 12 November.

Garrett Anderson, Elizabeth. 1874. 'Sex in mind and education. A reply', *Fortnightly Review*, vol. 15, pp. 582–94.

— 1877. Inaugural address, London School of Medicine, 1 October.

— 1899–1910. 'Puberty' and 'Menopause', in D. Chalmers Watson (ed.), *Encyclopaedia Medica*, 15 vols. London: Green & Sons.

Garrigues, Henry J. 1894. *A Textbook of the Diseases of Women*. Philadelphia, Pa: W. B. Saunders.

— 1896. 'Woman and the bicycle', *The Forum*, vol. 20, pp. 578–87.

Gasking, Elizabeth. 1967. *Investigations into Generation, 1651–1828*. Baltimore, Md: Johns Hopkins University Press.

Gathorne-Hardy, Jonathan. 1977. *The Public School Phenomenon, 1597–1977*. London: Hodder & Stoughton.

Gay, Peter. 1984. *The Bourgeois Experience: Victoria to Freud*, Volume I: *Education of the senses*. Oxford: Oxford University Press.

Geddes, Patrick. 1905. 'Adolescence', *The Paidologist*, vol. 7 (January), pp. 33–41.

— and Thompson, J. Arthur. 1889. *The Evolution of Sex*. London: Walter Scott.

Gibson, Mary Ellis. 1981. 'Review of Mary A. Hill (ed.), *Charlotte Perkins Gilman: the making of a radical feminist, 1860–1896*', *Signs*, vol. 7, pp. 753–7.

Gilbert, Sandra M., and Gubar, Susan. 1979. *The Madwoman in the Attic: the woman writer and the nineteenth-century imagination*. New Haven, Conn.: Yale University Press.

— 1988. *No Man's Land: the place of the woman writer in the twentieth century*, Volume I: *The war of words*. New Haven, Conn.: Yale University Press.

Gilman, Charlotte Perkins. 1883. 'The Providence Ladies' Gymnasium', *Providence Journal*, vol. 8 (23 May), p. 2.

— 1886. 'The Answer', *Woman's Journal*, vol. 17 (2 October), p. 313.

— 1892. 'The Yellow Wallpaper', *New England Magazine*, vol. 5, pp. 647–59.

— 1900. 'Mending morals by making muscles', *Saturday Evening Post*, 19 May, p. 1078.

— 1904. 'Housework and athletics', *Woman's Journal*, vol. 36 (5 March), p. 74.
— 1908. 'Three Women', *Success*, vol. II (August), pp. 490–1; 522–6.
— 1910. *The Home, Its Work and Influences*. New York: Charlton.
— 1911. *The Man-Made World of Our Androcentric Culture*. New York: Charlton.
— 1916. 'The unnatural mother', *The Forerunner*, vol. 7 (November), pp. 281–5.
— 1916. 'With her in Ourland', *The Forerunner*, vol. 7 (January), pp. 6–11; 7 (February), pp. 34–44; 7 (March), pp. 67–73; 7 (April), pp. 93–8; 7 (May), pp. 123–8, 7 (June), pp. 152–7; 7 (July), pp. 179–85; 7 (August), pp. 208–13; 7 (September), pp. 291–7; 7 (December), pp. 318–25.
— 1923. 'The Primal Power', *His Religion and Hers*. New York: Century.
— 1935. *The Living of Charlotte Perkins Gilman: an autobiography*. New York: D. Appleton.
— 1966 [1898]. *Women and Economics: a study of the economic relation between men and women as a factor in social evolution*. New York: Harper & Row.
— 1979 [1915]. *Herland: a lost feminist utopian novel*. New York: Pantheon Books.
— 1980 [1892]. 'The Yellow Wallpaper', in Ann J. Lane (ed.), *The Charlotte Perkins Gilman Reader*, pp. 3–21. New York: Pantheon Books.
Glover, J. W. 1921. *United States Life Tables, 1890, 1901, 1901–10*. Washington, DC: Bureau of the Census.
Goodell, William. 1882. *The Dangers and the Duty of the Hour*. Philadelphia, Pa.: S. M. Miller.
—, Thomas, T. Gaillard, Chadwick, James R., Mitchell, S. Weir, Starr, M. Allen, and Putnam, J. J. 1889. 'Co-education and the higher education of women – a symposium', *Medical News*, vol. 55, pp. 667–73.
Goodman, J. 1878. 'The cyclical theory of menstruation', *American Journal of Obstetrics*, vol. 11 (67), pp. 3–44.
Goodsell, Willystine. 1923. *The Education of Women: its social background and its problems*. New York: Macmillan.
Gordon, Linda. 1976. 'Voluntary motherhood: the beginnings of feminist birth control ideas in the United States', in Mary Hartman and Lois Banner (eds.), *Clio's Consciousness Raised: new perspectives on the history of women*, pp. 54–71. New York: Octagon Books.
— 1976. *Woman's Body, Woman's Right: a social history of birth control in America*. New York: Grossman.
Gorham, Deborah. 1982. *The Victorian Girl and the Feminine Ideal*. London: Croom Helm.
Gornick, Vivian. 1978. 'Twice told tales', *The Nation*, vol. 227 (9) (23 September), pp. 278–9.
Gosling, Francis G. 1985. 'Neurasthenia in Pennsylvania: a perspective on the origins of American psychotherapy, 1870–1910', *Journal of the History of Medicine and Allied Sciences*, vol. 40, pp. 188–206.
Gould, Stephen J. 1977. *Ever since Darwin: reflections on natural history*. New York: W. W. Norton.
— 1981. *The Mismeasure of Man*. New York: W. W. Norton.
Graaf, Regnier de. 1699. *Histoire anatomique des parties genitales de l'homme et de la femme*. Paris: Hilaire Baritel.
Graves, H., Hillier, G. L., and Malmesbury, Susan, Countess of. 1898. *Cycling*. London: Lawrence & Bullen.

References

Green, Charles M. 1892. 'The care of women in pregnancy', *Boston Medical and Surgical Journal*, vol. 126 (8), 25 February, pp. 186–90.

Green, Harvey. 1986. *Fit for America: health, fitness, sport and American society*. New York: Pantheon Books.

Grinder, Robert E. 1969. 'The concept of adolescence in the genetic psychology of G. Stanley Hall', *Child Development*, vol. 40 (June), pp. 355–69.

— and Strickland, Charles E. 1963. 'G. Stanley Hall and the social significance of adolescence', *Teachers College Record*, vol. 64 (February), pp. 390–99.

Grob, Gerald N. 1972. 'The social history of medicine and disease in America: problems and possibilities', *Journal of Social History*, vol. 3, pp. 391–409.

Gruman, Gerald A. 1961. 'The rise and fall of prolongevity hygiene', *Bulletin of the History of Medicine*, vol. 35 (3), pp. 221–9.

Gulick, Luther Halsey. 1904. 'The bicycle as a therapeutic agent', *Boston Medical and Surgical Journal*, vol. 150 (2), pp. 40–3.

— 1907. 'Play and democracy', *Proceedings of the First Annual Playground Congress*. New York: Playground Association of America, pp. 11–16.

Haber, Carole. 1983. *Beyond Sixty-Five: the dilemma of old age in America's past*. Cambridge: Cambridge University Press.

Haeckel, Ernest. 1879. *Evolution of Man*, 2 vols. London: Kegan Paul.

Haley, Bruce. 1978. *The Healthy Body and Victorian Culture*. Cambridge, Mass.: Harvard University Press.

Hall, G. Stanley, 1882. 'The education of the will', *Princeton Review*, vol. 10 (November), pp. 306–25.

— 1882. 'The moral and religious training of children', *Princeton Review*, vol. 10 (January), pp. 26–48.

— 1885. 'New departures in education', *North American Review*, vol. 140 (February), pp. 144–52.

— 1889. Address delivered at the opening of Clark University, *Clark University, Worcester, Massachusetts: opening exercises*. (Printed by the University), pp. 9–32.

— 1890. 'The educational state; or the methods of education in Europe', *Christian Register*, vol. 69 (November), p. 719.

— 1891. Editorial, *Pedagogical Seminary*, vol. 1 (December), pp. 311–26.

— 1891. 'The new movement in education', Address delivered to the School of Pedagogy, University of the City of New York, December.

— 1892. Editorial on health of school children', *Pedagogical Seminary*, vol. 2 (June), pp. 3–8.

— 1894. 'The new psychology as a basis of education', *The Forum*, vol. 17 (August), pp. 710–20.

— 1896. Address on Founder's Day at Mt Holyoke College, *Mount Holyoke News*, vol. 6 (November), pp. 64–72.

— 1897. 'A study of fears', *American Journal of Psychology*, vol. 8 (January), pp. 147–249.

— 1900. 'Child study and its relation to education', *The Forum*, vol. 29 (August), pp. 688–702.

— 1900. 'Some defects of the kindergarten in America', *The Forum*, vol. 28, pp. 579–91.

— 1901. 'The ideal school as based on child study', *The Forum*, vol. 32 (September), pp. 24–39.

References

— 1902. 'Christianity and physical culture', *Pedagogical Seminary*, vol. 9, pp. 374–8.

— 1902. 'The high school as a people's college', *Pedagogical Seminary*, vol. 9 (March), pp. 63–73.

— 1903. 'Co-education in the high school', *Proceedings of the National Educational Association*, n.p., pp. 446–51.

— 1904. *Adolescence, Its Psychology and Its Relation to Physiology, Anthropology, Sociology, Sex, Crime, Religion and Education*, 2 vols. New York: D. Appleton.

— 1905. Editorial, *New York Tribune* (5 February), p. 1.

— 1906. 'The feminist in science', *New York Independent*, 22 March, pp. 661–2.

— 1906. *Youth, Its Education, Regimen and Hygiene*. New York: D. Appleton.

— 1908. 'Feminization in school and home', *World's Work*, vol. 16 (May), pp. 1037–44.

— 1908. 'A glance at the phyletic background of genetic psychology', *American Journal of Psychology*, vol. 21, pp. 149–212.

— 1910. 'Education in sex hygiene', *Eugenics Review*, vol. 1 (January), pp. 242–53.

— 1911. *Educational Problems*, 2 vols. New York: D. Appleton.

— 1914. 'A synthetic genetic study of fear', *American Journal of Psychology*, vol. 25, pp. 149–200, 321–93.

— 1920. 'The fall of Atlantis', *Recreations of a Psychologist*, pp. 1–127. New York: D. Appleton.

— 1920. *Morale: the supreme standard of life and conduct*. New York: D. Appleton.

— 1923. *Life and Confessions of a Psychologist*. New York: D. Appleton.

— 1924. 'Can the masses rule the world?', *Scientific Monthly*, vol. 18, pp. 456–63.

Hall, H. J. 1905. 'The systematic use of work as a remedy in neurasthenia and allied conditions', *Boston Medical and Surgical Journal*, vol. 152, pp. 29–34.

Hall, Lucy M. 1885. 'Physical training of girls', *Popular Science Monthly*, vol. 26 (February), pp. 495–8.

— 1887. 'Higher education of women and the family', *Popular Science Monthly*, vol. 30 (March), pp. 612–18.

Hall, M. Ann, and Richardson, Dorothy A. 1982. *Fair Ball: towards sex equality in Canadian sport*. Ottawa: Canadian Advisory Council on the Status of Women.

Haller, John S. Jr. *American Medicine in Transition, 1840–1910*. Urbana, Ill.: University of Michigan Press.

— and Haller, Robin M. 1974. *The Physician and Sexuality in Victorian America*. Urbana, Ill.: University of Illinois Press.

Haller, Mark H. 1963. *Eugenics: hereditarian attitudes in American thought*. New Brunswick: Rutgers University Press.

Hammond, Graeme M. 1895. 'The influence of the bicycle in health and disease', *Medical Record*, vol. 47, pp. 129–33.

— 1906. 'Nerves and the American woman', *Harper's Bazaar*, vol. 40, pp. 590–2.

Haney-Peritz, Janice. 1986. 'Monumental feminism and literature's ancestral house: another look at "The Yellow Wallpaper" ', *Women's Studies*, vol. 12, pp. 113–28.

Hardaker, M. A. 1882. 'Science and the woman question', *Popular Science Monthly*, vol. 20 (March), pp. 577–84.

Hareven, Tamara. 1982. 'The life course and aging in historical perspective', in Tamara K. Hareven and Kathleen J. Adams (eds.), *Aging and Life Course*

Transitions: an interdisciplinary perspective, pp. 1–26. New York: Guildford Press.

Hargreaves, Jennifer. 1985. 'Playing like gentlemen while behaving like ladies: contradictory features of the formative years of women's sport', *British Journal of Sports History,* vol. 2 (1), pp. 40–52.

Harmond, Richard. 1971–72. 'Progress and flight: an interpretation of the American cycle craze of the 1890s', *Journal of Social History,* vol. 5 (2), pp. 234–57.

Harrison, Brian. 1978. *Separate Spheres: the opposition to women's suffrage in Britain.* London: Croom Helm.

— 1981. 'Women's health and the women's movement in Britain: 1840–1940', in Charles Webster (ed.), *Biology, Medicine and Society, 1840–1940,* pp. 15–71. Cambridge; Cambridge University Press.

Harrison, Fraser. 1977. *The Dark Angel: aspects of Victorian sexuality.* London: Sheldon Press.

Hartman, Mary and Banner, Lois (eds.) 1976. *Clio's Consciousness Raised: new perspectives on the history of women.* New York: Octagon Books.

Hatch, William C. 1897. 'Women and the bicycle', *Massachusetts Medical Journal,* vol. 17, pp. 10–15.

Haydon, Dolores. 1978. 'Two Utopian feminists and their campaigns for kitchenless houses', *Signs,* vol. 4 (2), pp. 274–90.

Hayes, Albert. 1869. *Physiology of Women.* Boston, Mass: Peabody Medical Institute.

Hedges, Elaine. 1973. 'Afterword', in Charlotte Perkins Gilman, *The Yellow Wallpaper* (ed. Elaine Hedges), pp. 37–63. Old Westbury, NY: Feminist Press.

Helsinger, Elizabeth K., Sheets, Robin Lauterback, and Veeder, William. 1983. *The Woman Question,* Volume I: *Defining voices 1837–1883;* Volume II: *Social issues 1837–1883.* New York: Garland Publishing.

Hersman, C. C. 1899. 'Relation of uterine disease to some of the insanities', *Journal of the American Medical Association,* vol. 33 (2), pp. 709–11.

Hewitt, M. 1958. *Wives and Mothers in Victorian Industry.* London: Rockcliffe.

Hicks, J. Braxton. 1877. 'The Croonian Lectures on the difference between the sexes in regard to the aspect and treatment of disease', *British Medical Journal,* vol. 11, pp. 473–6.

Hill, Mary A. 1980. *Charlotte Perkins Gilman: the making of a radical feminist, 1860–1896.* Philadelphia, Pa: Temple University Press.

— 1985. *Endure: the diaries of Charles Walter Stetson.* Philadelphia, Pa: Temple University Press.

Hitchcock, E. 1899. 'Some principles regarded as essential in the direction of the Department of Physical Education and Hygiene', in Isabel C. Barrow (ed.), *Report of the Discussions and Papers of the Physical Training Conference,* pp. 54–60. Boston, Mass: George H. Ellis.

Hofstadter, Richard. 1944. *Social Darwinism in American Thought, 1860–1915.* Philadelphia, Pa: University of Pennsylvania Press.

Holbrook, M. L. 1875. *Parturition without Pain: a code of directions for escaping from the primal curse.* New York: Wood & Holbrook.

Hollingworth, Leta Stetter. 1914. *Functional Periodicity: an experimental study of the mental and motor abilities of women during menstruation.* New York: Columbia University Press.

References

Holtzman, Eric. 1981. 'Science, philosophy and society', *International Journal of Health Services*, vol. 11 (1), pp. 123–49.

Holzner, Burkart, and Marx, John A. 1979. *Knowledge Application: the knowledge system in society*. Boston, Mass: Allyn & Bacon.

Horn, Margo. 1983. 'Sisters worthy of respect: family dynamics and women's roles in the Blackwell family', *Journal of Family History*, vol. 8 (4), pp. 367–82.

Horney, Karen. 1967. 'The problems of feminine masochism', *Feminine Psychology*. New York: W. W. Norton.

— 1973. 'The flight from womanhood: the masculinity complex in women as viewed by men and women', in Jean Baker Miller (ed.), *Psychoanalysis and Women*, pp. 5–20. Harmondsworth: Penguin Books.

Houston, Matilda. 1862. *Recommended to Mercy*. London: n.p.

Howard, William Lee. 1906. 'Athletics for young women', *New York Medical Journal*, vol. 83 (3 February), pp. 238–40.

Howe, Joseph W. 1883. *Excessive Venery, Masturbation and Continence*. New York: E. B. Trent.

Howe, Julia Ward (ed.) 1874. *Sex and Education: a reply to Dr Clarke's Sex in Education*. Boston, Mass.: Roberts Brothers. Reprinted New York: Arno Press, 1972.

Hubbard, Ruth. 1988. 'Science, facts and feminism', *Hypatia*, vol. 3 (1), pp. 5–17.

— and Lowe, M. (eds.) 1979. *Genes and Gender II: pitfalls in research on sex and gender*. Staten Island, NY: Gordian Press.

—, Henifin, Mary Sue, and Fried, Barbara (eds.) 1982. *Biological Woman: the convenient myth*. Cambridge, Mass: Schenkman.

Hudson, R. P. 1977. 'The biography of disease: lessons from chlorosis', *Bulletin of the History of Medicine*, vol. 51, pp. 440–63.

Hulse, Stewart H., and Green, Bert F. (eds.) 1986. *One Hundred Years of Psychological Research in America: G. Stanley Hall and the Johns Hopkins tradition*. Baltimore, Md: Johns Hopkins University Press.

Humphrey, George Murray. 1889. *Old Age: the results of information received respecting nearly nine hundred persons who had attained the age of eighty years including seventy-four centenarians*. Cambridge: Macmillan & Bowes.

Hunt, Harriet. 1852. *Proceedings of the Women's Rights Convention, October 1851*. Boston, Mass: n.p.

Hurd-Mead, Kate Campbell. 1933. *Medical Women of America*. New York: Froeben Press.

Huston, Nancy. 1986. 'The matrix of war: mothers and heroes', in Susan Rubin Suleiman (ed.), *The Female Body in Western Culture*, pp. 119–38. Cambridge, Mass: Harvard University Press.

Huxley, T. H. 1890. 'On the natural inequality of men', *Nineteenth Century*, vol. 27 (15) (January), pp. 1–3.

Icard, P. S. 1890. *La femme pendant la période menstruelle*. Paris: F. Alcan.

Illich, Ivan. 1977. *Medical Nemesis: the expropriation of health*. New York: Bantam Books.

Jackson, Wilson R. 1975. 'Essay review 1: Dewey's Hegelianism', *History of Education Quarterly*, vol. 14 (Spring), pp. 90–3.

Jacobi, Mary Putnam. 1874. 'Social aspects of the readmission of women into the medical profession', Paper and letters presented at the First Women's

Congress of the Association for the Advancement of Women, October. New York: n.p.

— 1874. 'Mental action and physical health', in Anna C. Brackett (ed.), *The Education of American Girls Considered in a Series of Essays*, pp. 255–306. New York: G. P. Putnams Sons.

— 1877. *The Question of Rest for Women during Menstruation*. New York: G. P. Putnam's Sons.

— 1882. 'Shall women practice medicine?', *North American Review*, vol. 134 (January), pp. 52–75.

— 1883. Annual Address delivered at the commencement of the Woman's Medical College of the New York Infirmary, 30 May. *Archives of Medicine*, vol. 10, pp. 59–71.

— 1890. 'Hysterical fever', *Journal of Nervous and Mental Disease*, vol. 15, pp. 373–88.

— 1891. 'On the opening of the Johns Hopkins Medical School to women', *Century Magazine*, vol. 411 (1) (February), pp. 632–7.

— 1891. 'Women in medicine', in Annie Nathan Meyer (ed.), *Women's Work in America*, pp. 139–205. New York: Henry Holt.

— 1929. 'Specialism in medicine', in Victor Robinson (ed.), *Pathfinders in Medicine*, pp. 673–4. New York: Medical Life Press.

Jacobus, Mary. 1981. 'Review of Sandra M. Gilbert and Susan Gubar's *The Madwoman in the Attic*', *Signs: Journal of Women in Culture and Society*, vol. 6 (3), pp. 518–23.

Jacques, D. H. 1890. *'Physical Perfection': or, the philosophy of human beauty; showing how to acquire and retain bodily symmetry, health and vigor, secure long life, and avoid the infirmities and deformities of old age*. New York: Fowler & Wells.

— 1890. *How to Grow Handsome*. New York: Fowler & Wells.

Jalland, Pat, and Hooper, John (eds.) 1986. *Women from Birth to Death: the female life cycle in Britain 1830–1914*. Brighton: Harvester Press.

James, J. 1896. 'The beneficial effects of cycling as an orthopaedic agent', *British Medical Journal*, vol. 2, pp. 942–8.

Jersey, Countess of. 1890. 'Ourselves and our foremothers', *Nineteenth Century*, vol. 27 (15), pp. 56–7.

Jewell, J. S. 1874. 'Influence of our present civilization in the production of nervous and mental energy', *Journal of Nervous and Mental Disease*, vol. 1, pp. 70–3.

Jex-Blake, Sophia. 1970 [1886]. *Medical Women: a thesis and a history*. New York: Source Book Press.

Jeye, Louise. 1895. (No title), *Lady Cyclist* (August), pp. 224–5.

Johanningmeier, E. V. 1971. 'Presbyterians, democracy and demography: essay review', *History of Education Quarterly*, vol. 11 (Summer), pp. 204–9.

Jones, E. L. 1897. *Chlorosis: the special anaemia of young women*. London: Ballière Tindall.

Karier, Clarence J. 1967. 'Elite views on American education', in W. Laqueur and G. L. Mosse (eds.), *Education and Social Structure in the Twentieth Century*. New York: Harper & Row.

— 1967. *Man, Society and Education: a history of American educational ideas*. Glenview, Ill: Scott, Foresman.

References

— 1983. 'G. Stanley Hall: a priestly prophet of a new dispensation', *Journal of Libertarian Studies*, vol. 7 (1), pp. 35–60.

Kaufert, Patricia A. 1982. 'Myth and the menopause', *Sociology of Health and Illness*, vol. 4 (2), pp. 141–66.

Kellogg, J. H. 1895. *Ladies' Guide in Health and Disease: girlhood, maidenhood, wifehood, motherhood*. Battle Creek, Mich.: Modern Medical Publishing.

— 1889. *Plain Facts for Old and Young*. Burlington, Io.: I. F. Segner.

— 1894. *Second Book on Physiology and Hygiene*. New York: American Books.

Kelly, Joan. 1986. *Women, History and Theory*. Chicago, Il.: University of Chicago Press.

Kelly-Gadol, Joan. 1976. 'The social relations of the sexes: methodological implications of women's history', *Signs: Journal of Women in Culture and Society*, vol. 1, pp. 809–23.

Kenealy, Arabella. 1896. 'Woman as athlete', *Nineteenth Century*, vol. 45, pp. 636–45.

— 1899. 'Woman as an athlete', *Living Age*, vol. 3, pp. 363–70.

— 1920. *Feminism and Sex Extinction*. London: T. Fisher Unwin.

Kennard, Jean E. 1981. 'Convention coverage or how to read your own life', *New Literary History*, vol. 13, pp. 69–88.

Kessler, Carol Farley (ed.) 1984. *Daring to Dream: utopian stories by United States women, 1836–1919*. Boston, Mass: Pandora Press.

Kett, Joseph. 1971. 'Adolescence and youth in nineteenth-century America', *Journal of Interdisciplinary History*, vol. 2 (Autumn), pp. 283–98.

King, A. F. A. 1875. 'A new basis for uterine pathology', *American Journal of Obstetrics*, vol. 8, pp. 237–56.

Kirp, David L., Yudolf, M. G., and Franks, M. S. 1986. *Gender Justice*. Chicago, Il.: University of Chicago Press.

Klaus, Patricia Otto. 1979. 'Women in the mirror: using novels to study Victorian women', in Barbara Kanner (ed.), *The Women of England from Anglo-Saxon Times to the Present*, pp. 296–344. Hamden, Conn.: Archon Books.

Koonz, Claudia. 1987. *Mothers in the Fatherland: women, the family and Nazi politics*. London: Jonathan Cape.

Lamarck, J. B. 1809. *Zoological Philosophy: an exposition with regard to the natural history of animals*. London: Macmillan.

Lane, Ann J. 1976. 'Woman in society: a critique of Frederick Engels' in Berenice A. Carroll (ed.), *Liberating Women's History: theoretical and critical essays*, pp. 4–25. Urbana, Ill.: University of Illinois Press.

— (ed.) 1979. Introduction to Charlotte Perkins Gilman, *Herland: a lost utopian novel*. New York: Pantheon Books.

— (ed.) 1980. *The Charlotte Perkins Gilman Reader*. New York: Pantheon Books.

Lange, Lynda. 1979. 'Rousseau: women and the general will', in L. M. G. Clark and L. Lange (eds.), *The Sexism of Social and Political Thought*, pp. 41–52. Toronto: University of Toronto Press.

Latimer, Caroline Wormeley. 1910. *Girl and Woman: a book for mothers and daughters*. New York: D. Appleton.

Leach, Gerald. 1970. *The Biocrats*. London: Jonathan Cape.

Leach, William. 1980. *True Love and Perfect Union: the feminist reform of sex and society*. New York: Basic Books.

References

Leavitt, Judith Walzer, and Numbers, Ronald L. (eds.) 1978. *Sickness and Health in America: readings in the history of medicine and public health*. Madison, Wisc.: University of Wisconsin Press.

Leibhardt, Laura. 1893. 'Our schoolgirl', *Women's Medical Journal*, vol. 1 (2), pp. 207–16.

Leonardo, R. 1944. *History of Gynecology*. New York: Froben.

Lerner, Gerda. 1986. *The Creation of Patriarchy*. Oxford: Oxford University Press.

Leslie, Murray. 1910–11. 'Women's progress in relation to eugenics', *Eugenics Review*, vol. 2, pp. 282–98.

Lewin, Ellen, and Olesen, Virginia (eds.) 1985. *Women, Health and Healing: toward a new perspective*. New York: Tavistock Publications.

Lewis, Dio, Stanton, Elizabeth Cady, and Chadwick, James Read. 1882. 'The health of American women', *North American Review*, vol. 135 (313), pp. 503–24.

Lewontin, R. C., Rose, Steven, and Kamin, Leon. 1984. *Not in Our Genes: biology, ideology and human nature*. New York: Pantheon Press.

Linton, Mrs E. Lynn. 1883. *The Girl of the Period, and Other Social Essays*, 2 vols. London: Richard Bentley.

Love, I. N. 1899. 'From a doctor's sentimental standpoint', *Journal of the American Medical Association*, vol. 32, pp. 1024–7.

Lovejoy, Esther Pohl. 1957. *Women Doctors of the World*. New York: Macmillan.

Lowe, Louisa. 1883. *The Bastilles of England: or the lunacy laws at work*. London: Crookenden.

Lowe, M., and Hubbard, R. (eds.) 1983. *Woman's Nature: rationalizations of inequality*. New York: Pergamon Press.

Lowell, Josephine. 1891. 'Open letter', *Century Magazine*, vol. 41 (1), p. 634.

McCleary, G. F. 1935. *The Maternity and Child Welfare Movement*. London: P. S. King & Son Ltd.

McCrone, Kathleen E. 1986. 'The "lady blue": sport at the Oxbridge women's colleges from their foundation to 1914', *British Journal of Sports History*, vol. 3 (2), pp. 191–215.

— 1987. ' "Play up! Play up! and play the game!" Sport at the late-Victorian girls' public schools', in J. A. Mangan and Roberta J. Park (eds.), *From 'Fair Sex' to Feminism: sport and socialization of women in the industrial and post-industrial eras*, pp. 97–129. London: Cass Publications.

— 1988. *Sport and the Physical Emancipation of English Women 1870–1914*. London: Routledge.

McGuigan, Dorothy. 1970. *A Dangerous Experiment: one hundred years of women at the University of Michigan*. Ann Arbor, Mich.: University of Michigan Press.

McIntosh, Peter C. 1952. *Physical Education in England since 1800*. London: G. Bell & Sons.

Mackern, Louie, and Boys, M. (eds.) 1899. *Our Lady of the Green* London: Lawrence & Bullen.

Mackie, M. 1986. 'Gender relations', in R. Hagedorn (ed.), *Sociology* (3rd edn), pp. 99–131. Toronto: Holt, Rinehart & Winston.

Maclaren, Angus. 1984. *Reproductive Rituals*. New York: Methuen.

MacPike, Loralee. 1975. 'Environment as psychological symbolism in "The Yellow Wallpaper" ', *American Literary Realism*, vol. 8 (3), pp. 286–8.

Mahowald, Mary B. 1987. 'Sex-role stereotypes in medicine', *Hypatia*, vol. 2 (2), pp. 21–38.

Malina, Robert M., Harper, Albert B., Avent, Henrietta H., and Campbell, Donald E. 1973. 'Age at menarche in athletes and non-athletes', *Medicine and Science in Sports*, vol. 5, pp. 11–13.

Malina, R. M., Spirduso, W. W., Tate, C., and Baylor, A. M. 1978. 'Age at menarche and selected menstrual characteristics in athletes at different competitive levels and in different sports', *Medicine and Science in Sports*, vol. 10, pp. 218–22.

Malmesbury, Susan, Countess of. 1900. 'Bicycling for women', in H. Peek and F. G. Aflulo (eds.), *The Encyclopedia of Sport* (standard edn), vol. A–EEL. London:Lawrence & Bullen.

Mangan, J. A., and Park, Roberta J. (eds.), *From 'Fair Sex' to Feminism: sport and socialization of women in the industrial and post-industrial eras*. London: Cass Publications.

Manton, Jo. 1965. *Elizabeth Garrett Anderson*. London: Methuen.

Manuel, Frank E., and Manuel, Fritzie P. 1982. *Utopian Thought in the Western World*. Cambridge, Mass: Belknap/Harvard University Press.

Marks, Cora Goldberg. 1986. 'In purity and love: an introduction to the Jewish attitudes towards marriage', *Lifestyles*, vol. 13, pp. 98–106.

Marland, Hilary (ed.) 1987. *Medicine and Society in Wakefield and Huddersfield 1780–1870*. Cambridge: Cambridge University Press.

Marrett, Cora Bagley. 1979. 'On the evolution of women's medical societies', *Bulletin of the History of Medicine*, vol. 53 (3), pp. 434–48.

Marshall, Maud. 1898. 'Lawn tennis', in Frances E. Slaughter (ed.), *The Sportswoman's Library*, vol. 2, pp. 315–17. London: Archibald Constable.

Martin, Emily, 1987. *The Woman in the Body: a cultural analysis of reproduction*. Boston, Mass: Beacon Press.

Martineau, Harriet. 1859. 'Female industry', *Edinburgh Review*. vol. 109, pp. 293–336.

Massachusetts Bureau of Labor Statistics. 1885. *Health Statistics of Female College Graduates*. Boston, Mass.

Maudsley, Henry. 1874. 'Sex in mind and education', *Fortnightly Review*, vol. 14, pp. 466–83.

Mead, Kate Campbell Hurt. 1933. *Medical Women of America: a short history of the pioneer medical women of America and a few of their colleagues in England*. New York: Froben Press.

Mead, Richard. 1765. *The Medical Works of Richard Mead*. Edinburgh: A. Donaldson & J. Reid.

Mechling, Jay. 1976. 'Author's response to comments on "Advice to historians on advice to mothers" ', *Journal of Social History*, vol. 10 (1), pp. 125–8.

Meigs, Charles D. 1879. *Females and Their Diseases*. Philadelphia, Pa: D. G. Brinton.

Mendeloff, John. 1983. 'Measuring elusive benefits: on the value of health', *Journal of Health Politics, Policy and Law*, vol. 8 (3), pp. 554–80.

Michelet, Jules. 1858. *L'Amour*. Paris: L. Hachette & Cie.

Mills, Charles K. 1888. 'The treatment of nervous and mental disease by systematized active exercises', *New York Medical Journal*, vol. 47 (4 February), pp. 129–37.

References

Mitchell, Silas Weir. 1869. 'Researches on the physiology of the cerebellum', *American Journal of Medical Science*, vol. 57, pp. 320–38.

— 1871. *Wear and Tear, or hints for the overworked*. Philadelphia, Pa: J. B. Lippincott.

— 1875. 'Rest in nervous disease: its use and abuse', in E. C. Seguin (ed.), *A Series of American Clinical Lectures*, vol. 1 pp. 83–102.

— 1877. *Fat and Blood: an essay on the treatment of certain forms of neurasthenia and hysteria* (10th edn). Philadelphia, Pa: J. B. Lippincott.

— 1885. *Lectures on Diseases of the Nervous System especially in Women*. Philadelphia, Pa: Lea Brothers.

— 1880. 'True and false palsies of hysterics', *Medical News and Abstract*, vol. 38 (February), pp. 63–71.

— 1888. *Doctor and Patient*. Philadelphia, Pa: J. B. Lippincott.

— 1900. *Fat and Blood and How to Make Them* (8th edn). Philadelphia, Pa: J. B. Lippincott.

— 1908. 'The treatment by rest, seclusion, etc., in relation to psychotherapy', *Journal of the American Medical Association*, vol. 50, pp. 2033–7.

Mitchinson, Wendy. 1984. 'Causes of disease in women: the case of late 19th century English Canada', in Charles G. Roland (ed.), *Health, Disease and Medicine*, pp. 381–95. Toronto: Hannah Institute for the History of Medicine.

Mishler, Elliot G. 1981. 'The health-care system: social contexts and consequences', in E. G. Mishler, L. AmaraSingham, S. Hauser, R. Liem, S. Osherson and N. E. Waxler, *Social Contexts of Health, Illness and Patient Care*, pp. 95–217. Cambridge: Cambridge University Press.

Moebius, Paul Julius. 1908. *Über den Physiologischen Schwachsinn des Weibes* (9th edn). Berlin, Halle a.d. S: C. Marhold.

Mohr, James C. 1984. 'Patterns of abortion and the response of American physicians, 1790–1930', in Judith Walzer Leavitt (ed.), *Women and Health in America: historical readings*, pp. 117–23. Madison, Wisc.: University of Wisconsin Press.

Moldow, Gloria. 1987. *Women Doctors in Gilded-Age Washington*. Urbana, Il.: University of Illinois Press.

Moore, William Withers, 1886. Presidential address, 54th Annual Meeting of the British Medical Association, Brighton, 1886, reported in *The Lancet*, vol. 2, p. 315.

Morantz, Regina Markell. 1976. 'The lady and her physician', in Mary Hartman and Lois Banner (eds.), *Clio's Consciousness Raised: new perspectives on the history of women*, pp. 38–53. New York: Octagon.

— 1977. 'Making women modern: middle-class women and health reform in nineteenth-century America', *Journal of Social History*, vol. 10 (4), pp. 490–507.

— 1978. 'The connecting link: the case for the woman doctor in 19th century America', in Judith Walzer Leavitt and Ronald L. Numbers (eds.), *Sickness and Health in America: readings in the history of medicine and public health*, pp. 117–28. Madison, Wisc.: University of Wisconsin Press.

— 1982. 'Feminism, professionalism and germs: the thought of Mary Putnam Jacobi and Elizabeth Blackwell', *American Quarterly*, vol. 34 (5), pp. 459–77.

— and Zschoche, Sue. 1980. 'Professionalism, feminism and gender roles: a comparative study of nineteenth-century medical therapeutics', *Journal of American History*, vol. 67 (3), pp. 568–88.

—, Pomerleau, Cynthia Stodola, and Fenichel, Carol (eds.) 1982. *In Her Own*

Words: oral histories of women physicians. Westport, Conn.: Greenwood Press.

Morantz-Sanchez, Regina Markell. 1985. *Sympathy and Science: women physicians in American medicine*. Oxford: Oxford University Press.

Mosedale, Susan Sleeth. 1978. 'Science corrupted: Victorian biologists consider the woman question', *Journal of the History of Biology*, vol. 11 (1), pp. 1–55.

Mosher, Clelia Duel. 1901. 'Normal menstruation and some of the factors modifying it', *Johns Hopkins Hospital Bulletin*, vol. 12 (April–May), pp. 178–9.

— 1911. 'Functional periodicity in women and some modifying factors', *California Journal of Medicine*, vol. 12 (January–February), pp. 1–21.

— 1914. 'A physiological treatment of congestive dysmenorrhea and kindred disorders associated with the menstrual function', *Journal of the American Medical Association*, Vol. 62 (25 April), pp. 1297–1301.

— 1923. 'Some of the causal factors in the increased height of college women', *Journal of the American Medical Association*, vol. 81, pp. 528–35.

— 1923 [1915]. *Women's Physical Freedom* (2nd edn). New York: Women's Press.

Mosher, Eliza M. 1888. 'The health of American women', in Benjamin Austin (ed.), *Woman: her character, culture and calling*, pp. 234–45. Brantford, Conn.: Book & Bible House.

— 1893. 'The influence of habitual posture on the symmetry and health of the body', *Proceedings of the American Association for the Advancement of Physical Education 1892*, pp. 116–33. Springfield, Mass: Press of the Springfield Printing and Binding Co.

— 1902. 'The better preparation of our women for maternity', *Women's Medical Journal*, vol. 12, pp. 205–8.

— 1916. 'The value of organization – what it has done for women', *Women's Medical Journal*, vol. 26, pp. 1–4.

Mosse, George L. 1964. *The Crisis of German Ideology*. New York: Grosset & Dunlap.

Mrozek, Donald J. 1983. *Sport and American Mentality, 1880–1910*. Knoxville, Tenn.: University of Tennessee Press.

Muirhead, J. H. 1905. 'The scope and object of child-study', *The Paidologist*, vol. 7 (January), pp. 66–73.

Muller, Herbert J. 1960. *Issues of Freedom*. New York: Harper & Row.

Mundé, Paul Fortunatus (ed.). 1891. *A Practical Treatise on the Diseases of Women*. Philadelphia, Pa: Lea's Son & Co.

Murray, Janet Horowitz. 1982. *Strong-Minded Women and Other Lost Voices from Nineteenth-Century England*. New York: Pantheon Books.

Murrell, Christine M. 1923. *Womanhood and Health*. London: Mills & Boon.

Napheys, George Henry. 1870. *The Physical Life of Women: advice to the maiden, wife and mother*. Philadelphia, Pa: G. Maclean.

Nash, Francis Smith. 1896. 'A plea for the new woman and the bicycle', *American Journal of Obstetrics*, vol. 33, pp. 556–60.

Negrier, Charles. 1840. *Recherches Anatomiques et Physiologiques sur les Ovaries dans l'espèce Humaine . . . .* Paris: Bechet & Labe.

Nett, Emily M. 1982. 'Midlife for women', unpublished paper presented at the Canadian Sociology and Anthropology Meeting, Ottawa, June.

Newcomer, Mabel. 1959. *A Century of Higher Education for American Women*. New York: Harper and Brothers.

References

Newman, Louise Michele (ed.) 1985. *Men's Ideas, Women's Realities: popular science, 1870–1915*. New York: Pergamon Press.

Nietzsche, F. L. 1969 [1883–91]. *Thus Spoke Zarathustra* (trans. R. J. Hollingdale). Harmondsworth: Penguin Books.

Nightingale, Florence. 1928. 'Cassandra', in Ray Strachey (ed.), *The Cause: a short history of the women's movement in Great Britain*. London. G. Bell & Sons.

Norton, Mary. 1979. 'The paradox of women's sphere', in Carol Ruth Berkin and Mary Norton (eds.), *Women of America: a history*, pp. 139–49. Boston, Mass: Houghton Mifflin.

Novak, E. 1916. 'The superstition and folklore of menstruation', *Johns Hopkins Hospital Bulletin*, vol. 27, pp. 270–4.

— 1921. *Menstruation and Its Disorders*. New York: D. Appleton.

O'Brien, Sharon. 1979. 'Tomboyism and adolescent conflict: three nineteenth-century studies', in Mary Kelley (ed.), *Woman's Being, Woman's Place: female identity and vocation in American history*, pp. 351–72. Boston, Mass: G. K. Hall.

Oglesby, Carole A. (ed.) 1978. *Women and Sport: from myth to reality*. Philadelphia, Pa: Lea & Febiger.

O'Neill, John. 1985. *Five Bodies: the human shape of modern society*. London: Cornell University Press.

Osherson, Samuel, and AmaraSingham, Lorna. 1981. 'The machine and metaphor in medicine', in E. G. Mishler, L. AmaraSingham, S. Hauser, R. Liem, S. Osherson and N. E. Waxler, *Social Contexts of Health, Illness and Patient Care*, pp. 218–49. Cambridge: Cambridge University Press.

Ostrow, A. C., and Dzewaltowski, D. A. 1981. 'Older adults' perceptions of physical activity participation based on age-role and sex-role appropriateness', *Research Quarterly for Exercise and Sport*, vol. 52 (2), pp. 216–27.

Oswald, Felix. 1881. 'Physical education', *Popular Science Monthly*, vol. 19 (May), pp. 7–24.

Oven, Bernard Van. 1853. *On the Decline of Life in Health and Disease*. London: John Churchill & Sons.

Packard, Alpheus. 1901. *Lamarck, the Founder of Evolution: his life and work*. New York: n.p.

Pancoast, S. 1859. *Ladies' Medical Guide to Mothers and Daughters of the United States of America*. Philadelphia, Pa: Keystone Publishing.

Park, Roberta J. 1977. 'The attitudes of leading New England Transcendentalists toward healthful exercise, active recreations and proper care of the body: 1830–1869', *Journal of Sport History*, vol. 4 (1), pp. 34–50.

— 1987. 'Edward M. Hartwell and physical training at the Johns Hopkins University, 1879–1890', *Journal of Sport History*, vol. 14 (1), pp. 108–19.

— 1987. 'Sport, gender and society in a transatlantic Victorian perspective', in J. A. Mangan and Roberta J. Park (eds.), *From 'Fair Sex' to Feminism: sport and socialization of women in the industrial and post-industrial eras*, pp. 58–93. London: Cass Publications.

Parker, W. W. 1892. 'Woman's place in the Christian world: superior morally, inferior mentally to man – not qualified for medicine or law – the contrariety and harmony of the sexes', *Transactions of the Medical Society of the State of Virginia*, Virginia, pp. 86–107.

Parry, Angenette. 1912. 'The relation of athletics to the reproductive life of women', *American Journal of Obstetrics and Diseases of Women and Children*, vol. 66 (3), pp. 341–57.

Parsons, Gail Pat. 1977. 'Equal treatment for all: American medical remedies for male sexual problems, 1850–1900', *Journal of the History of Medicine*, vol. 32, pp. 55–71.

Partridge, G. E. 1912. *Genetic Philosophy of Education: an epitome of the published educational writings of G. Stanley Hall of Clark University*. New York: Sturgis & Walton.

Peabody, L. G. 1901. 'The canoe and the woman', *Outing*, vol. 38, pp. 533–5.

Pearl, R. 1928. *The Rate of Living*. New York: Alfred A. Knopf.

Pearson, Carol. 1981. 'Coming home: four feminist utopians and patriarchal experience', in Marlene S. Barr (ed.), *Future Females: a critical anthology*, pp. 63–70. Bowling Green, Oh.: Bowling Green State University Popular Press.

Pearson, Karl. 1888. 'The woman question', *The Ethic of Free Thought*. London: T. F. Unwin.

— 1894 'Woman and labour', *Fortnightly Review*, vol. 329 (May), pp. 561–77.

Pearson, Ronald. 1969. *The Worm in the Bud: the world of Victorian sexuality*. Harmondsworth: Penguin Books.

Pegis, Anton C. (ed.) 1948. *Basic Writings of St Thomas Aquinus*. New York: Random House.

Pellegrino, E. D. 1963. 'Medicine, history and the ideas of man, medicine and society', *Annals of the American Academy of Political and Social Sciences*, vol. 346, pp. 9–20.

Perry, Ralph Barton. 1936. *The Thought and Character of William James*, Boston, Mass: Little, Brown.

Peterson, M. Jeanne. 1986. 'Dr Acton's enemy: medicine, sex and society in Victorian England', *Victorian Studies*, vol. 29 (4), pp. 569–90.

Pfister, G. 1981. 'The influence of women doctors on the origins of women's sports in Germany', *Medicine and Sport*, vol. 14, pp. 58–65.

Pfluger, E. P. F. 1865. *Über die Bedeutung und Ursache der Menstruation*. Berlin: n.p.

Pierce, R. V. 1908. *The People's Common Sense Medical Advisor* (new edn). Buffalo, NY: World's Dispensary Medical Association.

Piess, Kathy. 1986. *Cheap Amusements: working women and leisure in turn-of-the-century New York*. Philadelphia, Pa: Temple University Press.

Plato. [1945] *The Republic* (translated and edited by F. M. Cornford). New York: Oxford University Press.

Playfair, W. S. 1883. *The Systematic Treatment of Nerve Prostration and Hysteria*. Philadelphia, Pa: Henry C. Lea.

Pliny the Younger [Cajus Plinius Secundus] [1961] *Natural History* (translated by H. Rackham), Book 7. Cambridge, Mass.: Harvard University Press.

Poirier, Suzanne. 1983. 'The Weir Mitchell rest cure: doctors and patients', *Women's Studies*, vol. 10, pp. 15–40.

Pomeroy, Florence, Viscountess Harberton. 1882. 'Rational dress for women', *Macmillan's Magazine* reprinted in Janet Horowitz Murray, *Strong-Minded Women and other lost voices from nineteenth-century England*, New York: Pantheon Books, 1982, pp. 69–72.

Pope, Emily F., Call, Emma L., and Pope, C. Augusta. 1881. *The Practice of Medicine by Women in the United States*. Boston, Mass: Wright & Potter.

References

Posner, Judith. 1979. 'It's all in your head: feminist and medical models on menopause. (Strange bedfellows)', *Sex Roles*, vol. 5 (2), pp. 179–90.

Potter, William Warren. 1891. 'How should girls be educated?', *New York Medical Journal*, vol. 53 (21 March), pp. 321–6.

Power, John. 1831. *Essays on the Female Economy*. London: Burgess & Hill.

Prendergast, J. F. 1896. 'The bicycle for women', *American Journal of Obstetrics*, vol. 34 (2), pp. 245–53.

Preston, Ann. 1851. 'General Diagnosis', thesis, Medical College of Pennsylvania Archives.

— 1858. *Valedictory Address*. Philadelphia, Pa: A. K. Terrlinus.

Prior, Jerilyn, and Vigna, Yvette, 1983. 'Reproductive responses to endurance exercises in women: from corsets to shin splints', *Canadian Women's Studies*, vol. 4 (3), pp. 35–9.

Pruette, Lorine. 1926. *G. Stanley Hall: a biography of a mind*. New York: D. Appleton.

Quetelet, L. A. 1842. *A Treatise on Man and the Development of His Faculties*. Edinburgh: William & Robert Chambers.

Ravenhill, Alice. 1909–10. 'Eugenic ideals for motherhood', *Eugenics Review*, vol. 1, pp. 265–74.

Reed, James. 1979. 'Doctors, birth control and social values, 1830–1970', in Morris J. Vogel and Charles E. Rosenberg (eds.), *The Therapeutic Revolution: essays in the social history of human medicine*, pp. 109–33. Philadelphia, Pa: University of Pennsylvania Press.

Rensselaer, M. G. Van. 1892. 'The waste of woman's intellectual force', *The Forum*, vol. 13, pp. 614–17.

Report of the Inter-Departmental Committee on Physical Deterioration, vol. 1, Appendix and Index. 1904. London: HMSO.

Resek, C. 1960. *Lewis Henry Morgan: American scholar*. Chicago, Il.: University of Chicago Press.

Rice, J. M. 1892. 'Physiology and the prevention of disease', *Popular Science Monthly*, vol. 61, pp. 309–13.

Richards, Eugene. 1886. 'The influence of exercise upon health', *Popular Science Monthly*, vol. 29 (July), pp. 322–34.

Richardson, Sophia Foster. 1897. 'Tendencies in athletics for women in colleges and universities', *Popular Science Monthly*, vol. 50, pp. 517–26.

Riley, Glenda. 1986. *Inventing the American Woman: a perspective on women's history 1865 to the present*, 2 vols. Arlington Heights, Il.: Harlan Davidson.

Ritchie, David. 1909 [1890]. *Darwinism and Politics*. New York: Charles Scribner.

Robarts, James R. 1968. 'The quest for a science of education in the nineteenth century', *History of Education Quarterly*, vol. 8, pp. 431–46.

Roberts, C. 1883. 'Bodily deformities in girlhood', *Popular Science Monthly*, vol. 22 (January), pp. 322–8.

Robinson, Paul. 1976. *The Modernization of Sex: Havelock Ellis, Alfred Kinsey, William Masters and Virginia Johnson*. New York: Harper & Row.

Roebuck, J. 1984. 'The invisible woman is a little old lady: the need for change in assumptions and paradigms', paper presented at the 37th annual meeting of the Gerontological Society of America, San Antonio, Texas.

Romanes, George John. 1887. 'Mental differences between men and women',

Nineteenth Century, vol. 21 (123), pp. 654–72.

Roosevelt, Theodore. 1926. 'Birth reform, from the positive, not the negative side', *Complete Works of Theodore Roosevelt*, vol. 19, pp. 161–89.

Rosen, Lionel W., McKeag, Douglas B., Hough, David O., and Curley, Victoria. 1986. 'Pathogenic weight-control behaviour in female athletes', *The Physician and Sports Medicine*, vol. 14 (1), pp. 79–86.

Rosenberg, Charles E. 1962. 'The place of George M. Beard in nineteenth-century psychiatry', *Bulletin of the History of Medicine*, vol. 36 (3), pp. 245–59.

— 1966. 'Science and American social thought', in David D. Van Tassel and Michael G. Hall (eds.), *Science and Society in the United States*, pp. 135–62. Homewood, Ill.: Dorsey Press.

— 1976. *No Other Gods: on science and American social thought*. Baltimore, Md: Johns Hopkins University Press.

Rosenberg, Rosalind. 1982. *Beyond Separate Spheres: intellectual roots of modern feminism*. New Haven, Conn.: Yale University Press.

Ross, Dorothy. 1972. *G. Stanley Hall: the psychologist as prophet*. Chicago, Il.: University of Chicago Press.

Ross, Edwin A. 1901. 'The causes of racial superiority', *Annals of the American Academy of Political and Social Sciences*, vol. 18, pp. 85–6.

Ross, V. B. 1900. 'The human body as a machine', *Popular Science Monthly*, vol. 57 (September), pp. 491–9.

Rossi, Alice (ed.) 1971. *The Feminist Papers: from Adams to de Beauvoir*. New York: Bantam.

Rothstein, William G. 1972. *American Physicians in the Nineteenth Century: from sects to science*. Baltimore, Md: Johns Hopkins University Press.

Royce, Josiah. 1919. *Lectures on Modern Idealism*. New Haven, Conn.: Yale University Press.

Rubinstein, David. 1977. 'Cycling in the 1890s', *Victorian Studies*, vol. 21 (1), pp. 47–71.

Ruddock, Edward Harris. 1888. *The Common Diseases of Women* (6th edn). London: Jerrold & Sons.

Runge, Max. 1900. *Das Weib in Seiner Geschlechtliche Eigenart* (5th edn). Berlin: J. Springer.

Russ, Joanna. 1981. 'Recent feminist Utopias', in Marlene S. Barr (ed.), *Future Females: a critical anthology*, pp. 71–9. Bowling Green, Oh.: Bowling Green State University Popular Press.

Ruzek, Sheryl Burt. 1978. *The Women's Health Movement: feminist alternatives to medical control*. New York: Praeger.

Sahli, Nancy Ann. 1974. 'Elizabeth Blackwell: a biography', PhD thesis, University of Pennsylvania.

Saleeby, C. W. 1909. *Parenthood and Race Culture*. London: Mitchell Kennerley.

— 1909–10. 'The psychology of parenthood', *Eugenics Review*, vol. 1, pp. 37–46.

— 1911. *Woman and Womanhood*. New York: Mitchell Kennerley.

Sallis, James F. 1987. 'A commentary on children and fitness: a public health perspective', *Research Quarterly for Exercise and Sport*, vol. 58 (4), pp. 326–30.

Sandys, Edwyn. 1903. 'The place that woman occupies in sport', *Illustrated Sporting News*, vol. 2 (21 November), p. 11.

Sargent, Dudley Allen. 1882. *Handbook of Developing Exercises*. Boston, Mass:

References

Rand, Avery.

— 1889. 'The physical development of women', *Scribner's Magazine*, vol. 5, pp. 172–85.

Saur, Prudence B. 1891. *Maternity: a book for every wife and mother*. Chicago, Il.: L. P. Miller.

Sayers, Janet. 1982. *Biological Politics: feminist and anti-feminist perspectives*. London: Tavistock Publications.

Scharlieb, Mary. 1909–10. 'Adolescent girlhood under modern conditions, with special reference to motherhood', *Eugenics Review*, vol. 1 (April–January), pp. 174–83.

— 1915. *The Seven Ages of Woman: a consideration of the successive phases of a woman's life*. London: Cassell.

Scharnhorst, Gary. 1985. *Charlotte Perkins Gilman: a bibliography*. Metuchen, NJ: Scarecrow Press.

Schopp-Schilling, Beate. 1975. ' "The Yellow Wallpaper": a rediscovered realistic story', *American Literary Realism*, vol. 8, pp. 284–6.

Schramm, Sarah Slavin. 1979. *Plow Women rather than Reapers: an intellectual history of feminism in the United States*. Metuchen, NJ: Scarecrow Press.

Schwartz, B., Cumming, D. C., Riordan, E., Seyle, H, Yen, S. S. C., and Rebar, R. W. 1981. 'Exercise-associated amenorrhea: a distinct entity?', *American Journal of Obstetrics and Gynecology*, vol. 141, pp. 662–70.

Scott, Ingleby. 1860. 'Dr Elizabeth Blackwell', *Once a Week*, 16 June, p. 577.

Scovil, Elisabeth Robinson. 1889. *Preparation for Motherhood Manual*. Philadelphia, Pa: Henry Altemus.

Selye, H., and Prioreschi, P. 1960. 'Stress theory of aging', in N. W. Shock (ed.), *Aging, Some Social and Biological Aspects*. Washington, DC: American Association for the Advancement of Science.

Semmelweiss, Ignaz. 1983 (1861). *The Etiology, Concept and Prophylaxis of Childbed Fever* (translated and edited by K. Codell Carter). Madison, Wisc.: University of Wisconsin Press.

Shaffer, Elinor. 1980. 'Review of Michel Foucault's *The History of Sexuality, Volume I: An introduction*', *Signs: Journal of Women in Culture and Society*, vol. 5 (4), pp. 812–20.

Shaw, Anna Howard. 1915. *One Story of a Pioneer*. New York: Harper & Bros.

Shaw, George Bernard. 1913 [1891]. 'The Womanly Woman' from 'The quintessence of Ibsen' in *Collected Works*, vol. 1, London: Constable.

Shephard, R. J. 1985. 'Factors influencing the exercise behaviour of patients', *Sports Medicine*, vol. 2 (5), pp. 348–66.

Shirk, J. K. 1884. *Female Hygiene and Female Disease*. Lancaster, Pa: Lancaster Publishing.

Shorter, Edward. 1982. *A History of Women's Bodies*. New York: Basic Books.

Showalter, Elaine. 1977. *A Literature of Their Own*. Princeton, NJ: Princeton University Press.

— 1985. *The Female Malady: women, madness and English culture, 1830–1980*. New York: Penguin Books.

— and Showalter, English. 1970. 'Victorian women and menstruation', *Victorian Studies*, vol. 14 (1), pp. 83–9.

Shryock, Richard H. 1950. 'Women in American medicine', *Journal of the*

References

American Medical Women's Association, vol. 5 (9) (September), pp. 371–9.

— 1960. *Medicine and Society in America, 1660–1860*. New York: New York University Press.

Sicherman, Barbara. 1977. 'The uses of a diagnosis: doctor's patients and neurasthenia', *Journal of the History of Medicine and Allied Science*, vol. 32, pp. 33–54.

Siddall, A. C. 1982. 'Chlorosis: etiology reconsidered', *Bulletin of the History of Medicine*, vol. 56, pp. 254–60.

Sidgwick, Mrs Henry (Eleanor). 1890. *Health Statistics of Women Students of Cambridge and Oxford and of their Sisters*. Cambridge: Cambridge University Press.

Sidney, K. J., and Shephard, R. J. 1977. 'Perception of exercise in the elderly, effects of aging, modes of exercise and physical training', *Perceptual and Motor Skills*, vol. 44, pp. 999–1010.

Sigerist, Henry E. 1936. 'The history of medicine and the history of science', *Bulletin of the History of Medicine*, vol. 4, pp. 1–7.

Simons-Morton, Bruce, O'Hara, Nancy M., Simons-Morton, Denise, and Parcel, Guy S. 1987. 'Children and fitness: a public health perspective', *Research Quarterly for Exercise and Sport*, vol. 58 (4), pp. 295–302.

— 1988. ' "Children and fitness: a public health perspective": reaction to the reactions', *Research Quarterly for Exercise and Sport*, vol. 59 (2), pp. 177–9.

Sims, James Marion. 1884. *The Story of My Life*. New York: D. Appleton & Co.

Skene, Alexander. 1895. *Medical Gynecology*. New York: D. Appleton.

Sklar, Kathryn Kish. 1973. *Catharine Beecher: a study in American domesticity*. New Haven, Conn.: Yale University Press.

Sloan-Chesser, Elizabeth. 1912. *Perfect Health for Women and Children*. London: Methuen.

— 1913. *Woman, Marriage and Motherhood*. London: Methuen.

— 1914. *Physiology and Hygiene for Girls' Schools*. London: G. Bell & Sons.

Slocum, Henry W. Jr. 1889. 'Lawn tennis as a game for women', *Outing*, vol. 14 (April–September), pp. 289–300.

Smellie, William. 1766. *A Treatise on the Theory and Practice of Midwifery* (5th edn). 3 vols. London: Wilson.

Smith, Daniel Scott. 1976. 'Family limitations, sexual control and domestic feminism in Victorian America', in Mary Hartman and Lois Banner (eds.), *Clio's Consciousness Raised: new perspectives on the history of women*, pp. 119–36. New York: Octagon Books.

— 1979. 'Life course, norms and the family system of older Americans in 1900', *Journal of Family History*, vol. 14 (3), pp. 285–98.

Smith, Dorothy. 1974. 'A social construction of documentary reality', *Sociology Inquiry*, vol. 44 (4), pp. 257–67.

Smith, F. B. 1979. *The People's Health, 1830–1910*. London: Croom Helm.

Smith, N. J. 1980. 'Excessive weight loss and food aversion in athletes simulating anorexia nervosa', *Pediatrics*, vol. 66, pp. 139–42.

Smith, Robert A., 1972. *A Social History of the Bicycle: its early life and times in America*. New York: American Heritage Press.

Smith, Stephen. 1892. *Doctors in Medicine: and other papers on professional subjects*. New York: W. N. Wood.

Smith, W. Tyler. 1848. 'The climacteric disease in women', *London Medical Journal*, vol. 1 (July), pp. 601–9.

Smith-Rosenberg, Carroll. 1985. *Disorderly Conduct: visions of gender in Victorian America*. New York: Alfred A. Knopf.

Soranus. [1956] *Gynecology* (translated by Oswei Temkin). Baltimore, Md: Johns Hopkins University Press.

Speert, Harold. 1980. *Obstetrics and Gynecology in America: a history*. Baltimore, Md: Waverly Press.

Spencer, Herbert. 1861. *Education: intellectual, moral and physical*. London: Williams & Norgate.

— 1873. 'Psychology of the sexes', *Popular Science Monthly*, vol. 4 (November), pp. 30–8.

— 1864–67. *The Principles of Biology*. 2 vols. New York: D. Appleton.

— 1876–7. *The Principles of Sociology*, 3 vols. New York: D. Appleton.

Spring, Joel H. 1974. 'Mass culture and school sports', *History of Education Quarterly*, vol. 14, pp. 483–99.

Stables, Gordon. 1901. 'Health', *Girls' Own Paper*, in Wendy Forrester, *Great Grandmama's Weekly. A Celebration of The Girls' Own Paper 1880–1901*. Guildford and London; Lutterworth Press, 1980, pp. 18–19.

Stage, Sarah. 1979. *Female Complaints: Lydia Pinkham and the business of women's medicine*. New York: W. W. Norton.

Stansell, Christine. 1972. 'Elizabeth Stuart Phelps: a study in female rebellion', in Lee Edwards, Mary Heath and Lisa Baskin (eds.), *Woman: an issue*, pp. 239–59. Boston, Mass: Little, Brown.

Stanton, Elizabeth Cady. 1882. 'The health of American women', *North American Review*, vol. 135, pp. 503–24.

— 1895. No title. *Minneapolis Tribune*, 10 August.

— *et al.* (eds.) 1881–1922. *History of Women's Suffrage*, 6 vols. New York: Fowler & Wells.

Stearns, Peter N. 1980. 'Old women: some historical observations', *Journal of Family History*, vol. 5 (1), pp. 44–57.

Stephen, Barbara. 1927. *Emily Davies and Girton College*. London: Constable.

Stetson, Charlotte Perkins. 1885. 'On advertising for marriage', *Alpha*, vol. 2 (1), pp. 13–15.

— 1892. 'The Yellow Wallpaper', *New England Magazine*, vol. 5, pp. 647–59.

Stevens, W. L. 1883. *The Admission of Women to Universities*. Boston, Mass: Press of S. W. Green's Son.

Stocking, George W. Jr. 1962. 'Lamarckianism in American social science: 1890–1915', *Journal of the History of Ideas*, vol. 23, pp. 239–59.

Storer, Hortio Robinson. 1866. Letter to the Editor, *Boston Medical and Surgical Journal*, vol. 75, pp. 191–2.

Storey, W. 1878. Correspondence, *British Medical Journal*, (i), p. 324.

Strickland, Charles E. 1967. 'The child, the community and Clio: the uses of cultural history in elementary school experiments in the eighteen nineties', *Histor of Education Quarterly*, vol. 7, pp. 474–92.

— and Burgess, Charles. 1965. *Health, Growth and Heredity: G. Stanley Hall on natural education*. New York: Teachers College Press.

Strindberg, August. 1895. 'De l'inferiorité de la femme', *La Revue Blanche*

(January), pp. 14–20.

Sturrock, J. (ed.) 1979. *Structuralism and Since*. Oxford: Oxford University Press.

Suleiman, Susan Rubin (ed.) 1986. *The Female Body in Western Culture: contemporary perspectives*. Cambridge, Mass: Harvard University Press.

Sullivan, M. 1988. 'New studies link exercise to delays in menstruation – and less cancer', *New York Times*, 16 February, p. 3.

Swayze, G. B. H. 1875. 'Spermatorrhea', *Medical Surgery Report* (Philadelphia), vol. 33, pp. 27–32.

Swindells, Julia. 1985. *Victorian Writing and Working Women: the other side of silence*. Minneapolis, Minn.; University of Minesota Press.

Tait, R. L. 1889. *Disorders of Women*. Philadelphia, Pa: Lea.

Talmey, Bernard. 1906. *Woman*. New York: Stanley Press.

Taylor, Henry Ling. 1896. 'Exercise as a remedy', *Popular Science Monthly*, vol. 18 (March), pp. 625–36.

Taylor, J. Madison. 1896. 'Puberty in girls and certain of its disturbances', *Pediatrics*, n.v. (15 July), pp. 10–15.

— 1904. 'The conservation of energy in those of advancing years', *Popular Science Monthly*, vol. 64, pp. 541–9.

Taylor, Lloyd C. Jr. 1974. *The Medical Profession and Social Reform 1885–1945*. New York: St Martin's Press.

Taylor, Walter C. 1872. *A Physician's Counsels to Woman in Health and Disease*. Springfield, Mass: W. J. Holland.

Thomas, M. Carey. 1891. 'The Dean's office at Bryn Mawr College,' *Century Magazine*, vol. 41 (1), pp. 637–8.

Thompson, Helen Bradford. 1903. *The Mental Traits of Sex: an experimental investigation of the normal mind in men and women*. Chicago, Il.: University of Chicago Press.

Thorburn, John. 1884. *Female Education from a Medical Point of View*. Manchester: J. E. Cornish.

— 1885. *A Practical Treatise on the Diseases of Women*. London: John Churchill & Sons.

Thorndike, Edward L. 1928. 'Bibliography of the published writings of G. Stanley Hall', *Bibliographical Memoir of Granville Stanley Hall, 1846–1924*, vol. 12, pp. 150–80. Washington, DC: National Academy of Sciences.

Tilt, Edward. 1851. *On the Preservation of the Health of Women at the Critical Periods of Life*. London: John Churchill.

— 1857/1882. *The Change of Life in Health and Disease*. 2nd edn, London: John Churchill; 4th edn, New York: Bermingham.

— 1862. n.t., *The Lancet*, vol. 11, p. 480.

Todd, Margaret. 1918. *The Life of Sophia Jex-Blake*. London: Macmillan.

Tompkins, Lizzie A. 1889. 'Habit and saddle for ladies', *Outing*, vol. 14 (April–September), pp. 103–10.

Trecker, Janice Law. 1974. 'Sex, science and education', *American Quarterly*, vol. 26, pp. 352–66.

Truax, Rhoda. 1952. *The Doctors Jacobi*. Boston, Mass: Little, Brown.

Tuana, Nancy. 1988. 'The weaker seed: the sexist bias of reproductive theory', *Hypatia*, vol. 3 (1), pp. 35–59.

Turner, E. B. 1896a. 'A report on cycling in health and disease', *British Medical*

References

Journal (i) (30 May), pp. 1336–7.

— 1896b. 'Report on cycling', *British Medical Journal* (i) (27 June), p. 1564.

Tweedy, Alice B. 1892. 'Homely gymnastics', *Popular Science Monthly*, vol. 40, pp. 524–7.

Uhlenberg, Paul. 1969. 'A study of cohort life cycles: cohorts of native-born Massachusetts women, 1830–1920', *Population Studies*, vol. 23 (November), pp. 407–20.

Ultzmann, Robert. 1890. *The Neuroses of the Genito-Urinary System in the Male, with Sterlity and Impotence* (trans. Gardner A. Allen). Philadelphia, Pa: F. A. Davis.

Verbrugge, L. M. 1979. 'Female illness rates and illness behaviour: testing hypotheses about sex differences in health', *Women and Health*, vol. 4, pp. 61–79.

— 1980. 'Sex differences in complaints and diagnoses', *Journal of Behavioural Medicine*, vol. 3, pp. 327–55.

Verbrugge, Martha H. 1976. 'Women and medicine in nineteenth-century America', *Signs: Journal of Women in Culture and Society*, vol. 1 (4), pp. 957–73.

— 1979. 'The social meaning of personal health: the Ladies' Physiological Institute of Boston and vicinity in the 1850s', in Susan Reverby and David Rosner (eds.), *Health Care in America: essays in social history*, pp. 45–66. Philadelphia, Pa: Temple University Press.

— 1988. *Able-Bodied Womanhood; personal health and social change in nineteenth-century Boston*. Oxford: Oxford University Press.

Vertinsky, Patricia. 1979. 'Sexual equality and the legacy of Catharine Beecher', *Journal of Sport History*, vol. 6 (1), pp. 38–49.

— 1987. 'Biological determinism: medicine's accomplice in defining the exercise needs of women', paper presented at Aapherd (American Association for Physical and Health Education, Recreation and Dance), Las Vegas, April.

— 1987. 'Body shapes: the role of the medical establishment in informing female exercise and physical education in nineteenth-century North America', in J. A. Mangan and Roberta J. Park (eds.), *From 'Fair Sex' to Feminism: sport and the socialization of women in the industrial and post-industrial eras*, pp. 256–81. London: Cass Publications.

— 1987. 'Exercise, physical capability and the eternally wounded woman in late-nineteenth-century North America', *Journal of Sport History*, vol. 14 (1), pp. 7–27.

— and Auman, J. 1988. 'Elderly women's barriers to exercise, Part I: perceived risks', *Health Values*, vol. 12 (4), pp. 13–20.

— and — 1988. 'Elderly women's barriers to exercise, Part II: the physician's role', *Health Values*, vol. 12 (4), pp. 20–25.

Vicinus, Martha (ed.) 1972. *Suffer and Be Still: women in the Victorian age*. Bloomington, Ind.: Indiana University Press.

Vosselmann, Fritz. 1935. *La Menstruations, Légendes, Coutumes et Superstitions*. Bourg: Imprimerie Berthold. (Thesis: University of Lyon.)

de Wachter, Frans. 1985. 'The symbolism of the healthy body: a philosophical analysis of the sportive imagery of health', *Journal of the Philosophy of Sport*, vol. 11, pp. 56–62.

Wainwright, J. W. 1906. 'Exercise', *Medical Record*, 5 May, pp. 706–9.

Walker, Alexander. 1892. *Beauty in Women, Analysed and Classified*. London: Simpkin, Marshall.

References

Walker, William B. 1954. Luigi Cornaro, a Renaissance writer on personal hygiene', *Bulletin of the History of Medicine*, vol. 28, pp. 525–34.

Walsh, Mary Roth. 1977. *Doctors Wanted, No Women Need Apply: sexual barriers in the medical profession, 1835–1975*. New Haven, Conn.: Yale University Press.

— 1979. 'The rediscovery of the need for a feminist medical education', *Harvard Educational Review*, vol. 49 (4), pp. 447–66.

— 1983. 'The quirls of a woman's brain', in Ruth Hubbard, Mary Sue Henifin and Barbara Fried (eds.), *Biological Woman: the convenient myth*, pp. 241–63. Cambridge, Mass: Schenkman.

Walter, Richard D. 1970. *S. Weir Mitchell MD, Neurologist: a medical biography*. Springfield, Il.: Charles C. Thomas.

Ward, Lester Frank. 1888. 'Our better halves', *The Forum*, vol. 6 (November), pp. 266–75.

Warker, Ely Van De. 1874. 'The genesis of women', *Popular Science Monthly*, vol. 5 (June) pp. 269–77.

Warner, L. 1875. *A Popular Treatise on the Functions and Diseases of Women*. New York: Manhattan Publishing Co.

Warren, M. P. 1980. 'The effects of exercise on pubertal progression and reproductive function in girls', *Journal of Clinical Endocrinology and Metabolism*, vol. 51, pp. 1150–57.

Webster, Charles (ed.) 1981. *Biology, Medicine and Society, 1840–1940*. Cambridge: Cambridge University Press.

Webster, J. C. 1892. *Puberty and the Change of Life: a book for women*. London: n.p.

Weideger, Paula. 1975. *Menstruation and Menopause: the physiology and psychology, the myth and the reality*. New York: Alfred A. Knopf.

Wells, Christine L. 1985. *Women, Sport and Performance: a physiological perspective*. Champaign, Il.: Human Kinetics.

Wells, Robert V. 1979. 'Women's lives transformed: demographic and family patterns in America, 1600–1970', in Carol Ruth Berkin and Mary Norton (eds.), *Women of America: a history*, pp. 16–33. Boston, Mass: Houghton Mifflin.

Whetham, Catherine. 1917. *The Upbringing of Daughter*. London: Longman Green.

Whetham, William, and Whetham, Catherine. 1909. *The Family and the Nation* London: Longman Green.

— and — 1912. *Heredity and Society*. London: Longman Green.

Whipple, G. C. 1917. *State Sanitation*, 2 vols. Cambridge, Mass: Harvard University Press.

White, John S. 1889. 'The new athletics', *Proceedings of the American Association for the Advancement of Physical Education*, vol. 3, pp. 46–52.

White, J. William. 1887. 'A physician's view of exercise and athletics', *Lippincott's Magazine*, vol. 39, pp. 1008–33.

White, S. P. 1890. 'Modern mannish maidens', *Blackwoods Magazine*, vol. 147, pp. 254–5.

Whitaker, N. C. 1907. 'The health of American girls', *Popular Science Monthly*, vol. 71, pp. 234–45.

Whorton, James C. 1978. 'The hygiene of the wheel: an episode in Victorian sanitary science', *Bulletin of the History of Medicine*, vol. 52 (1), pp. 61–8.

— 1982. 'Athlete's heart: the medical debate over athleticism, 1870–1920', *Journal of Sport History*, vol. 9 (1), pp. 30–52.

— 1982. *Crusaders for Fitness: the history of American health reformers*. New York: Princeton University Press.

Wiebe, Robert. W. 1967. *The Search for Order, 1877–1920*. New York: Hill & Wang.

Willard, Frances. 1889. *How to Win: a book for girls*. New York: Funk & Wagnalls.

— 1895. *A Wheel within a Wheel*. New York: F. H. Revell Co.

Williams, J. Sir. 1875–76. *Obstetrical Journal of Britain and Ireland*, vol. 3, pp. 496–507.

Wilmore, J. H. Brown, C. H., and Davis, J. A. 1977. 'Body physique and composition of the female distance runner', *Annals of the New York Academy of Sciences*, vol. 32, pp. 764–76.

Wilson, Christopher P. 1986. 'Charlotte Perkins Gilman's steady burghers: the terrain of Herland', *Women's Studies*, vol. 12, pp. 271–2.

Wilson, Dorothy Clarke. 1970. *Lone Woman: the story of Elizabeth Blackwell, the first woman doctor*. Boston, Mass: Little, Brown.

Wilson, E. O. 1975. *Sociobiology: the new synthesis*. Cambridge, Mass: Harvard University Press.

Wilson, J. T. 1885. 'Menstrual disorder in schoolgirls', *The Texas Sanitarium* (June), pp. 17–19.

Wilson, Robert A., and Wilson, Thelma H. 1965. 'The facts of the non-treated post-menopausal woman: a plea for the maintenance of adequate estrogen from puberty to the grave', *Journal of the American Geriatric Society*, vol. 11, pp. 351–6.

Winslow, Forbes. 1878. *Mad Humanity: in forms apparent and obscure*. London: C. A. Pearson.

Woloch, Nancy. 1984. *Women and the American Experience*. New York: Alfred A. Knopf.

Wood, Ann Douglas. 1976. ' "The fashionable diseases": women's complaints and their treatment in nineteenth-century America', in Mary Hartman and Lois Banner (eds.), *Clio's Consciousness Raised: new perspectives on the history of women*, pp. 1–22. New York: Octagon Books.

Wood, Mrs Henry (Ellen). 1865. *Mildred Arkell*. London: Tunsley Bros.

Woolf, Virginia. 1957 [1929]. *A Room of One's Own*. New York: Harbinger Books.

Woodworth, Robert. 1939. 'Psychiatry and experimental psychology', *Psychological Issues: selected papers of Robert S. Woodworth*. New York: Columbia University Press.

Woodward, John, and Richards, David (eds.) 1977. *Health Care and Popular Medicine in Nineteenth-Century England: essays in the social history of medicine*. London: Croom Helm.

Woody, Thomas. 1974 (1929). *A History of Women's Education in the United States*, 2 vols. New York: Octagon Books.

Woolson, Abba Gould. 1873. *Women in American Society*. Boston, Mass: Roberts.

Wright, Will. 1982. *The Social Logic of Health*. New Brunswick, NJ: Rutgers University Press.

Zita, Jacquelyn N. 1988. 'The premenstrual syndrome: "dis-easing" the female cycle', *Hypatia*, vol. 3 (1), pp. 77–99.

Index

Note: Only those authors writing in the nineteenth century *and* quoted by name in the text are included in the index. Please see chapter notes and the 'References' section for a complete list.

275